Principles of Pediatric Neurosurgery

Series Editor: Anthony J. Raimondi

Principles of Pediatric Neurosurgery

Head Injuries in the Newborn and Infant

The Pediatric Spine I: Development and the Dysraphic State
The Pediatric Spine II: Developmental Anomalies
The Pediatric Spine III: Cysts, Tumors, and Infections

Edited by Anthony J. Raimondi, Maurice Choux,
and Concezio Di Rocco

The Pediatric Spine I
Development and the Dysraphic State

Edited by Anthony J. Raimondi,
Maurice Choux, and Concezio Di Rocco

With 108 Figures

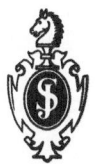

Springer-Verlag
New York Berlin Heidelberg
London Paris Tokyo

ANTHONY J. RAIMONDI, M.D., 37020 Gargagnago (Verona), Italy

MAURICE CHOUX, M.D., Hôpital des Enfants de la Timone, Rue Saint Pierre, 13005 Marseille, France

CONCEZIO DI ROCCO, M.D., Istituto di Neurochirurgia, Università Cattolica del Sacro Cuore, Largo Gemelli 8, 00168 Rome, Italy

Library of Congress Cataloging-in-Publication Data
The Pediatric spine.
  (Principles of pediatric neurosurgery)
  Includes bibliographies and index.
  Contents: 1. Development and the dysraphic state.
  1. Spine—Diseases. 2. Spine—Abnormalities.
3. Spine—Surgery. 4. Pediatric neurology.
I. Raimondi, Anthony J. II. Choux, M. (Maurice)
III. Di Rocco, C. (Concezio) IV. Series.
[DNLM: 1. Spinal Diseases—in infancy and childhood.
2. Spine—growth & development. WE 725 P3711]
RD768.P36 1989   618.92′73   88-24822

Printed on acid-free paper.

Typeset by Caliber Design Planning, Inc., New York, New York.

9 8 7 6 5 4 3 2 1

ISBN-13:978-1-4613-8822-7   e-ISBN-13:978-1-4613-8820-3
DOI: 10.1007/978-1-4613-8820-3

Series Preface

It is estimated that the functionally significant body of knowledge for a given medical specialty changes radically every 8 years. New specialties and "subspecialization" are occurring at approximately an equal rate. Historically, established journals have not been able either to absorb this increase in publishable material or to extend their readership to the new specialists. International and national meetings, symposia and seminars, workshops and newsletters successfully bring to the attention of physicians within developing specialties what is occurring, but generally only in demonstration form without providing historical perspective, pathoanatomical correlates, or extensive discussion. Page and time limitations oblige the authors to present only the essence of their material.

Pediatric neurosurgery is an example of a specialty that has developed during the past 15 years. Over this period, neurosurgeons have obtained special training in pediatric neurosurgery, and then dedicated themselves primarily to its practice. Centers, Chairs, and educational programs have been established as groups of neurosurgeons in different countries throughout the world organized themselves respectively into national and international societies for pediatric neurosurgery. These events were both preceded and followed by specialized courses, national and international journals, and ever-increasing clinical and investigative studies into all aspects of surgically treatable diseases of the child's nervous system.

Principles of Pediatric Neurosurgery is an ongoing series of publications, each dedicated exclusively to a particular subject, a subject which is currently timely either because of an extensive amount of work occurring in it, or because it has been neglected. The two first subjects, "Head Injuries in the Newborn and Infant" and "The Pediatric Spine," are expressive of those extremes.

Volumes will be published continuously, as the subjects are dealt with, rather than on an annual basis, since our goal is to make this information available to the specialist when it is new and informative. If a volume becomes obsolete because of newer methods of treatment and concepts, we shall publish a new edition.

The chapters are selected and arranged to provide the reader, in each instance, with embryological, developmental, epidemiological, clinical, therapeutic, and psychosocial aspects of each subject, thus permitting each specialist to learn what is current in his field and to familiarize himself with sister fields of the same subject. Each chapter is organized along classical lines, progressing from introduction through symptoms and treatment, to prognosis, for clinical material; and introduction through history and data, to results and discussion, for experimental material.

Contents

Contributors

ENRICO BERTINI
Associate Professor, Pediatric Neurology, "Bambino Gesú" Hospital, Rome, Italy

FRANCOIS BONNEL
Chirurgien des Hôpitaux á la Faculté de Médecine de Montpellier, Montpellier, France

MASSIMO CALDARELLI
Assistant Professor, Department of Neurosurgery, Catholic University Medical School, Rome, Italy

LUCIANO S. DIAS
Associate Professor, Department of Orthopaedic Surgery, Northwestern University Medical School, Chicago, Illinois, USA

MATTEO DI CAPUA
Assistant Professor, Pediatric Neurology, "Bambino Gesú" Hospital, Rome, Italy

ALAIN DiMEGLIO
Professeur, Chirurgien des Hôpitaux á la Faculté de Médecine de Montpellier, Montpellier, France

RONALD J. LEMIRE
Professor, Department of Pediatrics, University of Washington School of Medicine, Seattle, Washington, USA

RITA P.M. LUCIANO
Division of Neonatology, Institute of Pediatrics, Division of Neonatology, Università Cattolica del S. Cuore, Roma, Italy

DAVID C. McCULLOUGH
Professor, Neurosurgery, George Washington University School of Medicine, Washington, D.C., USA

DAVID G. MCLONE
Professor of Surgery (Neurosurgery), Northwestern University Medical School, Chicago, Illinois, USA

THERESA CUNNINGHAM MEYER
Unit Coordinator, Neuroscience Unit, Children's Memorial Hospital, Chicago, Illinois, USA

GIOVANNI NERI
Professor of Medical Genetics, Department of Biology and Genetics, Università G. D'Annunzio, Chieti, Italy

SONYA OPPENHEIMER
Professor of Clinical Pediatrics, Department of Pediatrics, Cincinnati Center Developmental Disorder, University of Cincinnati, Cincinnati, Ohio, USA

ANTHONY J. RAIMONDI
Northwestern University Medical School, Chicago, Illinois, USA (Emeritus) and Dipartimento di Neurochirurgia, Universita degli Studi, Verona, Italy

EDGARDO SCHIJMAN
Children's Hospital, Buenos Aires, Argentina

FRANCESCO VELARDI
Assistant Professor, Institute of Neurosurgery, Università Cattolica, Rome, Italy

FEDERICO VIGEVANO
Assistant Professor, Pediatric Neurology, "Bambino Gesú" Hospital, Rome, Italy

CHAPTER 1

Comparative Anatomy of the Spine in the Newborn, Infant, and Toddler

Edgardo Schijman

The vertebral column is a flexible structure composed of a series of 33 vertebrae, which extend from the base of the skull, where they articulate with the occipital bone, down to the pelvis, where they articulate with the ileum. The spine consists of seven cervical vertebrae, 12 thoracic vertebrae, five lumbar vertebrae, five sacral vertebrae (these latter fuse, forming a single structure, the sacrum) and four coccygeal vertebrae (also fused in the adult to form a single bone, the coccyx).

The individual anatomic features of these vertebrae remain unchanged from the time of their formation during the embryonic stages of life, since the subsequent changes undergone by vertebrae and articulations are structural, inasmuch as they relate to the child's growth and development. Therefore, although the anatomy is unchanged, modifications take place due to incomplete ossification of vertebral bodies and arches, as well as pronounced viscoelasticity of the ligaments, in the newborn. Whereas in the adult spinal stability depends mainly on vertebral bodies and articular processes, in the child additional osseous structures are also involved, such as laminae and spinous processes, which provide insertion for paraspinal muscles. Accordingly, structural alterations of the spine, such as those arising from infant laminectomy with loss of posterior spinal arch support, may lead to undue stress on anterior support structures, progressive compression of the anterior portion of the vertebral bodies, and excessive looseness in intervertebral spaces. The final outcome is often kyphosis, anterior subluxation, and instability of the spine.

General Features of Cervical, Dorsal, and Lumbar Vertebrae

The spine is composed of a series of vertebrae joined by fibrocartilaginous intervertebral discs. Within, it lodges and protects the spinal cord and its covering inside the spinal canal, formed by a succession of spinal foramina. Although vertebrae exhibit distinct individual features in the various regions of the spine, they are all made up of a body (centrum), and a vertebral arch (formed by pedicles, laminae, spinous processes, articular processes, and transverse processes).

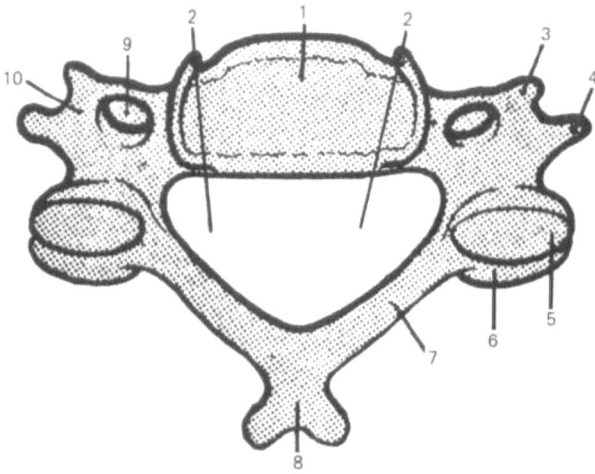

Figure 1.1. Upper view of a cervical vertebra: 1, body; 2, vertebral foramen; 3, anterior tubercle of the transverse process; 4, posterior tubercle of the transverse process; 5, upper articular process; 6, lower articular process; 7, laminae; 8, spinous process; 9, transverse foramen; 10, transverse process.

The vertebral body, cylindrical in shape, has flat upper and lower aspects and concave anterior and lateral surfaces, all with openings for vascular structures. Its posterior aspect is also flat and shows larger openings for veins communicating with the epidural spinal plexus.

In the cervical level the bodies are small, but increase progressively in size caudally. The spinal foramen is relatively large and corresponds to a thicker spinal cord at this level. The body's transverse diameter is large in comparison to the height and anteroposterior length (Figs. 1.1 and 1.2).

In the thoracic level, the bodies are wedge-shaped; their posterior borders are higher than the anterior, contributing thus to shape the dorsal kyphosis. The size decreases from the second to the fourth or fifth thoracic vertebrae to increase again toward lower thoracic and lumbar levels. In the most posterior and lateral portions of their upper and lower borders, thoracic vertebrae present two articular demifacets which, supplemented by similar demifacets belonging to neighboring vertebrae, allow the ribs to articulate with the vertebral bodies. The spinal foramen is relatively small at this level but easily lodges the spinal cord which is narrower than in the cervical level (Figs. 1.3 and 1.4).

In the lumbar levels, the vertebral bodies are more voluminous and have lower posterior than anterior borders, contributing thus to lumbar lordosis. The spinal foramen, in turn, is intermediate in size, smaller than in the cervical level but larger than the thoracic level (Figs. 1.5 and 1.6).

The pedicles, which are short, arise in the postero-external portions of the body. They limit the upper and lower intervertebral notches which, together with

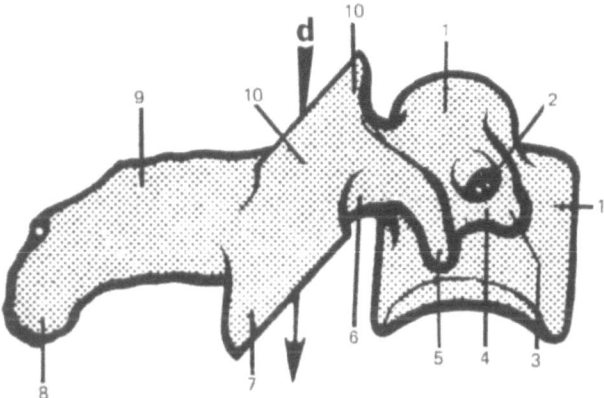

Figure 1.2. Lateral view of a cervical vertebra: 1, body; 2, transverse foramen; 3, anterior tubercle of the transverse process; 4, transverse process; 5, posterior tubercle of the transverse process; 6, lower notch; 7, lower articular process; 8, spinous process; 9, laminae; 10, upper articular process; Arrow, vertebral foramen.

pedicles belonging to adjacent vertebrae, define the intervertebral foramina for the passage of spinal nerves and vessels.

The laminae are plane quadrilateral structures, joined anteriorly and laterally to the pedicles, while posteriorly and along their common midline they close the spinal foramen from the rear.

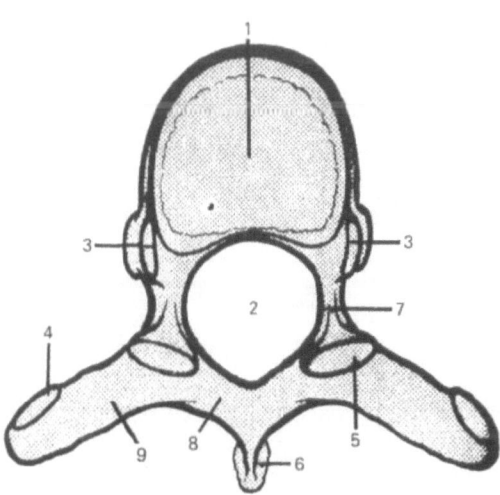

Figure 1.3. Upper view of a thoracic vertebra: 1, body; 2, vertebral foramen; 3, demifacet for rib head; 4, facet for rib tubercle; 5, upper articular process; 6, spinous process; 7, pedicle; 8, laminae; 9, transverse process.

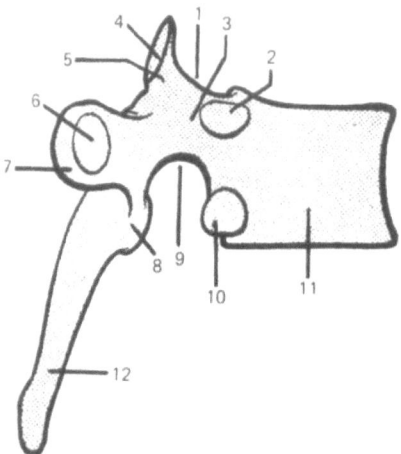

Figure 1.4. Lateral view of a thoracic vertebra: 1, upper vertebral notch; 2, upper demifacet for rib head; 3, pedicle; 4, upper articular facet; 5, upper articular process; 6, facet for rib tubercle; 7, transverse process; 8, lower articular process; 9, lower vertebral notch; 10. lower demifacet for rib head; 11, body; 12, spinous process.

Articular processes are both superior and inferior. They are positioned vertically and arise from the junction of the pedicles with the laminae. The superior ones present an articular facet in the posterior aspect which joins a similar facet located in the anterior aspect of the inferior articular process belonging to the vertebra immediately above. At the cervical level, these facets are tilted in such a way that the superior ones face posteriorly and cephalad, whereas the inferior ones face anteriorly and caudally. On the other hand, at the thoracic level, the superior ones mainly face posteriorly and the inferior ones, anteriorly.

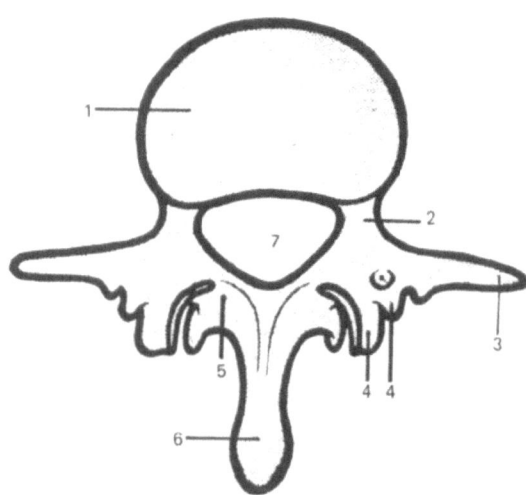

Figure 1.5. Upper view of a lumbar vertebra: 1, body; 2, pedicle; 3, transverse process; 4, upper articular process; 5, laminae; 6, spinous process; 7, vertebral foramen.

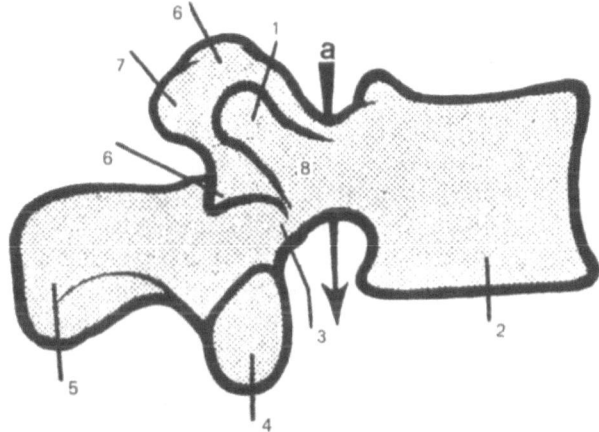

Figure 1.6. Lateral view of a lumbar vertebra: 1, transverse process; 2, body; 3, laminae; 4, lower articular process; 5, spinous process; 6, upper articular process; 7, mammillar tubercle; 8, pedicle. Arrow, vertebral foramen.

At the lumbar level the articular processes are more prominent: their superior articular facets face posteriorly and medially and their inferior ones, anteriorly and laterally.

The transverse processes project laterally from the sides of the vertebral arch. They are quite short at the cervical level, where they hold, just outside the pedicles, the vertebral foramina which allow the passage of the vertebral artery, except at the seventh cervical vertebra. On emerging from the intervertebral foramina, the spinal nerves pass behind the vertebral vessels. Distal to this foramen, the upper aspect of the transverse processes holds a sulcus, or canal, whose anterior and posterior borders come to an end at the anterior and posterior tubercles. The most prominent of these is the sixth cervical anterior tubercle. These features of the transverse cervical processes are not found at other levels. In the thoracic region of the spine, the transverse processes have in the outermost part of their anterior aspect an articular facet for the ribs. This facet is not found in the lumbar vertebrae, and may even be absent in the last two or three thoracic vertebrae. At the lumbar level, in contrast to the voluminous vertebral bodies, the transverse processes are slenderer and weaker than their thoracic counterparts.

The spinous processes arise at the junction of the two laminae, and are directed posteriorly. At the cervical level they are small and bifid; only the spinous processes of the last two cervical vertebrae may be palpated, particularly the one belonging to the seventh cervical vertebra, longer than the others and known as *vertebra prominens*. On the other hand, at the thoracic level, the spinous processes are longer and directed posteriorly and inferiorly so they become almost vertical. At the lumbar level, they are shorter, thicker, and stronger, having a quadrilateral profile.

General Features of Intervertebral Articulations

Intervertebral discs are fibrocartilaginous formations adhering to a thin layer of hyaline cartilage between the upper and lower aspects of neighboring vertebral bodies. In their peripheral portion, the annulus fibrosus predominates, forming concentric sheets placed in oblique bundles running in opposite directions in successive layers. Their central elastic portion, named *nucleus pulposus*, is normally located somewhat nearer the posterior than the anterior border of the disc. The latter changes constantly with age, as will be described later on, so that in the elderly the *nucleus pulposus* cannot be distinguished from the *annulus fibrosus*. The discs are quite thick at the cervical level, especially along their anterior border, conforming to the cervical lordosis.

Other structures, though less important than the discs, may also be observed in intervertebral articulations (Fig. 1.7). The anterior longitudinal ligament descends along the spine's anterior aspect from the anteroinferior aspect of the basilar process of the occipital bone to the anterior aspect of the sacrum, attached firmly to the intervertebral discs and to the borders of neighboring vertebrae. From the rear, the posterior longitudinal ligament follows the posterior aspect of the vertebral bodies in the spinal canal's anterior wall. It extends from the clivus or posterosuperior aspect of the occipital's basilar process to the sacrum. Like the anterior ligament, it broadens and adheres closely to the intervertebral discs and to the adjacent portion of the vertebral bodies. In its narrower portions, it is separated from the posterior aspect of the vertebral bodies by the emergence of their intrinsic veins.

The *ligamenta flava* extend from the inferior-ventral surface of a given lamina to the superior-dorsal surface of the lamina immediately below. Laterally, they merge with the capsular ligament, a fibrous capsule covering the articulation between adjacent upper and lower articular processes, while medially they are slightly separated from the contralateral *ligamentum flavum* by the passage of veins communicating with the intra- and extraspinal plexuses.

The intertransverse ligaments, of minor importance, extend vertically from the lower border of the upper transverse process to the upper border of the transverse process immediately below. The interspinous ligaments, as weak as the previous ones, present a similar pattern, extending from the lower border of the spinous process above to the upper border of the spinous process immediately below. Lastly, the supraspinous ligaments extend between the vertices of neighboring spinous processes. Stronger than the previous ones, they are especially developed at the cervical level, where they make up the posterior cervical ligament.

Special Features of Certain Vertebrae and Articulations

A number of vertebrae present very distinctive features within the general anatomic outline given above.

One of them is the *atlas*, the first cervical vertebra, which lacks a vertebral body (Fig. 1.8). It presents two cylindrical lateral masses whose bases make up

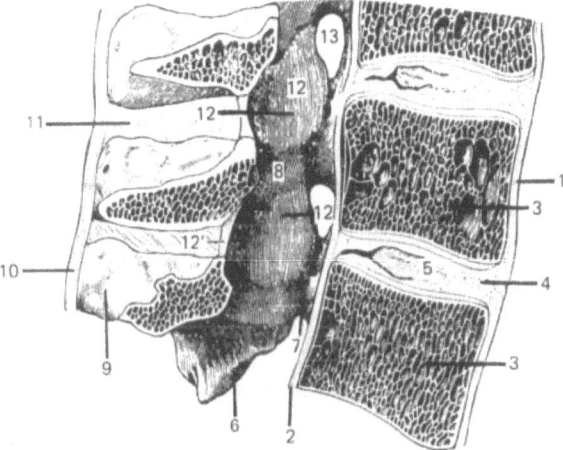

Figure 1.7. Median section of the spine: intervertebral joints; 1, anterior common ligament; 2, posterior common ligament; 3, vertebral body; 4, intervertebral disc; 5, nucleus pulposus; 6, lower articular process; 7, pedicle; 8, laminae; 9, spinous process; 10, supraspinous ligament; 11, interspinous ligament; 12, ligamentum flavum; 13, intervertebral foramen.

the lower articular facets, slightly concave, directed caudally and somewhat medially which, posteriorly articulate with the axis. In the outer portion of their superior aspect the lateral masses present the superior articular facet, oriented superiorly and medially, which provides articulation for the occipital condyle. Medially, the facet exhibits a prominence for the insertion of the transverse ligament.

The atlas also presents a short, almost straight anterior arch, extending between the anterior aspect of both lateral masses. There is a prominence in the middle portion of its anterior aspect, the anterior tubercle. In the middle portion of its posterior aspect there is an articular facet for the odontoid process of the axis. In the upper aspect of this anterior arch is inserted the anterior atlanto-occipital ligament, which extends superiorly to the anterior border of the foramen magnum.

The transverse processes are short and thick, but do not come to an end at the anterior and posterior tubercles as the remaining cervical vertebrae. They present a vertebral foramen somewhat more lateral than the lower vertebrae; hence, the vertebral vessels must describe an outwardly convex curve when passing from the second to the first cervical vertebra. Once they cross the vertebral foramen, they turn again, medially and posteriorly, following a canal in the posterior aspect of the lateral masses and in the upper aspect of the posterior arch before entering the skull through the foramen magnum.

The posterior arch, longer than the anterior, extends between the posterior aspect of both lateral masses. In the middle portion of its posterior aspect is found the posterior tubercle of the atlas, akin to the spinous processes at other levels,

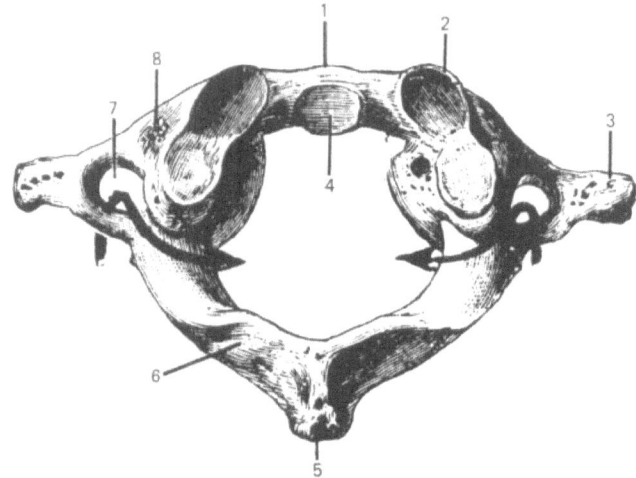

Figure 1.8. Upper view of the atlas: 1, anterior arch; 2, articular facet for the occipital bone; 3, transverse process; 4, articular facet for the odontoid process; 5, posterior tubercle; 6, posterior arch; 7, transverse foramen for the vertebral artery; 8, lateral masses. Arrows, path of the vertebral artery.

which provides insertion for the powerful *ligamentum nuchae*. Further caudad, the lower border of the same posterior arch provides insertion for the uppermost *ligamentum flavum*, whereas above, in the upper border, is the insertion for the posterior atlanto-occipital ligament which extends superiorly to the foramen magnum's posterior border.

The transverse ligament is a strong fibrous band extending transversely between the inner tubercles or prominences of the atlas' lateral masses (Fig. 1.9). In the middle of its anterior aspect, it presents a cartilaginous facet for the posterior aspect of the odontoid process. In this way, the transverse ligament divides the great ring defined by the anterior and posterior arches, and by the lateral masses of the atlas, in two portions: a smaller anterior one, intended for the odontoid process of the axis; and a larger posterior one, an extension of the spinal canal, which lodges the spinal cord and its meningeal coverings.

Except for the significant modifications in its upper aspect the *axis* follows the anatomic pattern described for the vertebrae in general and for the cervical vertebrae in particular. Although its spinous process is rather short, its transverse processes present no tubercles at their ends. Its articular processes are more voluminous (Fig. 1.10). The body of the axis extends superiorly to form the odontoid process. Its base, which narrows slightly, presents in its posterior aspect an articular facet for the transverse ligament. In its anterior aspect there is another articular facet for the anterior arch of the atlas.

There are two articulations between the atlas and the axis: one is the atlanto-odontoid articulation, located in the midline in the anterior compartment of the

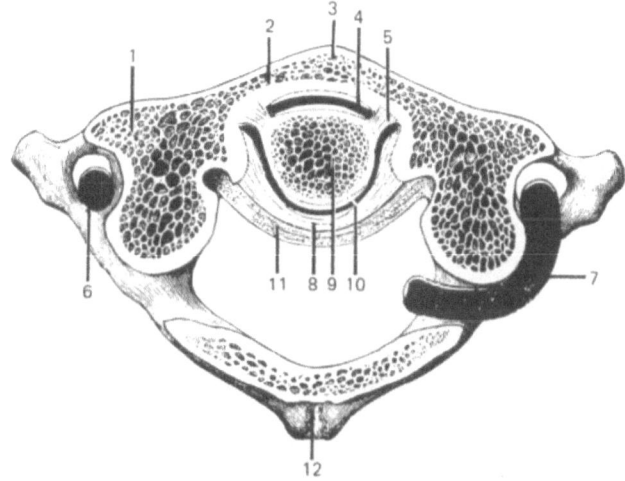

Figure 1.9. Upper view of the atlanto-odontoid joint: 1, lateral masses; 2, anterior arch; 3, anterior tubercle; 4, atlanto-odontoid joint; 5, fibrous tissue between anterior and posterior synovial cavities; 6, transverse foramen for the vertebral artery; 7, vertebral artery running in a groove on the posterior arch; 8, transverse ligament; 9, odontoid process; 10, joint between the odontoid process and the transverse ligament; 11, posterior common ligament; 12, posterior arch.

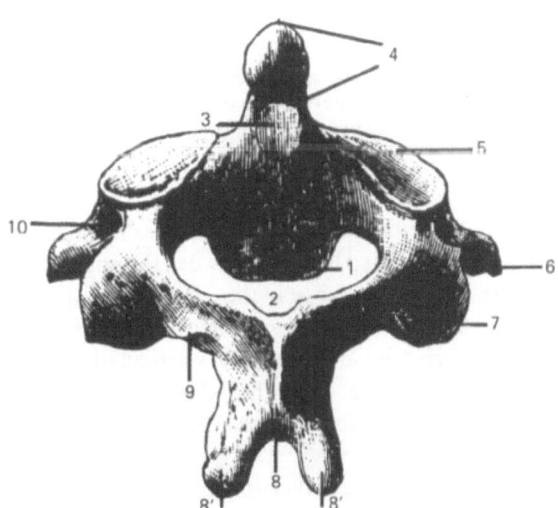

Figure 1.10. Upper view of the axis: 1, body; 2, vertebral foramen; 3, articular facet for the transverse ligament; 4, odontoid process; 5, upper articular process; 6, transverse process; 7, lower articular process; 8, spinous process; 8, prima, tubercles of the spinous process; 9, laminae; 10, transverse foramen.

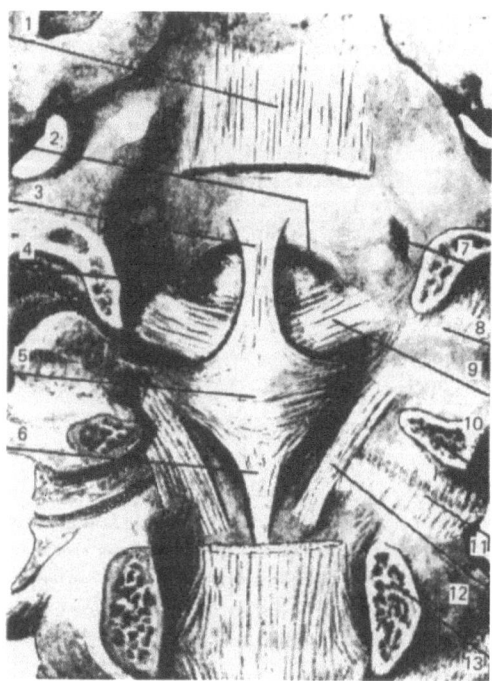

Figure 1.11. The ligaments of the occipit, the atlas, and the axis; posterior view showing the vertebral canal: 1, posterior longitudinal ligament; 2, anterior border of foramen magnum; 3, upper longitudinal band of the cruciform ligamen; 4, anterior atlanto-occipital ligament; 5, transverse ligament; 6, lower longitudinal band of the cruciform ligament; 7, anterior condylar foramen; 8, capsular ligament of the atlanto-occipital joint; 9, alar ligament of the odontoid process; 10, posterior arch of the atlas; 11, capsular ligament of the atlanto-axial joint; 12, accessory atlanto-axial ligament; 13, laminae of axis.

atlas' ring between its anterior arch and the transverse ligament; the other is the atlanto-axial articulation, located laterally between the upper articular processes of the axis and the lower articular facets of the atlas. These articulations allow the rotation of the head and the atlas as regards the remainder of the spine. As happens at other spinal levels, the articular facet's articulation is enveloped in an articular capsule of fibrous tissue, strengthened at this level by the atlanto-axial accessory ligament extending from the atlas' lateral masses and the posterior aspect of the axis' body.

Besides those mentioned above, other important ligaments are found in this region (Fig. 1.11). The *ligamentum suspensorium*, or apical ligament, of the odontoid process extends from the latter's vertex to the foramen magnum's anterior border. The odontoid or check ligaments rise laterally to their insertion in the occipital condyles' inner aspect. The cruciform ligament is made up of a horizontal portion, the transverse ligament, already described, and a vertical

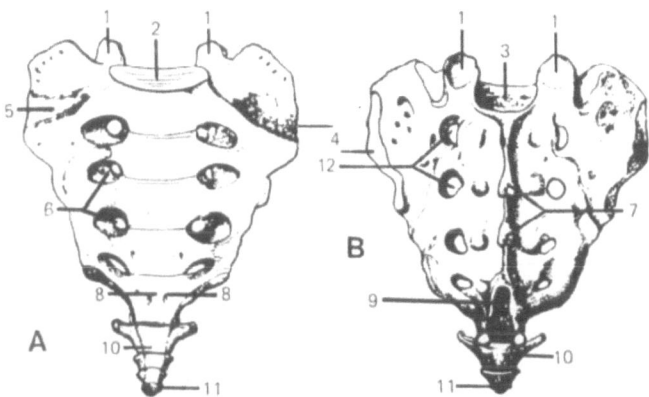

Figure 1.12. A: Anterior aspect of the sacrum and coccyx; **B**: Posterior aspect of the sacrum and coccyx; 1, upper articular process; 2, articular surface for the fifth lumbar vertebra; 3, sacral canal; 4, auricular surface; 5, alae; 6, pelvic sacral foramen; 7, median sacral crest; 8, tip of the sacrum; 9, sacral hiatus; 10, base of the coccyx; 11, tip of the coccyx; 12, dorsal sacral foramen.

portion, the transverse-occipital ligament or superior longitudinal band of the cruciform ligament extending from the transverse ligament to the foramen magnum's anterior border, and the transverse-axial ligament or inferior longitudinal band of the cruciform ligament extending, in turn, from the transverse ligament to the posterior aspect of the axis' body. These ligaments are covered along their posterior aspect by the highest portion of the posterior common ligament extending up to the posterosuperior aspect of the clivus, where they fuse with the dura mater.

The *sacrum* also presents unique features which distinguish it from the remaining vertebrae (Fig. 1.12). It is made up of the union of five sacral vertebrae separated from one another in the child, but fused in the adult. Its anterior aspect, smooth, concave, and directed caudally and anteriorly, exhibits four transverse lines defined by the intervertebral discs, later ossified, which separate the various sacral vertebrae. The sacrum's base, actually its upper aspect, resembles the body of a lumbar vertebra, tilting anteriorly and caudally, its anterior border forming the so-called promontory upon articulating with the lower aspect of the fifth lumbar vertebra.

As at other levels, the posterior aspect of the sacral vertebral bodies make up the spinal canal's anterior wall, here called the sacral canal. Along the posterior border of its upper opening is inserted the lowest *ligamentum flava*. Its lower opening is not closed at the rear due to the lack of fusion along the midline of the fifth and sometimes also the fourth sacral vertebral laminae. This is known as the sacral hiatus. Within the sacral canal lodges the lowest portion of the cauda equina and its meningeal coverings. The subarachnoid space comes to an end at the second sacral level.

The intervertebral foramina are found, four on each side, in the sacral canal's lateral walls, where the sacral nerves emerge. The fifth sacral pair emerges from the sacral hiatus together with the *filum terminalis* which comes to an end in the posterior aspect of the coccyx. Behind the sacral canal, and forming its posterior wall, are found the laminae that make up an ample irregular surface, where the spinal muscles are inserted. The midline of its posterior aspect presents the sacral crest with three or four spinous tubercles. Laterally there are other prominences arising from the fusion of the articular processes, called posterointernal sacral tubercles.

The lateral portions of the sacrum are known as lateral masses. Between the latter and the vertebral bodies, at the ends of the transverse lines representing the intervertebral discs, are found, anteriorly, the anterior or pelvic sacral foramina, and posteriorly, the smaller posterior or dorsal sacral foramina. Laterally from the latter the postero-external sacral tubercles may be seen. Through these anterior and posterior sacral foramina course, respectively, the anterior and posterior branches of the sacral nerves which emerge from the sacral canal through the intervertebral foramina. The sacral alae are lateral to the pedicles, the articular processes, and the body of the first sacral vertebra, making up the base of the sacrum. In the upper portion, at the level of the first two sacral vertebrae, the bone's lateral borders present an articular facet for the ileum, below which the lateral borders thin out quickly to serve as an insertion site, like the sacrum's anterior and posterior aspects, for major muscles and ligaments of the region.

The coccyx, small in size and pyramidal in shape, is made up by the fusion of four coccygeal vertebrae. The first one presents in its upper aspect an articular facet that forms the base of the coccyx and provides articulation with the sacrum. Laterally, the first coccygeal vertebra exhibits two small transverse processes and two small coccygeal horns that rise slightly from its posterior aspect.

Comparative Anatomy of the Spine in the Newborn, Infant, and Toddler

The vertebral column grows during the first months and years of life, starting from some 20 cm in length from the occipital bone to the promontory in the newborn and reaching 45 cm at the age of 2 years. Growth then slackens, and the total length reaches 50 cm in adolescence and 60 to 75 cm at the age of 22 to 24 years. This development of the spine is proportional to the longitudinal growth of the body, representing some 40% both in the newborn and the adult, as compared to 75% at 2 months of intrauterine life.

At birth, the column presents a single, anteriorly concave curvature following its marked flexion during fetal life. This curvature persists permanently in the thoracic and sacral regions, but other inflections in the same sagittal plane appear later as the human adapts to the biped position; namely, the lordosis, or posterior concavity presenting at the cervical level around the age of 3 months, when the child raises the head and at the lumbar level around the age of 6 months, when the child adopts the seated and standing positions.

Curvatures in the coronal plane are also secondary, as they are absent in the newborn and during infancy, appearing at the age of 7 years and developing progressively thereafter. In right-handed individuals, these curvatures are convex toward the right at the thoracic level and, in compensation, convex toward the left at the cervical and lumbar levels. Curvatures in both the sagittal and coronal planes arise from the remodelling of the intervertebral discs by changes in the height of their anterior, posterior, or lateral borders.

The developing spine undergoes a process of initial mesenchymal anatomic conformation in a pre-cartilaginous stage, followed by one of chondrification starting around 2 months of embryonic life and one of ossification starting at the third month. The ossification proceeds very slowly: only partial at birth, reaching completion as late as at 25 or 30 years of age.

In the newborn, the cartilaginous pattern persists in articular, transverse, and spinous processes, as well as in the last one or two sacral and coccygeal vertebrae. As hyaline cartilage, it also persists in the upper and lower aspects of the vertebral bodies. The latter are almost entirely ossified, starting from the body's primary ossification nucleus, called centrum, sparing only the cartilages of polar growth and the neurosomatic ones.

A lateral spinal x-ray film, taken at this time, shows that the bodies are notched anteriorly by the intersegmental artery, still patent at birth, which supplies the body's ossification nucleus. The development of this primary ossification nucleus parallels the vascularization received from the branches of these intersegmental arteries, the polar arteries irrigating the nucleus' upper and lower portions and the equatorial arteries supplying its equator. This abundant vascularization appears between 2 and 4 years of age, together with considerable irrigation of the primary ossification centers of the neural arches.

Later, from 4 to 9 years of age, there is a reinforcement of blood vessels from both the vertebral body and the neural arches toward the innermost portion of the neurosomatic cartilage, contributing thus to its ossification. In children from 9 to 12 years of age, blood vessels are dilated to the maximum, forming vascular lacunae in the bodies' polar zones below the apophysial cartilages and in the neural arches. These vascular structures start their involution at puberty, around 13 years of age.

Venous anatomy, though less regular and consistent than arterial, follows the latter in general lines.

In the newborn and infant, the height of the intervertebral spaces seems to be less than that of the intervertebral discs and the radiologic space between ossified vertebral bodies is increased by the translucent image of the disc plus the non-ossified portion of adjacent vertebral bodies. The union between the intervertebral disc and the body's non-ossified portion, called the polar cartilaginous lamina, is so solid that in case of fracture with displacement, the body's ossified nucleus breaks away from the cartilaginous lamina, but there is no separation between the vertebral body as a whole and the intervertebral disc. Therefore, it may be said that the body and the neural arches are almost entirely ossified at the time of birth.

Although the growth and development of the various structures making up the spine thereafter follow a common pattern, both the general and the unique features presented by the vertebrae during their evolution at various spinal levels will be described. Except for the first two, the development of the cervical vertebrae is mainly uniform. In the atlas, the anterior arch at birth may have an active ossification nucleus, on occasion bifid, or a purely cartilaginous arch with the nucleus appearing during the first year of life (Fig. 1.13). In some cases, this nucleus is absent throughout life, so that the structures formed by this center persist in the cartilaginous state, namely the anterior arch and the greater portion of the lateral masses. In other instances, their growth may be arrested in early infancy so that these structures arise mainly from the anterior extension of the ossification centers for the neural arches.

Individually, each neural arch possesses its own primary ossification center, already present at birth, and ossifies between 6 and 12 months of age, forming a synchondrosis at the level of the atlas' posterior tubercle, which closes when both neural arches fuse around the age of 3 years, on occasion preceded by the appearance of a secondary ossification center. In some cases, the atlas' posterior arch remains bifid throughout the entire lifetime.

The neurocentral synchondrosis that joins the neural arches to the anterior arch, and whose cartilage is responsible for the growth of the pedicles and of the dorsolateral portion of the lateral masses, closes around the age of 7 years. Its complete ossification is sometimes delayed until puberty. Its presence in anterior view x-ray films, transoral projection, may be mistaken for a fracture. Besides the secondary ossification center already mentioned at the level of the atlas' posterior tubercle, others may be observed for the anterior tubercle and for the tip of the transverse process.

At birth, the axis presents four ossification centers (Fig. 1.13B): one for each neural arch, one for the body, on occasion a double center, and one for the odontoid process. Accordingly, the various portions of the axis are already partially ossified at the time of birth and are separated from one another by cartilaginous tissue. Both neural arches fuse with one another by ossification of the synchondrosis, between 2 and 3 years of age. The synchondrosis between the body and the odontoid process, a true growth cartilage of the latter, and the synchondrosis between the body and both neural arches, neurocentral synchondrosis, close at 3 to 6 years of age, so that their visible radiotransparent images should disappear from transoral x-ray films by that time. On occasion, growth cartilage may persist in the odontoid process until around the age of 11 years, and is seen at radiology as a thin transparent line mimicking a nondisplaced linear fracture. This cartilage is a homologue of the intervertebral discs at other levels. Its ossification, as with the sacral vertebral discs, starts peripherally but the central portion remains cartilaginous until middle age. Odontoid process ossification develops in concentric rings, so that cartilaginous tissue may persist in its central area until advanced age.

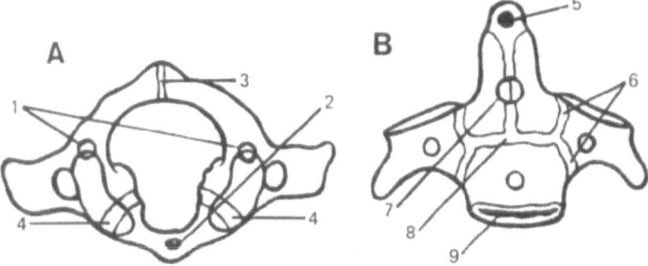

Figure 1.13. A: Postnatal development of the atlas: 1, primary center in the neural arch; 2, primary center in the anterior arch; 3, junction of the two neural arch centers; 4, neurocentral joint. **B**: Postnatal development of the axis: 5, secondary center at the tip of the odontoid process; 6, neurocentral joint; 7, junction of the primary centers in the odontoid process; 8, junction between the odontoid process and body of axis; 9, lower marginal epiphysial ring of the axis.

The vertex of the odontoid process is not ossified at birth, but is bifid and Y-shaped. At this level, a small secondary ossification center appears at 3 to 6 years of age to complete odontoid ossification by fusing to the process around the age of 12 years. Its independent and separate persistence from the odontoid process is known as *ossiculum terminale*. The ossification center of the axis cartilaginous endplates, located in its lower aspect, appears at puberty and fuses with the body of the axis around the age of 25 years.

As stated above, the development of the remaining cervical vertebrae is more regular (Fig. 1.14). At birth, both the vertebral body and each neural arch are almost fully ossified, starting from the respective ossification centers. The neural arches close with one another at 2 to 3 years, whereas the neurocentral synchondrosis closes at 3 to 6 years of age.

The anterior segment, called costal, of the seventh cervical vertebra's transverse process may develop from an independent ossification center present at the time of birth, one that fuses with the transverse process' main ossification center around the age of 6 years. Its failure to fuse gives rise to a supernumerary cervical rib.

Secondary ossification nuclei for the tips of the bifid spinous processes and transverse processes appear during puberty, around 15 to 16 years of age, and fuse to the main nucleus at the age of 25 years.

Toward the end of childhood and beginning of adolescence, the radiologic appearance of the cervical column changes with the development of cartilaginous end, epiphyseal, plate ossification nuclei in the upper and lower aspects of the vertebral bodies. This ossification starts in the periphery, hence the name epiphyseal ring, whereas the central portion remains in the cartilaginous state. The peripheral portion fuses with the remainder of the vertebral body formed from the centrum or main nucleus around the age of 20 years.

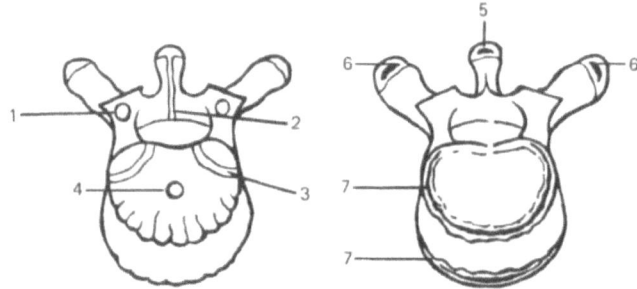

Figure 1.14. Postnatal development of vertebrae: 1, primary center in the neural arch; 2, junction of the two neural arch centers; 3, neurocentral joint; 4, primary center in the vertebral body (centrum) 5, secondary center at the tip of the spinous process; 6, secondary center at the tip of the transverse process; 7, upper and lower marginal epiphysial rings.

The so-called unco-vertebral articulations seen in adults are not found in children's cervical spine: the *annulus fibrosus* completely fills the peripheral portion of the intervertebral space without histologic evidence of a synovial joint.

Thoracic and lumbar vertebrae follow the same general developmental pattern as cervical vertebrae, presenting at birth partially ossified bodies and neural arches, each one from an independent ossification center. The resultant synchondrosis between both neural arches closes somewhat earlier at dorsal than at cervical levels, and even later at the lumbar level.

Around the age of 14 to 16 years, secondary ossification centers appear for the tips of the transverse and spinous processes, cartilaginous until then, which fuse to the main nucleus in the mid-30s.

Besides the given features common to cervical, dorsal, and lumbar vertebrae, the latter may present two secondary centers of late appearance, at the level of the mammillar tubercles, small prominences located on the posterolateral aspects of the upper articular processes. On occasion, the first lumbar vertebra's transverse processes present a secondary ossification center, also of late appearance, which gives rise to a supernumerary lumbar rib, a homologue of its cervical counterpart, should it fail to fuse to the main nucleus.

At birth the sacrum is mostly cartilaginous, its primary ossification centers for the body and neural arches already present, although their growth is very slow (Fig. 1.15). As at other levels, cartilaginous tissue separates the vertebral bodies from one another, the vertebral arches from one another, and also the arches from the bodies themselves. At 6 to 8 months of life, costal ossification centers appear on the sacrum's lateral surface, three or four in number, representing the costal rudiments of the first three or four sacral vertebrae. These lateral ossification areas fuse to the vertebral arches around the age of 6 years and with one another rather later, when puberty begins.

During infancy the sacral vertebral bodies are separated from one another by fibrocartilaginous intervertebral discs. The two lower ones ossify at around 18 years of age and the remainder do so later. The vertebral arches fuse to the

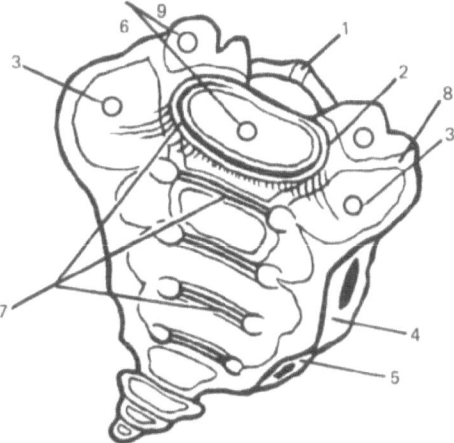

Figure 1.15. Postnatal development of the sacrum: 1, junction of the two neural arch primary centers; 2, neurocentral joint; 3, costal center in the first sacral vertebra; 4, secondary center in the auricular process; 5, secondary center in the lateral border of the sacrum; 6, primary center in the body (centrum); 7, marginal epiphysial ring; 8, junction of the neural arch and the costal element in the first sacral vertebra; 9, primary center in the neural arch.

vertebral body at the age of 2 years in the case of the lower sacral vertebrae and at 6 years for the upper ones. The dorsal union of the vertebral arches takes place later, between 8 and 16 years of age. However, this never happens for the fifth sacral vertebra and only occasionally for the fourth, thus giving rise to the sacral hiatus.

The upper and lower aspects of the cartilaginous surfaces presented by each sacral segment, the so-called polar or epiphyseal cartilaginous laminae, develop as at other levels, a secondary ossification center appearing around the age of 16 years, first in the lower ones and later in the upper. Lastly, the sacrum's lateral aspects present their secondary ossification centers at 18 to 20 years of age. Accordingly, the ossification of the sacrum is completed around the age of 25 years. Cartilaginous areas may persist, throughout life, in the central portion of the intervertebral discs.

At birth, the coccyx is often made up of four rudimentary cartilaginous vertebrae, arising from the six original coccygeal vertebrae in prenatal life by fusion of the more distal ones. The ossification process starts after birth from an ossification center for each coccygeal segment, which appears at 1 to 4 years of age in the first vertebra, at 5 to 10 in the second, at 10 to 15 in the third, and at 14 to 20 in the fourth. Lastly, around the age of 30 years, the coccyx completes its ossification and fuses to the sacrum.

The arrangement of intervertebral disc components in the adult, namely a central portion or nucleus pulposus and a peripheral portion or annulus fibrosus, is already present in the child, although morphologic features of both portions change with age. In the newborn, the nucleus pulposus contains collagenous fibrous tissue which develops from its fibrocartilaginous covering in the mucoid material, formed by the degeneration of mesenchymal cells derived from the notochord, with a progressive disappearance of these cells, accompanied by a steady increase in mucoid substance from 5 months of life. Up to that age, there is a great proliferation of cells from the notochord at the nucleus pulposus level, so that the latter initially grows more than the *annulus fibrosus*. Concurrently, notochord cells disappear from the vertebral bodies. Thereafter, the growth of the disc is at the expense of fibrous elements. Besides, the *nucleus pulposus* is increasingly invaded by cartilaginous tissue in the mucoid substance, as well as undergoing a progressive loss of liquid content.

Each intervertebral disc is composed of, in addition, the cartilage plates which cover the upper and lower surfaces of the intervertebral bodies, where secondary ossification centers appear as already described, around the age of 13 years. On fusing to the vertebral body around 17 years of age, they stop its development, together with the growth of the entire vertebral column. These ossification centers do not form endochondral bone, which instead arises from the upper and lower portion of the cartilage adjacent to the vertebral body's primary ossification center.

The fourth component of the intervertebral discs is the *annulus fibrosus*, composed of concentric layers of fibrous tissue that adhere firmly to the borders of adjacent vertebrae. The *annulus fibrosus* is homologous to the capsular ligament found in the limbs and its fibrous tissue is formed from the fibroblasts located in the peripheral portion of the intervertebral spaces.

The vascular supply to the intervertebral discs and its relationship to the structural changes they present is of great interest. Studied by microangiography, this vascularization follows a process of involution, starting soon after birth and developing progressively, so that by 18 to 20 years of age almost all the blood vessels irrigating the intervertebral discs have disappeared and nutrition takes place by diffusion through the cartilaginous laminae. This process is, therefore, the main cause of the gradual loss of the discs' gelatinous consistency. Its transformation into a fibrous structure is likewise the principal reason for the progressive loss of the vertebral column's elasticity.

Summary

Although the vertebral column follows a process of growth and development during infancy and adolescence that does not significantly modify newborn anatomy, important structural changes contribute to maintain its stability.

A knowledge of spinal anatomy and biomechanics in childhood is essential to understand its neurologic and orthopedic alterations, to plan suitable surgical treatment when indicated and to avoid the severe deformities that all too often are the unwanted sequela to vertebral column anomalies in infancy.

Bibliography

1. Bailey DK: Normal cervical spine in infants and children. Radiology 59:712, 1952.
2. Bradford FK, Spurling RG: The Intervertebral Disc. Charles C Thomas, Springfield, IL, 1941.
3. Breathnach AS: Frazer's anatomy of the Human Skeleton. 5th. Edit. J. and H. Churchill, London, 1958.
4. Caffey J: Pediatric X-Ray Diagnosis, 5th edit., Yearbook Medical Publishers: Chicago, 1967.
5. Compere EL, Keyes DC: Roentgenological studies of the intervertebral disc. A discussion of the embryology, anatomy, physiology, clinical and experimental pathology. Am J Roentgenol 29:774, 1933.
6. Draper Mineiro J: The ontogenesis of the human spine. IOeme. Congres de la Societe Internationale de Chirurgie Ortopedique et de Traumatologie, 1966.
7. England MA: A colour Atlas of Life before Birth (normal fetal development). Wolfe Medical Publications, London, 1983.
8. Ferguson W: Some observations on the circulation in fetal and infant spines. J Bone Joint Surg 32(A): 640, 1950.
9. Fielding JW: Anatomia de la columna vertebral. Acta Ortoped Latinoamer I(I):7, 1974.
10. Gooding CA, Neuhauser EBD: Growth and development of the vertebral body in the presence and absence of normal stress. Am J Roentgenol 93:398, 1965.
11. Gray H: Anatomy, descriptive and surgical. Henry C Lea, Philadelphia.
12. Joplin RJ: The intervertebral disc: embryology, anatomy, physiology and pathology. Surg Gynecol Obstet 61:591, 1935.
13. Lockhart RD, Hamilton GF, Fyfe FW: Anatomy of the human body. Faber & Faber Limited, London, 1959.
14. Noback C: Some gross structural and quantitative aspects of the developmental anatomy of the human embryonic, fetal and circumnatal skeleton. Anat Rec 87:29, 1943.
15. Noback C: The developmental anatomy of the human osseous skeleton during the embryonic, fetal and circumnatal periods. Anat Rec 88:91, 1944.
16. Orts Llorca F: Anatomía Humana, Tomo I, 5ta. Edición. Editorial Científica Médica, Barcelona, 1981.
17. Raimondi AJ, Gutierrez FA, DiRocco C: Laminotomy and total reconstruction of the posterior spinal arch for spinal canal surgery in children. J Neurosurg 45:555, 1976.
18. Rothman RH, Simeone FA: The Spine. W.B. Saunders, Philadelphia.
19. Sherk HH: Developmental anatomy of the cervical spine. In: Instructional Course Lectures. The American Academy of Orthopaedic Surgeons. Vol XXVII, Chapter 13;C.V. Mosby, St. Louis, 1978.
20. Testut L: Traite d'anatomie humaine. 9e. Ed., G. Doin & Cie., Paris 1948-49.
21. Tondury G: Le developpement de la colonne vertebrale. Revue de Chirurgie Orthopedique 39:558, 1953.
22. Yasuoka S, Peterson H, Laws ER Jr., MacCarty CS: Pathogenesis and prophylaxis of post-laminectomy deformity of the spine after multiple level laminectomy: difference between children and adults. Neurosurgery 9:145, 1981.

CHAPTER 2

Intrauterine Development of the Vertebrae and Spinal Cord

Ronald J. Lemire

Introduction

The early development of the vertebrae and spinal cord in humans has been extensively studied. Perhaps the most helpful format for the recording of these important events is the staging of human embryos that has been used over the past decades. Every developing system can be mapped against the morphologic stages devised by Streeter,[1-5] Streeter et al.,[6] and Heuser and Corner[7] and revised and extended by O'Rahilly[8] and O'Rahilly and Müller.[9] The 23 stages of human embryonic development begin with fertilization and extend to the 60th day (2 months after conception) when the embryo is about 33 mm in crown–rump (CR) length.[10,11] Each stage is 2 to 2½ days in length and development of various organs and structures can be expected to be identical within a given stage. Beyond the embryonic period there are not yet specific stages and most references during the latter 7 months of intrauterine development are made to the lengths of the fetus, e.g., CR, crown–heel (CH), and foot length (FL)[12-15] or organ weights.[16,17]

Although the present chapter is mainly a discussion of intrauterine development of vertebrae and spinal cord, it will also include information about the meninges which are intimately related to both systems. Table 2.1 shows the relationships of the varying stages of embryonic development to size, gestational age, and selected early events of vertebral, spinal cord, and meningeal differentiation. These few notations in the table provide only a brief framework of comparative phases of development. It is apparent that development of the meninges occurs much later than that of either the vertebrae or spinal cord.

Review of the Literature

Vertebral Column

During the early years of this century Charles Bardeen[18-20] published a series of articles describing the development of the vertebrae in man. He reviewed the literature prior to that time and noted that excellent studies relating to compara-

Table 2.1. General relationships of vertebrae, spinal cord, and meninges during embryonic stages

Stage	CR length (mm)	Age (days)	Selected general features	Early differentiation of Vertebrae–spinal cord–meninges
1	–	1	Fertilization	
2	–	2–3	2–16 cell size	
3	–	4–5	Blastocyst	
4	–	5–6	Blastocyst attachment to walls of uterus	
5	0.1–0.2	7–12	Implantation	
6	0.2	13–15	Primitive streak	
7	0.4	15–17	Notochordal process	Notochordal process
8	1.0–1.5	17–19	Primitive pit; notochordal canal; neurenteric canal	Neural plate; neural folds
9	1.5–2.5	19–21	Dorsal concavity (lordosis); otic disc; foregut	Neural groove; 1–3 somites
10	2–3.5	22–23	Two endothelial tubes fuse and heart develops "S" curve	Neural folds fuse; 4–12 somites; sclerotomic cells migrate ventromedially
11	2.5–4.5	23–26	Mandibular and hyoid bars. primordia of thyroid and liver	13–20 somites
12	3–5	26–30	Three branchial bars divided into dorsoventral parts; primary lung diverticulum	Posterior neuropore closes; 21–29 somites; spinal ganglia anlage
13	4–6	28–32	Arm and leg buds; mesonephric duct opens into urogenital sinus; heart chambers distended	Intrasclerotomic fissures; vertebrae distinguishable from meninx primitiva
14	5–7	31–35	Invagination of lens; myocardium in layers; trachea separated from esophagus, Rathke's pouch	Mantle layer differentiating; perichordal sheath on notochord; brachial and lumbar plexuses developing
15	7–9	35–38	Metanephros; germ cells; primary intestinal loop; first indication of aorta and pulmonary artery division	Spinal nerves formed from dorsal and ventral roots
16	8–11	37–42	Nostrils; auricular hillocks; interventricular septum begins; hepatic ducts; common bile duct	Closure membrane; disc anlage marked by notochordal thickenings; meninx primitiva prominent
17	11–14	42–44	Digital rays in hands; aorta and pulmonary artery separate; dorsal and ventral pancreas fuse	Dens (axis) distinguishable; dorsal rami of spinal nerves
18	13–17	44–48	Tertiary bronchi; müllerian duct; interventricular septum complete	Cervical and lumbar flexures; cartilage in vertebral lamina

Table 2.1. (*Continued*)

Stage	CR length (mm)	Age (days)	Selected general features	Early differentiation of spinal Vertebrae–spinal cord–meninges
19	16–18	48–51	Toe rays; arms and legs extend straight forward	Pedicles condrified
20	18–22	51–53	Arms bent at elbows; vascular plexus low on scalp; spoon-shaped Bowman's capsules	Dura mater differentiates
21	22–24	53–54	Hands flexed at wrists; vascular plexus midway to vertex	Stratification of closure membrane; neuroblasts and glioblasts differentiated
22	23–28	54–56	Hands overlap; vascular plexus three-fourths way to vertex; large glomeruli	Dura mater in lumbar region
23	27–31	56–60	Head erect; vascular plexus near vertex	Epidural space; dura mater complete around cord

tive differentiations were available. Bardeen's first article[18] described the development of the thoracic vertebrae as divided into three overlapping periods: (1) membranous (or blastemal), (2) chondrogenous, and (3) osseogenous. This was accompanied[19] by a description of the lumbar, sacral, and coccygeal vertebrae and finally 3 years later[20] the cervical vertebrae. Much of this material is also available in his chapter in the highly regarded embryologic collections of Keibal and Mall.[21] Early ossification data on vertebrae were provided by Mall.[22]

Calkins and Scammon[23] published a table of linear growth data for the fetal spine (and its components) between 25 and 550 mm CH length. As for Scammon cited above, these data are also available in more extensive format in their book on fetal growth published 2 years later.[13]

Because it will be apparent that somites play an important role in vertebral development the work of Arey[24] is mentioned here. The first four somites are actually incorporated into the occipital bone rather than the vertebral column and therefore the segmentations relative to vertebral level will be different than those relative to the somite level.

Scholarly attempts to correlate embryonic–fetal development with clinical and pathologic problems have been made and will be recognized by citing the work of Ehrenhaft,[25] who briefly reviewed vertebral development, presented several good photomicrographs of the embryonic vertebral column, and correlated these with some clinical entities. Perhaps one of the most succinct articles on embryonic and fetal vertebral column development published during the 1940s was that of Wyburn,[26] whose block diagrams (in addition to photomicrographs) are very understandable. Peacock[27] later provided information of development of the intervertebral disc. The classics, however, are the works of Sensenig,[28,29] who utilized the embryonic material in the Carnegie Institution in detailed studies that provided the descriptive basis for vertebral column development for the past 35 years.

Recent publications by O'Rahilly and Meyer,[30] who review all the important aspects of differentiation of the vertebral column during the embryonic stages, and O'Rahilly et al.,[31,32] who markedly extended the information about the vertebral column in stage 23 (the final embryonic stage), are excellent recent resources.

Spinal Cord

The early literature on spinal cord development is well referenced in the work of Streeter in 1912,[33] whose chapter still seems unsurpassed in its scope. Because the brain and spinal cord originate from the early axial orientation of the embryo some of the work relative to induction and later organization should be mentioned, although it is predominately in the experimental realm. Spemann[34] is an excellent reference source of this work in addition to Spratt,[35-39] Gaertner,[40] Saxen and Toivonen,[41] Seichert and Jelínek,[42] Toivonen and Saxen,[43] Klika and Jelínek,[44] Jelínek et al.,[45] Schroeder,[46] and Karfunkel.[47] Relationships between notochord and spinal cord have been studied.[9,48,49] Finally information relative to early caudal human spinal cord development is available.[50-56]

Malínský and Malínská[57] described spinal cord development in "15 stages," some of which overlap with the previously mentioned stages of embryonic development. Earlier studies by Bardeen[18] and Lassek and Rasmussen[58,59] provided general growth evaluation of the spinal cord, while Langworthy[60] and Yakovlev and Lecours[61] discussed patterns of myelination.

Meninges

Most of the information on the development of the meninges has focused on intracranial aspects because of the complexities of the dural reflections and venous sinuses. One descriptive study by Sensenig[62] on spinal meningeal differentiation is still current and available.

Early Axial Determinants

Primitive Streak and Notochord

The neurospinal axis orientation is provided by the primitive streak and node in embryonic stage 6 (0.2 mm CR; 13 to 15 days). During stage 7 (0.4 mm CR; 15 to 17 days) cells that will become the notochord migrate rostrally from the primitive node; shortly thereafter in stage 8 these notochord cells are in contact with the overlying ectoderm which thickens and becomes the neural plate.[9] This process is also found in subhuman species and the manner in which these and other tissues later interact in an inductive way is a classic model of experimental embryology.[34-47] The notochord activates the neuroectoderm and secondarily the latter is transformed into the neural plate. The rostral notochord seems to induce more neural structures and caudal notochord, mesodermal structures.[41.43] In humans the embryonic notochord also develops a canal and a transient neuro-enteric canal is formed in the region of the primitive pit when some of the ventral notochordal tissue breaks down. The significance of this early event is unknown.

The primitive streak, primitive node, and notochord are therefore the determinants of the early rostral–caudal axis. The notochord continues to play an important role but the primitive streak is incorporated into the embryonic tail which shows regression during the subsequent stages of embryonic development.

Neurulation

The neural plate, formed in human embryonic stage 8 (1.0 to 1.5 mm CR; 17 to 19 days), is transformed into neural folds/neural groove during stage 9 (1.5 to 2.5 mm CR; 19 to 21 days). This early event is critical for the later development of the vertebrae as during stage 9 the first three somites are formed. While these somites are eventually incorporated into development of the occipital bone, the pattern of early embryonic vertebral segmentation is probably in part determined at this time, especially the craniovertebral junction and the first two cervical vertebrae. Anlage of both spinal cord and vertebrae are present during this time with the process of neurulation continuing through stage 12 when the posterior (caudal) neuropore closes (3 to 5 mm CR length; 26 to 30 days). Stage 12 is also characterized by 21 to 29 somite pairs and therefore at the end of this stage the segmentation is complete through the lumbar region (subtracting four occipital segments). An important concept to consider is the fact that the human, much like lower species, does not seem to complete neural tube formation by the process of neurulation. Changes in rostral somites are taking place during the period of neurulation whereas caudal somite differentiation tends to lag behind. Also, the overall configuration of the embryo is undergoing changes in that the cranial flexure occurs during stage 10 followed by the pontine and cervical flexures in stage 13 (4 to 6 mm CR; 28 to 32 days) just after neurulation is completed.

Cellular Kinetics and Myelination

The mechanisms by which neurulation takes place are complex and not well understood in humans. In experimental animals there are excellent studies that implicate changes in cellular shape, regional stratification, and intracellular microtubules and microfilaments.[47] Equally important in early as well as subsequent development of the neural tube is the interkinetic germinal cell cycle. Cells undergoing mitosis are located at the lumen but exit in a pseudostratified manner.[63-73] Nuclei of these cells migrate toward, then away from, the lumen in a regular pattern in the ependymal layer. The relative position depends on whether they are synthesizing DNA or dividing. Shortly after neural tube closure the mantle layer is formed as some of thes germinal cells escape to differentiate into neuroblasts. The manner in which this is done has been studied but is complex and not well understood.[57,72,74] Whether or not the same cell lines also have the ability to differentiate into glioblasts or whether separate cell lines exist to contribute the latter is still debated. The marginal layer consists of axons and glial cells, the former of which become myelinated by oligodendroglia in the central nervous system. One oligodendrocyte can myelinate more than one central axon as opposed to peripheral axons which are myelinated by a single Schwann cell. Central myelination is preceded by proliferation of oligodendrocytes ("myelination gliosis") and an increase in vascularization in that area. The mantle layer formation is a relatively late event in the human spinal cord, beginning somewhere around 75 to 100 mm CR length as determined by electron microscopy.[57]

Developoment of Caudal Neural Tube

It is unclear how the human neural tube forms caudal to the posterior neuropore but this process apparently has a mechanism different than that of neurulation. The area involved is the embryonic tail, where the notochord blends with a mass of undifferentiated cells. In experimental animals and probably humans this region is where the primitive node and streak has undergone regression[35-40,75,76] and the only adjacent structures are the hindgut and mesonephros. The manner in which elongation of the neural tube takes place is different in avians[40,42,44,45] and humans.[50,53,54] Somehow within this "caudal cell mass" cavities appear, coalesce, then connect with the existing central canal to provide elongation of neural tube. This process is termed "canalization" and around the development lumina the cells orient themselves radially and differentiate to resemble neuroepithelium. In human embryos the process is quite imperfect and many acessory channels are formed.[53,54]

Because the posterior neuropore closes in stage 12 this secondary process of postneurulation caudal neural tube development must begin in stage 13 (4 to 6 mm CR; 28 to 32 days) but evidence for the specific changes mentioned actually becomes prominent during stage 14 (5 to 7 mm CR; 31 to 35 days) and continues until approximately stage 20 (18 to 22 mm CR; 51 to 53 days).

Final shaping of caudal neural tube and surrounding vertebrae begins about this time and continues until late in gestation—and in part even during infancy. An organized regression of this recently formed neural tube takes place in such a precise manner that it has been termed "retrogressive differentiation" by Streeter.[51] Arising out of this process are the conus medullaris, ventricular terminalis, filum terminale, and coccygeal medullary vestige.[51,52] Segmentation of the sacral and coccygeal vertebrae and ascent of the spinal cord within the spinal canal occur during this period.[55]

Vertebral Development

The early aspects of development of the notochord have been previously discussed, as have the somites as their numbered pairs relate to the embryonic stages. These structures are the first recognizable components of the vertebral

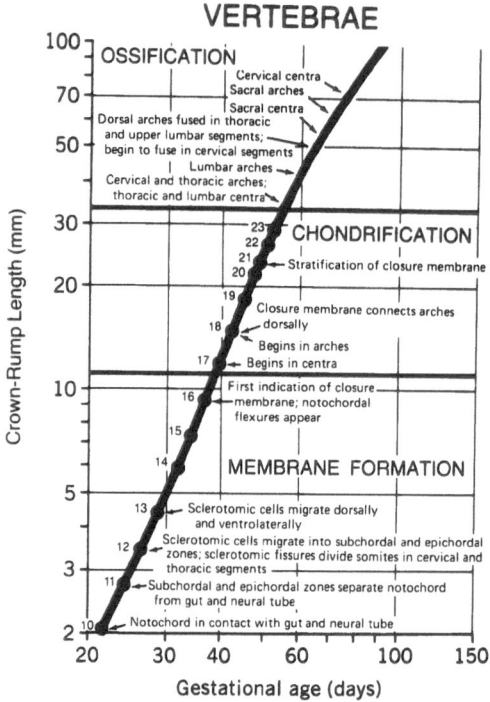

Figure 2.1. Selected features in the development of the vertebral column as correlated with embryonic stage, CR length, and gestational age. Three periods exist consisting of membrane formation, chondrification, and ossification. (Adapted from ref. 56.)

column. A rostral–caudal gradient of differentiation prevents a simple discussion of all vertebrae at a point in time. Also there are anatomic differences in the regional and individual vertebrae. A framework for discussion of vertebral development has been provided by Sensenig[28] which applies to the early differentiation of most vertebrae. He divided the sequence into three periods: (1) membrane formation within which there are three stages, (2) cartilage formation, and (3) bone formation (Figure 2.1).

Period of Membrane Formation

The first indication of vertebrae encompasses embryonic stages 10 through 12. During this time the notochord is in contact with both the foregut ventrally and the neural tube dorsally. Laterally, a cavity (myocele) divides the somites into medial and lateral components, whereas intersegmental fissures delineate the rostral and caudal boundaries. In the cervical region, epichordal and subchordal zones are created as the notochord begins to lose its contact with the neural tube and foregut. Sclerotomic cells then migrate into these epi- and subchordal zones and the cells that are close to the notochord surround it to form a perichordal tube. Other cells from the sclerotome begin migration dorsally toward the region that will become neural arch.

The final segmental composition of a vertebra does not correspond to a somite and it is during this early period that the sclerotomic fissures arise to initiate the change. These fissures separate the somite into rostral and caudal components and the vertebrae are formed when the rostral portion of one somite unites with the caudal portion of another. As with the previous sequencing, sclerotomic fissures are present in the cervical and upper thoracic vertebrae first and then are found in a progression caudally.

During the period of membrane formation there is also ventrolateral migration of sclerotomic cells to become the primordia of the ribs. This starts during embryonic stage 13 (4 to 6 mm CR; 28 to 32 days). Dorsal migration of other sclerotoic cells becomes more prominent as the space between the sensory ganglia and myotomes increases. Most of these migrating cells originate from the caudal portion of the sclerotome. Because the sensory ganglia lie medial to the rostral portion of the sclerotome the spatial relationship allows adequate room for cellular migration during stage 14 (5 to 7 mm CR; 31 to 35 days).

Stages 15 (7 to 9 mm CR; 35 to 38 days) and 16 (8 to 11 mm CR; 37 to 42 days) are marked by an increase in the number of cells migrating; and the initial formation of the "closure membrane" dorsally over the neural tube is identifiable. The notochord is also showing significant change at this time with flexures and furrows being found opposite intervertebral discs and vertebral bodies anlage. With all of the above changes the final delineation of the vertebrae has not yet occurred as intersegmental and sclerotomic fissures still are present. However, the period of membrane formation is completed during this time.

Period of Cartilage Formation

Embryonic stage 17 (11 to 14 mm CR; 42 to 44 days) denotes the onset of chondrification which is first found in the vertebral bodies. Cartilage next develops in portions of the arches during stage 18 (13 to 17 mm CR; 44 to 48 days). Also during the latter stage the dorsal closure membrane is continuous with the neural arches laterally and is part of a two-layer cover. The tips of the arches have a cellular proliferation that contributes to the eventual dorsal neural arch and the inner aspect of the closure membrane will eventually form dura mater. The process is dynamic and by stage 23 (27 to 31 mm CR; 56 to 60 days) the neural arch tips have deflected medially.

Period of Bone Formation

Ossification overlaps with chondrification with evidence of it found at the beginning of the fetal period in the cervical and thoracic regions (at 33 mm CR length) followed by lumbar (41 mm CR length) and sacrum (50 mm CR length). This period extends into postnatal life.

Selected Considerations

Every vertebrae is different and yet the development of most have enough similarities that they do not need to be discussed individually. Because of "regional" differences there are some selected concepts of differentiation that are worthy of comment. These mainly occur at both ends of the spine, the occipitocervical and sacrococcygeal areas.

The first cervical intersegmental artery is within the fissure dividing the 4th and 5th somites. The primordium of the proatlas is formed by the rostral portion of the 5th somite, whereas the caudal portion of this somite combines with the rostral portion of the 6th to become the atlas. The fact that the first four somites become part of the occipital bone is indicative of the nature of the early development in this region. During stages 17 (11 to 14 mm CR) and 18 (13 to 17 mm CR) the odontoid process primordium develops. Also cartilage is present in the cervical vertebral bodies and the pedicles of the atlas at this time. Shortly thereafter (stages 19 to 20), the atlantooccipital articulations appear.

A few comments will be made regarding the caudal spine, although most of the basic aspects have been previously discussed under postneurulation development of the caudal neural tube. The process of "retrogressive differentiation" is the manner in which the caudal vertebral column arises as well as the spinal cord. Thirty-eight segments are usually formed with seven or eight being in the embryonic tail, beyond which is a portion referred to as the nonvertebrated tail. The iliac blastema is located opposite the 25th to 26th primitive vertebrae (S1−2) during stage 17 (11 to 14 mm CR). The lateral aspect of the 25th through the 29th segments fuses into a solid mass with the membranous coccyx making up the next six to seven segments. It is not known what happens to the extra segments. In stage 22 (23 to 28 mm CR) the coccyx begins to curve between the 30th and 31st vertebral segments and reaches 90° by 37 mm CR length.

Spinal Cord Development

General Features

Staging of the development of the spinal cord has been done by Malínský and Malínská,[57] but these do not coincide with the embryonic stages (Table 2.2). The first six of their stages cover embryonic stages 10 to 23, with their stage 7 being an overlap between stages in the transition from embryonic to fetal development.

Most of the early development of spinal cord has been previously discussed in this chapter as it pertains to neurulations and postneurulation development of the caudal neural tube. Other methods of noting growing of spinal cord pertains to length,[19,55,59] cross-sectional area,[58,59,77] and myelination.[60,61] Overall the central canal starts large but rapidly decreases in size to become a small hole by 80 mm CR length (about 80 days gestational age). Myelination of spinal cord also begin about this time.

Cellular Differentiation

With the possible exception of precursors of Clark's column which appears at 32 mm CR,[78] most cell groups within fetal spinal cord are found by 90 mm CR

Table 2.2. Selected features in human spinal cord development

Embryonic stage or CR length (mm)	Malínský and Malínská (1970)		Spinal cord development
	Stage	Age (days)	
10	1	17–21	Ependymal zone only; neural groove and first fusion of neural folds
11–12	2	21–25	Neuropores close
13–14	3	25–29	Lateral walls thicken; dorsoventral axis of central canal greater than lateral; groups of cells in basal lamina begin to differentiate; marginal zone present
15–17	4	29–35	Sulcus limitans divides ependymal zone into two symmetric halves; marginal zone present in several areas
18–20	5	35–41	Sulcus limitans more ventrally placed; first indication of obliteration of central canal in dorsal part
21–23	6	41–49	Neuroblasts and glioblasts can be classified in the basal lamina; contralateral funiculi not yet fused in medial plane
26–38 mm	7	49–57	Marginal zone around entire spinal cord with some glial cells migrating into it; first groups of large motor neurons in basal lamina
38–55 mm	8	57–67	Ependymal zone much thinner; central canal small and pentagonal
55–75 mm	9	67–77	Increase in marginal zone greater than increase in mantle zone; thin glial layer is first indication of posterial median septum
75–105 mm	10	77–91	Greater volume of white matter than gray matter; first myelin formation by EM; first synapses
105–145 mm	11	91–112	Posterior columns more flattened and elongated; myelin sheaths visible through light microscope
145–180 mm	12	112–140	Fetal cord has similar shape and ultrastructural features of postnatal cord
180–265 mm	13	140–189	Thoracic cord over 60% white matter
265–340 mm	14	189–term	All cells in gray and white matter can be classified
340	15	Newborn	—

From ref. 56.

length and tend to cluster until about 150 mm CR.[79] Well-defined groups are present between 150 and 200 mm CR after which there is dispersion and overlap, the adult pattern being reached somewhere about the fourth month of gestation.[80]

One indication of early development is that tracts and sensory fibers cross the anterior commissure and others connect with the anterior horn cells at 36 mm CR length. A portion of the dorsal commissure appears shortly thereafter (40 mm CR length) and the dorsal spinocerebellar tract has been identified in a 53-mm CR specimen.[78]

Transitory unipolar and bipolar sensory ganglia cells have been found within cord proper as early as 16 mm CR length[81,82] and within the central canal as

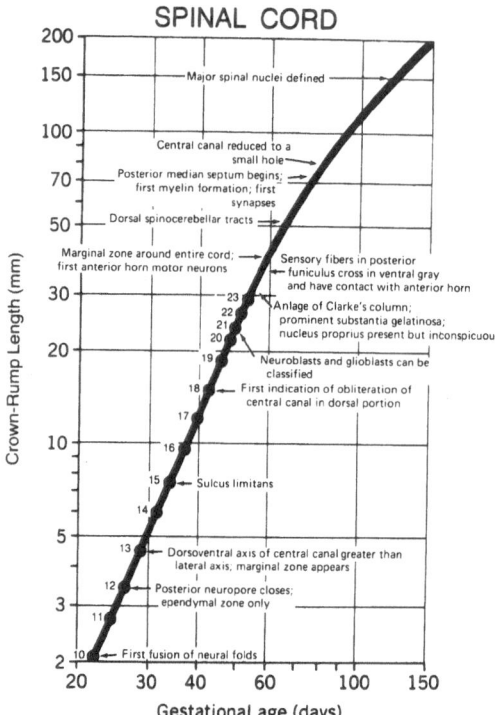

Figure 2.2. Selected features in the development of the spinal cord as correlated with embryonic stage, CR length, and gestational age. (Adapted from ref. 56.)

well.[83] Most are found in the lumbosacral area. Selected features of spinal cord development are shown in Figure 2.2.

Spinal Nerves

Early spinal cord development involves differentiation of the spinal nerves. Neural crest cells in clusters are the first indication of spinal ganglia and these are seen in embryonic stage 12 (3 to 5 mm CR; 26 to 30 days).[62] During stages 13 (4 to 6 mm CR; 28 to 32 days) through 15 (7 to 9 mm CR; 35 to 38 days) these ganglia enlarge and migrate ventrally. Motor nerve roots emerge from the ganglia tips shortly thereafter, and by stage 18 (13 to 17 mm CR; 44 to 48 days) they enter the intervertebral foramina. They lie completely within these foramina by stage 23 (27 to 31 mm CR; 56 to 60 days). The sensory component seems to be present during stage 14 when connections with the ganglia are present in some presumptive cervical segments.[33] In stage 15 some of these sensory fibers mix with the ventral motor fibers and a spinal nerve is formed. Distribution of the sensory nerves has been studied and the cutaneous distribution mapped in late embryonic and early fetal specimens.[84] Complex sensory nerve endings have been found in fetal muscle at 20 weeks gestation and terminal knobs at 28 weeks.[85]

All motor roots (through S2) are present with intersegmental anastomoses by stage 15. They blend with sensory fibers as noted above.[86-88] Motor end-plate development continues throughout fetal life.[85,89]

Figure 2.3. Selected features in the development of the motor nerves of the spinal cord as correlated with embryonic stage, CR length, and gestational age. (Adapted from ref. 56.)

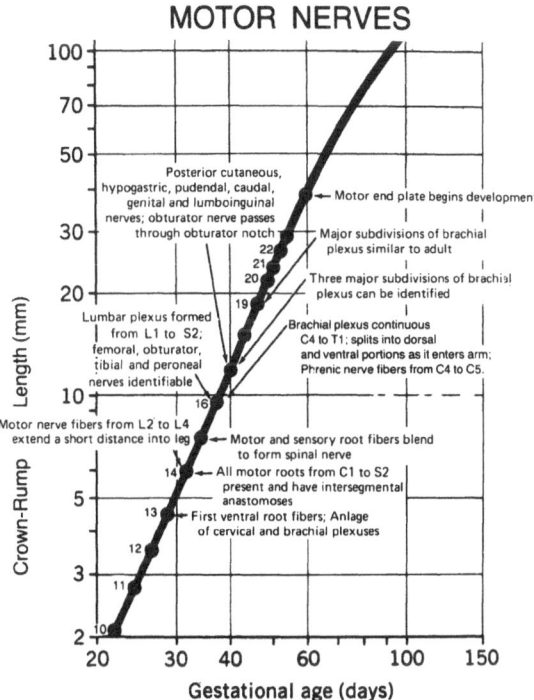

Figure 2.4. Selected features in the development of the sensory nerves of the spinal cord, as correlated with embryonic stage, CR length, and gestational age. (Adapted from ref. 56.)

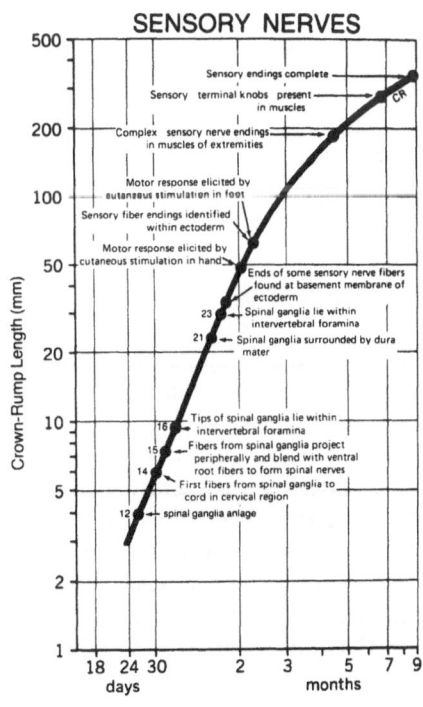

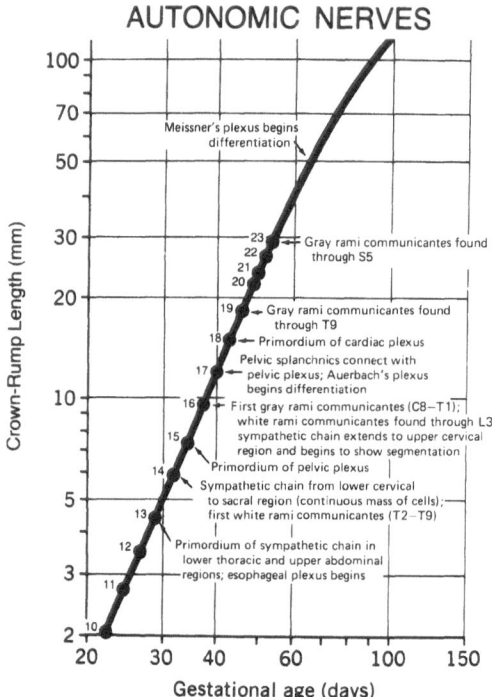

Figure 2.5. Selected features in the development of the autonomic nerves of the spinal cord, as correlated with embryonic stage, CR length, and gestational age. (Adapted from ref. 56.)

A detailed description of all nerves and their peripheral connections has been previously discussed by Lemire et al.[56] Numerous studies have been done on various aspects of development of nerves to the limbs,[86,87,90,91] the sympathetic chain,[92,93] esophageal and cardiac plexuses,[92] and pelvic plexus[94,95] for those wishing more in-depth knowledge in these areas. Selected features of motor, sensory, and autonomic nerve development are shown in Figures 2.3, 2.4, and 2.5.

Development of the Meninges

While numerous studies are available the work of Sensenig (1951) on the spinal meninges is still an excellent and current treatise on their development as related to embryologic staging (Fig. 2.6).

A sparsely cellular network exists between the somites, notochord, and neural tube. Although it is not actually a true meninx, the "meninx primitiva" provides a matrix in which cells migrate and condense to contribute to early development of vertebrae and meninges. It is first found in stage 15 (7 to 9 mm CR; 35 to 38 days), and then extends around the entire neural tube in stage 16 (8 to 11 mm CR; 37 to 42 days). In stage 18 (13 to 17 mm CR; 44 to 48 days) it stratifies and in stage 19 (16 to 18 mm CR; 48 to 51 days) cavitates. Within this matrix neural crest cells that began a ventral migration earlier (stage 13) and spinal ganglia (previously discussed) are situated. Although contributions to all meningeal

Figure 2.6. Selected features in the development of the meninges, as correlated with embryonic stage, CR length, and gestational age. (Adapted from ref. 56.)

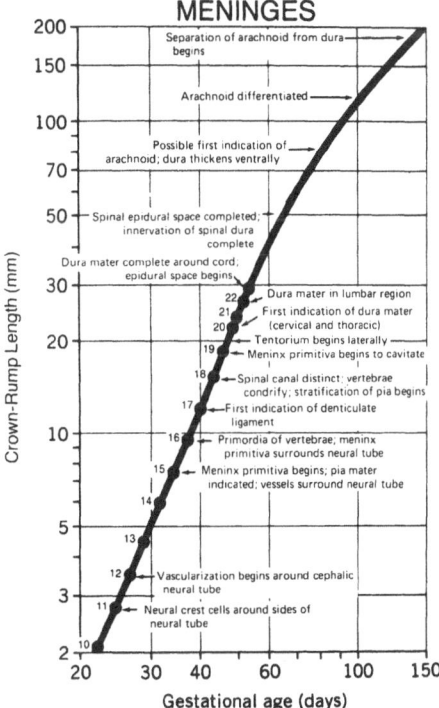

MENINGES

layers are somewhat interlinked it is important to realize that the pia mater and dura mater originate from the above framework, whereas the arachnoid follows somewhat later.

Dura Mater

Mesodermal cells originating from sclerotome and/or meninx primitiva form precursor of dura mater in stages 19 and 20 (18 to 22 mm CR; 51 to 53 days). This is first found in cervical and thoracic regions ventral to the cord. Shortly thereafter (stage 22) the dura mater blends with cells of the vertebral bodies and intervertebral discs, and surrounds the spinal ganglia. At the end of the embryonic period (stage 23) the dura mater surrounds the neural tube; and, although mainly continuous with perichondrium, has some areas of separation. At 50 mm CR length the dura mater and perichondrium have separated, and at 80 mm CR have assumed many of the characteristics found in the newborn.

Pia Mater

Most of the pia mater originates from meninx primitiva but there is some contribution from neural crest. The latter is found in stage 11 (2.5 to 4.5 mm CR; 23 to 26 days) as a single layer of cells around the neural tube. By stage 15 (7 to

9 mm CR; 35 to 38 days), identifiable pia mater is located along the lateral and ventral aspects of the cord, and, during stage 17 (11 to 14 mm CR; 42 to 44 days), denticulate ligament precursors are present.

The two layers of pia mater are suggested in stage 18 (13 to 17 mm CR; 44 to 48 days) and by 50 mm CR length there is a definite plexus of vessels in the epipial tissue.

Arachnoid

Differentiation of arachnoid is complex and its origin is uncertain. It is most likely derived from mesoderm and develops from the inner aspect of the dura mater. As previously mentioned, it is the last of the meninges to differentiate and is first found at 80 mm CR length (80 days gestational age). Delamination from the dura occurs much later with the first indications coming at 200 mm CR length.[56]

Acknowledgments. The author gratefully acknowledges the help in manuscript preparation by Marjorie Clausing, and illustrations by Cheryl Herndon.

References

1. Streeter GL: Developmental horizons in human embryos. Description of age group XI, 13 to 20 somites and age group XII, 21 to 29 somites. Contrib Embryol 30:211–245, 1942.
2. Streeter GL: Developmental horizons in human embryos. Description of age group XIII embryos about 4 or 5 millimeters long, and age group XIV, period of indentation of the lens vesicle. Contrib Embryol 31:27–63, 1945.
3. Streeter GL: Developmental horizons in human embryos. Description of age groups XV, XVI, XVII and XVIII, being the third issue of a survey of the Carnegie collection. Contrib Embryol 33:149–167, 1948.
4. Streeter GL: Developmental horizons in human embryos (fourth issue). A review of the istogènesis of bone and cartilage. Contrib Embryol 33:149–167, 1949.
5. Streeter GL: Developmental Horizons in Human Embryos. Age Groups XI–XXIII. Embryology Reprint, Vol. II. Carnegie Institute, Washington DC, 1951.
6. Streeter GL, Heuser CH, Corner GW: Developmental horizons in human embryos. Description of age groups XIX, XX, XXI, XXII and XXIII, being the fifth issue of a survey of the Carnegie collection. Contrib Embryol 34:165–196, 1951.
7. Heuser CH, Corner GW: Developmental horizons in human embryos. Description of age group X, 4 to 12 somites. Contrib Embryol 36:29–39, 1957.
8. O'Rahilly R: Developmental Stages in Human Embryos, Part A: Embryos of the First Three Weeks (Stages 1 to 9). Carnegie Institute, Washington DC, 1973.
9. O'Rahilly R, Müller F: The first appearance of the human nervous system at stage 8. Anat Embryol 163:1–13, 1981.
10. Iffy L, Shepard TH, Jakobovits A, Lemire RJ, Kerner P: The rate of growth in young human embryos of Streeter's Horizons XIII–XXIII. Acta Anat (Basel) 66:178–186, 1967.
11. Jirásek JE: Development of the Genital System and Male Pseudohermaphroditism. Cohen MM Jr (ed). Johns Hopkins University Press, Baltimore, 1971.

12. Scammon RE: Two simple nomographs for estimating the age and some of the major external dimensions of the human fetus. Anat Rec 68:221–255, 1937.

13. Scammon RE, Calkins LA: The Development and Growth of the External Dimensions of the Human Body in the Fetal Period. University of Minnesota Press, Minneapolis, 1929.

14. Streeter GL: Weight, sitting height, head size, foot length and menstrual age of the human embryo. Contrib Embryol 11:143–170, 1920.

15. Trolle D: Age of foetus determined from its measures. Acta Obstet Gynecol Scand 27:327–337, 1948.

16. Gruenwald P, Minh HN: Evaluation of body and organ weights in perinatal pathology: I. Normal standards derived from autopsies. Am J Clin Pathol 34:247–253, 1960.

17. Tanimura T, Nelson T, Hollingsworth RR, Shepard TH: Weight standards for organs from early human fetuses. Anat Rec 171:227–236, 1971.

18. Bardeen CR: The development of the thoracic vertebrae in man. Am J Anat 4:163–174, 1905a.

19. Bardeen CR: Studies on the development of the human skeleton. Am J Anat 4:265–302, 1905b.

20. Bardeen CR: Early development of the cervical vertebrae and the base of the occipital bone in man. Am J Anat 8:181–186, 1908.

21. Bardeen CR: The development of the skeleton and of the connective tissues. Part II. The morphogenesis of the skeletal system. In: Manual of Human Embryology, Vol. I. Keibal F, Mall FP, (ed.), JB Lippincott, Philadelphia 1910, pp. 316–366.

22. Mall FP: On ossification centers in human embryos less than one hundred days old. Am J Anat 5:433–458, 1906.

23. Calkins LA, Scammon RE: The growth of the spinal axis of the human body in prenatal life. Proc Soc Exp Biol Med 24:300–303, 1927.

24. Arey LB: The history of the first somite in human embryos. Contrib Embryol 27:235–269, 1938.

25. Ehrenhaft JL: Development of the vertebral column as related to certain congenital and pathological changes. Surg Gynecol Obstet 76:282–292, 1943.

26. Wyburn GM: Observations on the development of the human vertebral column. J Anat 78:94–102, 1944.

27. Peacock A: Observations on the development of the intervertebral disc in man. J Anat 85:260–274, 1951.

28. Sensenig EC: The early development of the human vertebral column. Contrib Embryol 33:23–41, 1949.

29. Sensenig EC: The development of the occipital and cervical segments and their associated structures in human embryos. Contrib Embryol 36:141–152, 1957.

30. O'Rahilly R, Meyer DB: The timing and sequence of events in the development of the human vertebral column during the embryonic period proper. Anat Embryol 157:167–176, 1979.

31. O'Rahilly R, Müller F, Meyer DB: The human vertebral column at the end of the embryonic period proper. 1. The column as a whole. J Anat 131:565–575, 1980.

32. O'Rahilly R, Müller F, Meyer DB: The human vertebral column at the end of the embryonic period proper. 2. The occipitocervical region. J Anat 136:181–195, 1983.

33. Streeter GL: The development of the nervous system. In: Keibel F, Mall FP (eds). Manual of Human Embryology, Vol. II. JB Lippincott, Philadelphia, 1912, pp. 1–156.

34. Spemann H: Embryonic Development and Induction. Yale University Press, New Haven, 1938.

35. Spratt NT Jr: Regression and shortening of the primitive streak in the explanted chick blastoderm. J Exp Zool 104:69–100, 1947.

36. Spratt NT Jr: Localization of the prospective neural plate in the early chick blastoderm. J Exp Zool 120:109–130, 1952.

37. Spratt NT Jr: Analysis of the organizer center in the early chick embryo. I. Localization of prospective notochord and somite cells. J Exp Zool 128:121–163, 1955.

38. Spratt NT Jr: Analysis of the organizer center in the early chick embryo. II. Studies of the mechanics of notochord elongation and somite formation. J Exp Zool 134:577–612, 1957a.

39. Spratt NT Jr: Analysis of the organizer center in the early chick embryo. III. Regulative properties of the chorda and somite centers. J Exp Zool 135:319–353, 1957b.

40. Gaertner RA: Development of the posterior trunk and tail of the chick embryo, J Exp Zool 111:157–174, 1949.

41. Saxen L, Toivonen S: The two-gradient hypothesis in primary induction: the combined effect of two types of inductors mixed in different ratios. J Embryol Exp Morphol 9:514–533, 1961.

42. Seichert V, Jelínek R: Tissue shifts in the end and tail bud of the chick embryo. Folia Morphol (Praha) 16:436–446, 1968.

43. Toivonen S, Saxen L: Morphogenetic interaction of presumptive neural and mesodermal cells mixed in different ratios. Science 159:529–540, 1968.

44. Klika E, Jelínek R: The structure of the end and tail bud of the chick embryo. Folia Morphol (Praha) 17:29–40, 1969.

45. Jelínek R, Seichert V, Klika E: Mechanism of morphogenesis of the caudal neural tube in the chick embryo. Folia Morphol (Praha) 17:355–357, 1969.

46. Schroeder TE: Neurulation in *Xenopus laevis*: An analysis and model based upon light and electron microscopy. J Embryol Exp Morphol 23:427–462, 1970.

47. Karfunkel P: The mechanisms of neural tube formation. Int Rev Cytol 38:245–271, 1974.

48. Duncan D: Electron microscope study of the embryonic neural tube and notochord. Tex Rep Biol Med 15:367–377, 1957.

49. Jurand A: The development of the notochord in chick embryos. J Embryol Exp Morphol 10:602–621, 1962.

50. Kunitomo K: The development and reduction of the tail and the caudal end of the spinal cord. Contrib Embryol 8:161–198, 1918.

51. Streeter GL: Factors involved in the formation of the filum terminale. Am J Anat 25:1–11, 1919.

52. Kernohan JW: The ventriculus terminalis: its growth and development. J Comp Neurol 38:107–125, 1925.

53. Bolli P: Sekundäre Lumenbildungen im Neuralrohr und Rückenmark menschlicher Embryonen. Acta Anat 64:48–81, 1966.

54. Lemire RJ: Variations in development of the caudal neural tube in human embryos (Horizons XIV–XXI) Teratology 2:361–369, 1969.

55. Barson AJ: The vertebral level of termination of the spinal cord during normal and abnormal development. J Anat 106:489–497, 1970.

56. Lemire RF, Loeser JD, Leech RW, Alvord EC Jr: Normal and Abnormal Development of the Human Nervous System. Harper & Row Hagerstown, 1975.

57. Malínský J, Malínská J: Developmental stages of prenatal spinal cord in man. Folia Morphol (Praha) 18:228–235, 1970.

58. Lassek AM, Rasmussen GL: A quantitative study of the newborn and adult spinal cords of man. J Comp Neurol 69:371–379, 1938.

59. Lassek AM, Rasmussen GL: A regional volumetric study of the gray and white matter of the human prenatal spinal cord. J Comp Neurol 70:137–151, 1939.

60. Langworthy OR: Development of behavior patterns and myelinization of the nervous system in the human fetus and infant. Contrib Embryol 24:1–57, 1933.

61. Yaklovlev PI, Lecours AR: The myelogenetic cycles of the regional maturation of the brain. In: Minkowski A (ed): Regional Development of the Brain in Early Life. Blackwell, Oxford, 1967, pp. 3–70.

62. Sensenig EC: The early development of the meninges of the spinal cord in human embryos. Contrib Embryol 34:145–157, 1951.

63. Sauer FC: Mitosis in the neural tube. J Comp Neurol 62:377–405, 1935a.

64. Sauer FC: The cellular structure of the neural tube. J Comp Neurol 63:13–23, 1935b.

65. Sauer FC: The interkinetic migration of embryonic epithelial nuclei. J Morphol 60:1–11, 1936.

66. Sauer FC: Some factors in the morphogenesis of vertebrate embryonic epithelium. J Morphol 61:563–579, 1937.

67. Sauer ME, Walker BE: Radioautographic study of interkinetic nuclear migration in the neural tube. Proc Soc Exp Biol Med 101:557–560, 1959.

68. Watterston RL: Structure and mitotic behavior of the early neural tube. Organogenesis. In: DeHaan RL, H Ursprung (eds). New York, Holt, Rinehart and Winston, New York, 1965, pp. 129–159.

69. Sidman RL: Cellular proliferation and migration in the developing brain. Drugs and Poisons in Relation to the Developing Nervous System. Public Health Service Publication No. 1791, 1967, pp. 5–11.

70. Sidman RL, Miale IL, Feder N: Cell proliferation and migration in the primitive ependymal zone; an autoradiographic study of histogenesis in the nervous system. Exp Neurol 1:322–333, 1959.

71. Fugita S: Kinetics of cellular proliferation. Exp Cell Res 28:52–60, 1962.

72. Martin A, Langman J: The development of the spinal cord examined by autoradiography. J Embryol Exp Morphol 14:25–35, 1965.

73. Rakic P, Sidman RL: Supravital DNA synthesis in the developing human and mouse brain. J Neuropathol Exp Neurol 27:246–276, 1968.

74. Martin AH: Significance of mitotic spindle fiber orientation in the neural tube. Nature 216:1133–1134, 1967.

75. Grabowski CT: The effects of the excision of Henson's node on the early development of the chick embryo. J Exp Zool 133:301–344, 1956.

76. Rosenquist GC: A radioautographic study of labeled grafts in the chick blastoderm. Development from primitive-streak stages to Stage 12. Contrib Embryol 38:71–110, 1966.

77. Lemire FJ, Shepard TH, Alvord EC Jr: Caudal myeloschisis (lumbosacral spina bifida cystica) in a five millimeter (Horizon XIV) human embryo. Anat Rec 152:9–16, 1965.

78. Hogg ID: The development of the nucleus dorsalis (Clarke's column) J Comp Neurol 81:69–95, 1944.

79. Elliott HC: Studies on the motor cells of the spinal cord: II. Distribution in the normal human fetal cord. Am J Anat 72:29–38, 1943.

80. Romanes GJ: Cell columns in the spinal cord of a human foetus of fourteen weeks. J Anat 75:145–152, 1941.

81. Humphrey T: Primitive neurons in the embryonic human central nervous system. J Comp Neurol 81:1–45, 1944.

82. Youngstrom KA: Intramedullary sensory type ganglion cells in the spinal cord of human embryos. J Comp Neurol 81:47–53, 1944.

83. Humphrey T: Sensory ganglion cells within the central canal of the embryonic human spinal cord. J Comp Neurol 86:1–35, 1947.
84. Hogg ID: Sensory nerves and associated structures in the skin of human fetuses of 8 to 14 233ks of menstrual age correlated with functional capability. J Comp Neurol 75:371–410, 1941.
85. Hewer EE: The development of nerve endings in the human foetus. J Anat 69:369–379, 1935.
86. Bardeen CR, Lewis WH: Development of the limbs, body-wall and back in man. Am J Anat 1:1–35, 1901.
87. Lewis WH: The development of the arm in man. Am J Anat 1:145–183, 1902.
88. Streeter GL: The development of the cranial and spinal nerves in the occipital region of the human embryo. Am J Anat 4:83–116, 1904.
89. Cuajunco F: Development of human motor end plate. Contrib Embryol 30:127–152, 1942.
90. Streeter GL: The peripheral nervous system in the human embryo at the end of the first month (10 mm). Am J Anat 8:285–301, 1908.
91. Bardeen CR: Development and variation of the nerves and musculature of the inferior extremity and of the neighboring regions of the trunk in man. Am J Anat 6:259–390, 1907.
92. Kuntz A: The development of the sympathetic nervous system in man. J Comp Neurol 32:173–229, 1921.
93. Pearson AA, Eckhardt AL: Observations on the gray and white rami communicantes in human embryos. Anat Rec 138:115–127, 1960.
94. Kuntz A: Origin and early development of the pelvic neural plexus. J Comp Neurol 96:345–357, 1952.
95. Kimmel DL, McCrea E: The development of the pelvic plexuses and the distribution of the pelvic splanchnic nerves in the human embryo and fetus. J Comp Neurol 110:271–298, 1958.

CHAPTER 3

Growth of the Spine

A. DiMeglio and F. Bonnel

Introduction

Three periods characterize the growth of the spine: (1) the *embryonic period* during which all vertebral column and cord elements become identifiable; (2) the *fetal period*, corresponding to the onset of the vertebral ossification; (3) the *postnatal period*, characterized by the progression of ossification, and musculo-skeletal growth and development.

Vertebral growth is *growth by endochondral ossification*, a three-phase process by which the vertebral column forms: (1) a mesenchymal stage, which corresponds approximately to the embryonic period; (2) a cartilaginous stage, which acts as the matrix of the third stage; (3) ossification. The growth of the posterior arch, the closure of which is partly linked to the presence of the neural tube, is different from the growth of the vertebral body which behaves like a long bone. The growth velocity is different, not only from one level of the spine to another, but also at each vertebral level, and morphology at the end of growth is the result of the synchronized development of more than 100 growth plates.

All of spinal pathology depends on the dynamics of these growth plates; consequently, every affection intermingles sooner or later with growth plate pathology. Consequently the growth of the spine is complex and hierarchized. Actually, it is the result of multiple microgrowths: the growth of the vertebral body; the growth of the posterior arch; the growth of the cord and of its roots. Each component has its own growth rate but they are all synchronized and progress according to perfectly programmed timing.

The Three Distinct Periods

An embryonic period, a fetal period, a postnatal period all overlap and mingle regularly in time. The mesenchymal stage is just completed when the cartilaginous stage starts. And as soon as the cartilage stage is formed, ossification begins. But, the ossification process, which starts as soon as the second month of intrauterine life, is a slow process which proceeds throughout the growing years, to age 18.

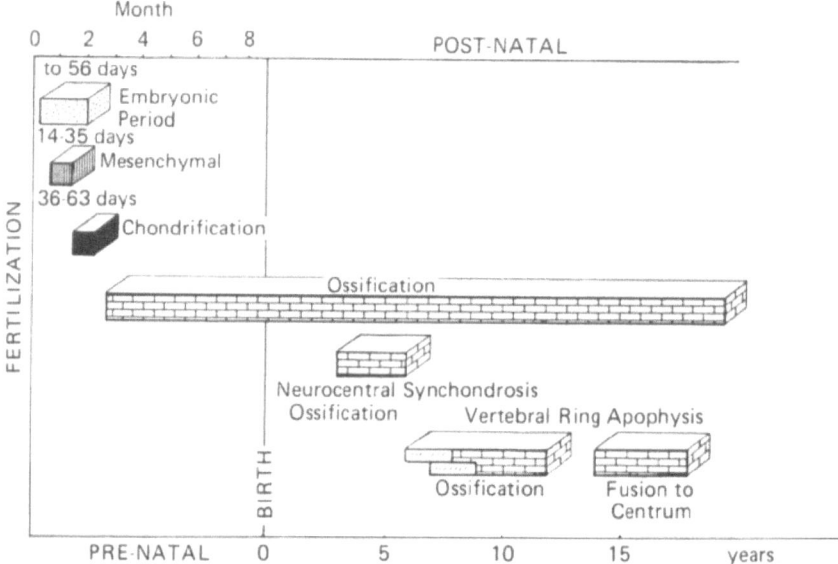

Figure 3.1. Developmental periods of vertebra. (After Tsou: Embryology of Kyphosis Clin Orthop 128:18–25, 1977)

The Embryonic Period

The embryonic period, from day 0 to day 60, is the time during which the cord and its roots on one side, and the vertebra on the other side, become fully identifiable structures. Misdirections or disturbances of most any sort lead to a malformation. The essential factors are the role of the notochord, the redistribution of the sclerotomes, and the closure of the posterior arch, which is linked to the closure of the spinal cord.

Two layers are face-to-face: the ectoblast, representing the future spinal cord, and the mesoblast, representing the future vertebrae. Then, the ectoblast invaginates as the mesoblast thickens. The somites appear, then somites split as the sclerotomes appear. These latter migrate laterally and fuse around the chord. Then the sclerotomes, after fusion, divide into segments (decisive period) before the vertebral anlage appears. All these events during the embryonic period develop at an exponential rate. Many congenital spinal malformations occur during this segmentation process, during which the caudal pole of a sclerotome meets the underlying proximal pole.

Charles Rivard's experimental work on mice embryos showed that it was possible to induce a congenital spinal malformation. Since the sclerotome and the notochord form an inductive complex, it appears that the notochord controls the migration of the sclerotomic cells and, also, their differentiation in the vertebrae.

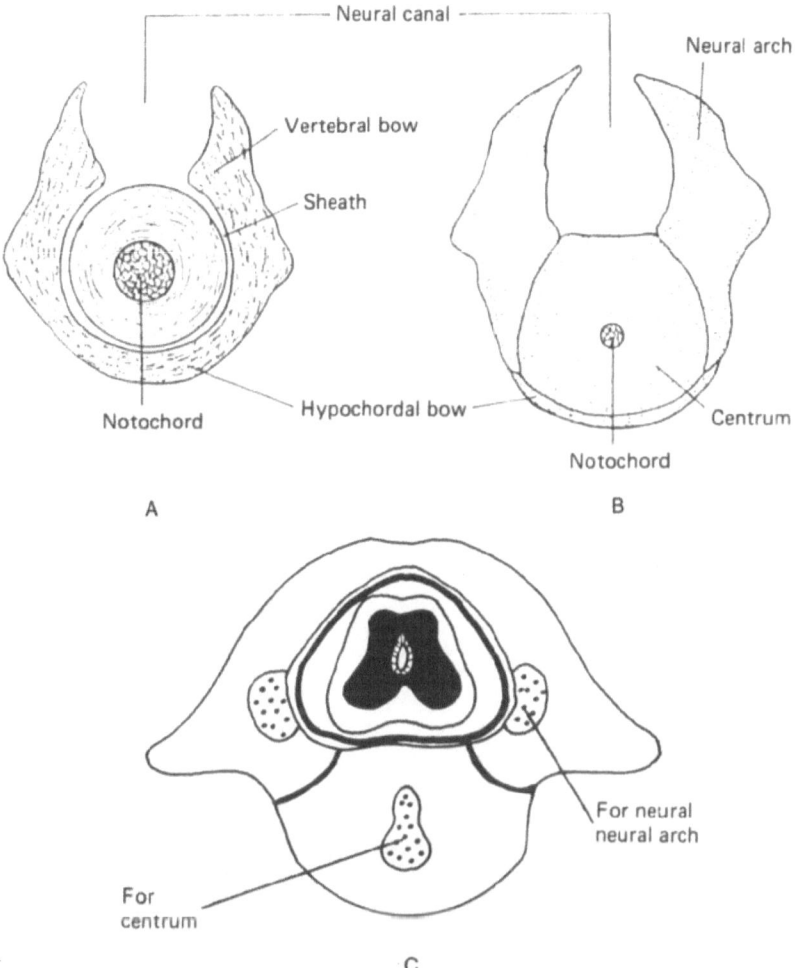

Figure 3.2. Stages in the development of a vertebra. A: Membranous stage. B: Cartilaginous stage. C: Chondrification centers appear in the mesenchymatous outline of a vertebra (sixth embryonic week). Some investigators state that only one chondrification center appears in the centrum while the majority favor the formation of two chondrification centers laterally, which rapidly fuse, in the regions surrounding the notochord.

The glucosaminoglycans seem to play a significant biochemical part. Thus it could be that the congenital vertebral malformations occur before the fetal period, even before the cartilaginous phase. Since these developmental stages overlap considerably, a child may be born with some spina bifida and a malformation of the vertebral bodies.

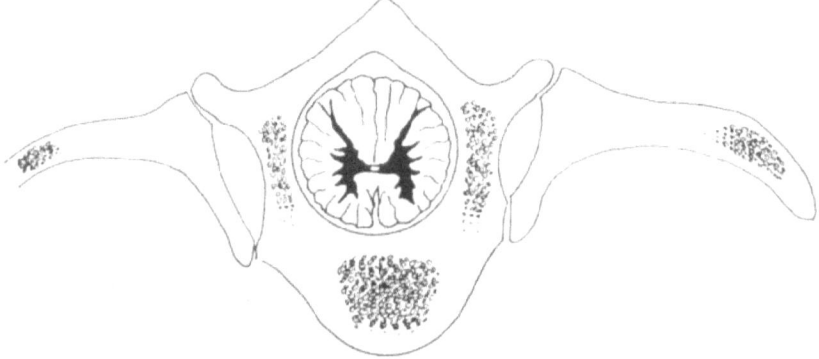

Figure 3.3. Ossification of the vertebral column. Neural arch (7th–8th week)–Centrum (8th week).

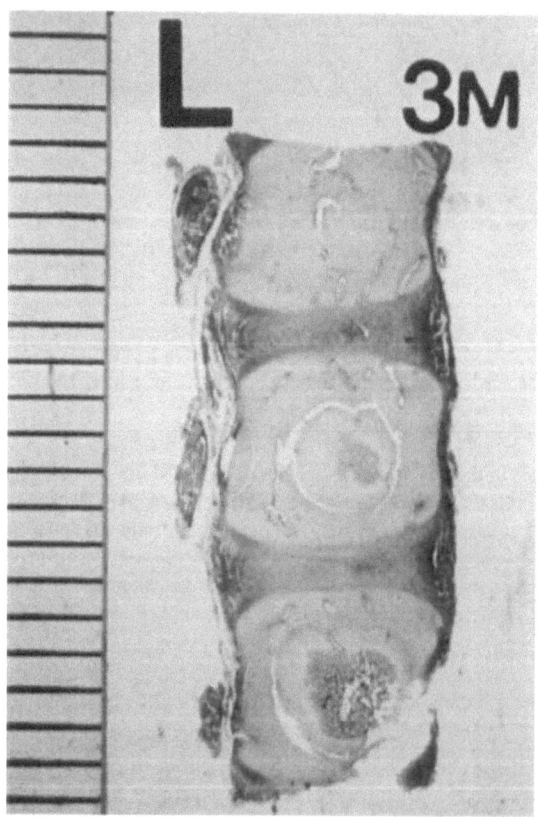

Figure 3.4. At 3 months, ossification starts in the vertebral body.

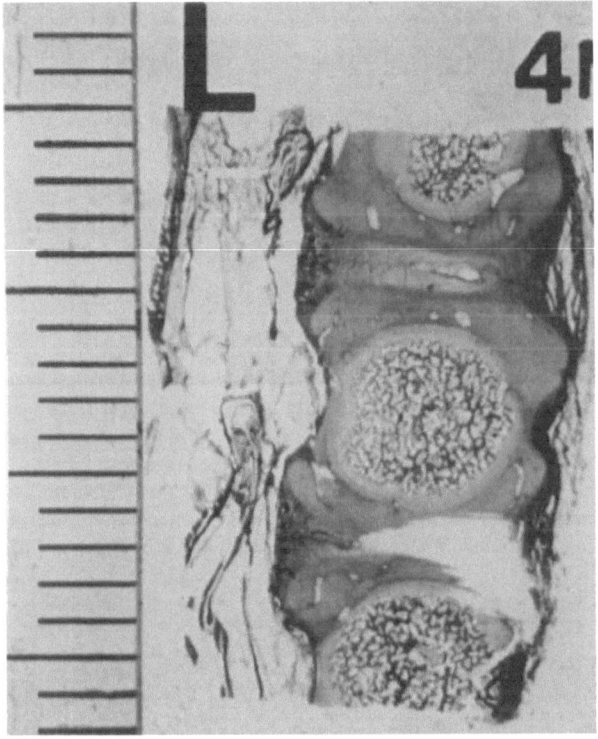

Figure 3.5. At 4 months, progression of the ossification is very spectacular.

The Fetal Period

The fetal period, from day 60 to birth, corresponds to the very beginning of the ossification of the vertebral body. The mesenchymal phase is brief, and very quickly followed by the cartilaginous phase. Cartilage is present in the pedicles, the laminae, and the transverse apophyses (from 30 to 35 mm). Hypertrophied cartilage centers appear very soon during the fetal period, not only in the arches, but also in the centrum (at about 36 mm). Ossification follows rapidly.

About the third month (week 12, size: 80 mm), the cartilaginous posterior arches fuse backward, allowing one to suppose that spina bifida occurs before this period. As soon as the cartilaginous processes of the posterior arches fuse, a spinous process becomes visible (120 mm). During this period, the proportions change. At month 2 of intrauterine life, the vertebral column represents about three-fourths of the body length, a proportion that changes progressively as the lower limbs develop. At month 5 of intrauterine life, the spine length represents only three-fifths of the fetus' total length, and then only two-fifths at birth.

Vertebral ossification does not progress simultaneously and symmetrically in all the parts of the vertebral column. Rather, its progress is radial:

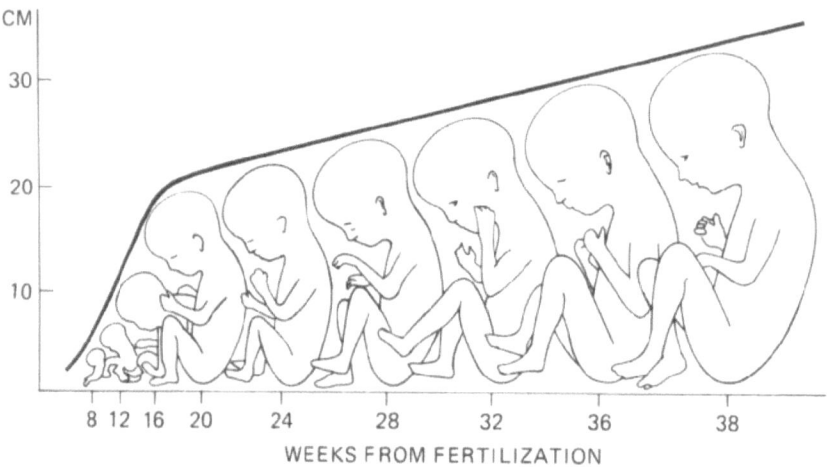

Figure 3.6. Curve of the vertex–coccyx segment in the fetus. At month 3, it is about 10 cm long, and reaches 25 cm at month 4. Thus, the growth rate is very significant during the fourth month. At month 5, it is 30 cm long and will reach 34 cm at birth.

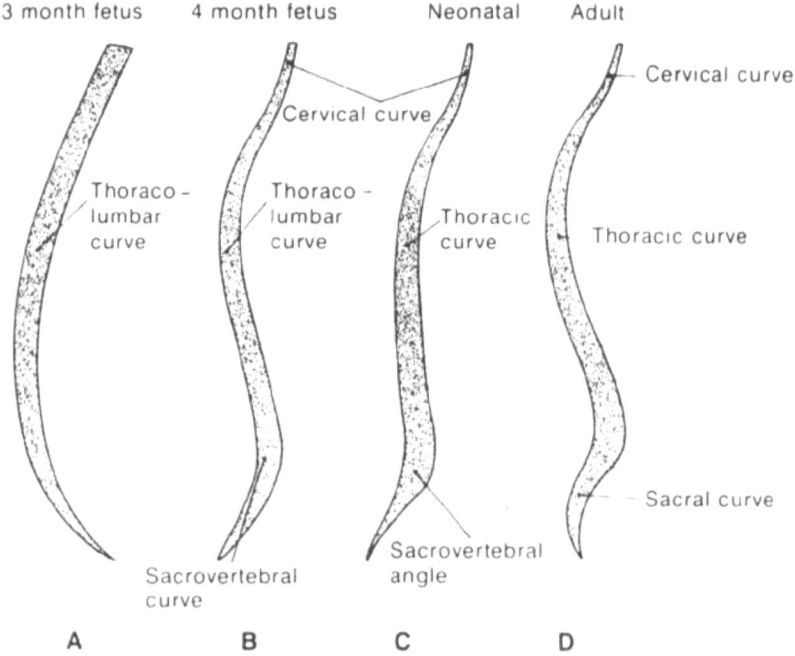

Figure 3.7. Evolution of the spinal curvatures. A: Three months fetus with C-shaped curve. B: Four-month fetus. C: Neonate. D: Adult with normal cervical lordosis, thoracic kyphosis, and lumbar lordosis. (After Gehweiler J, Osborne R, Becker F: The radiology of vertebral trauma. Saunders, Philadelphia, 1980.)

Figure 3.8. Vertebral ossification at birth. The cervical spine is still cartilaginous. Ossification is more important in the thoracic area, and then progresses toward the lumbar and cervical areas.

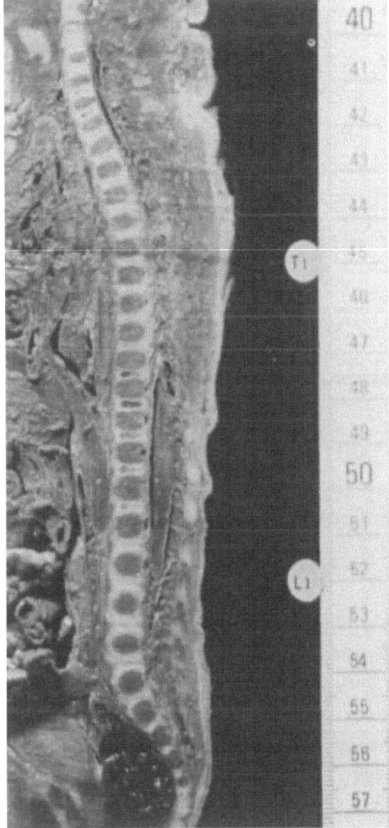

Backward, at the laminar level, this ossification starts in the cervical area and then regularly progresses from top to bottom until the coccyx.

Forward, at the vertebral body level; it appears first in the thoracic area and then progresses toward the lumbar and cervical areas.

The spinal curvatures are not primitive but acquired. During the first period of intrauterine life, the vertebral column is nearly rectilinear or slightly concave forward. At month 5, the sacral–vertebral angle begins to form, delimiting respectively the lumbar area and the sacral area. But even at birth there is nearly no trace of the inflections that characterize the cervical area and the lumbar area.

From Birth to Adulthood

At birth, two new elements play an essential part: neurological maturation and the sitting height (the development of which reflects vertebral growth). At birth, the vertebrae present three ossification centers: one for the central anterior part,

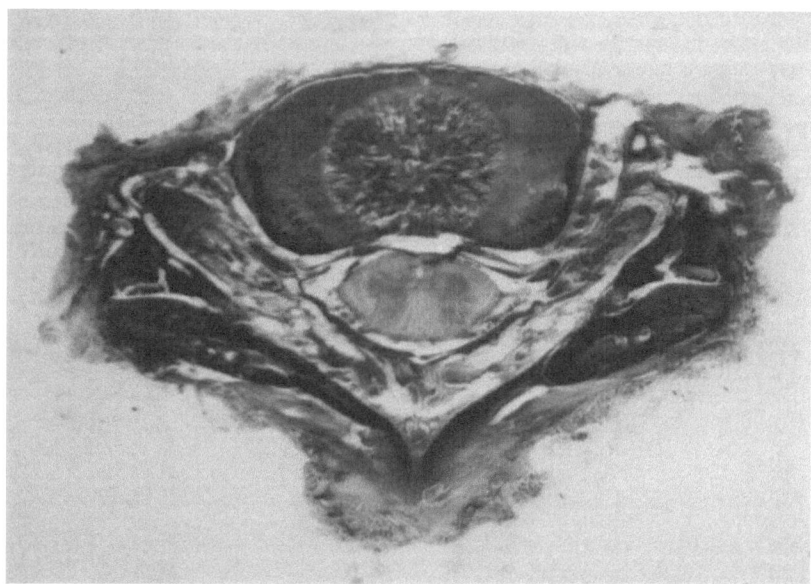

Figure 3.9. At birth, the vertebra presents three ossification centers: one for the central anterior part, one for each of the posterior arches. On this view of a cervical vertebra, note the neuro–central synchondrosis: the neural synchondrosis fuses in the cervical region at 3 years. This union proceeds caudally and is usually complete in the sacrum by age 7. The neural arch forms the vertebral arch and contributes a tiny portion to the centrum on each side to form the vertebral body. During the first year of life, the two neural arches join dorsally. This union first occurs in the lumbar region, shortly after birth, and extends cranially into the thoracic and cervical regions by the second year.

and one for each of the posterior arches. The vertebral column is approximately 24 cm long at this time. Its length will nearly triple within the end of growth (about 70 cm). Only 30% of the spine is ossified at this time, there are no significant differences from one vertebra to another, and the vertebral body of a thoracic vertebra is about 7.6 mm thick, 8 mm for a lumbar vertebra (height). The sitting height is 35 cm.

The first year of life is marked by two events: (1) the development of the spinal cord within its container and (2) the constitution of the cervical, dorsal, and lumbar curves subsequent to assumption of the upright position. Once in the upright position, about age 1, the cervical and lumbar lordotic curves appear, a result of the "cephalo–caudal" influence of neuromotor development and neurologic maturation.

The vertebral body may include two ossification centers. The coronal cleft, which is sometimes visible at birth, disappears through the first year of life. However, the radiologic image, which should be considered a variation of endochondral ossification, may persist until age 4.

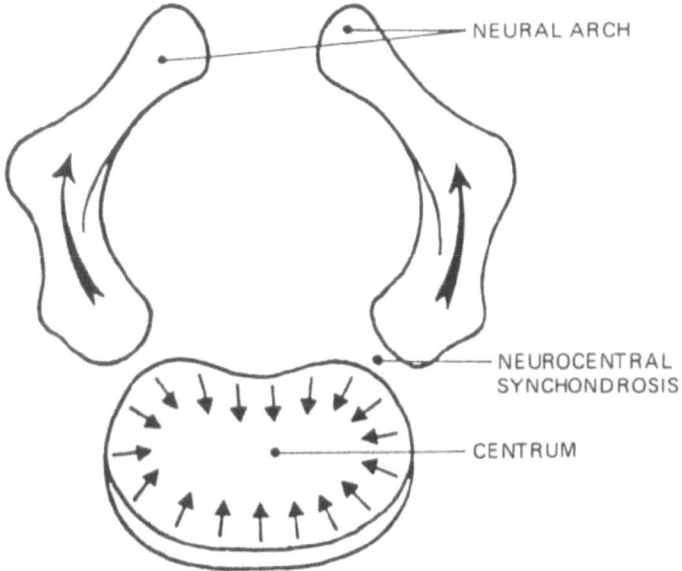

Figure 3.10. A vertebra at birth.

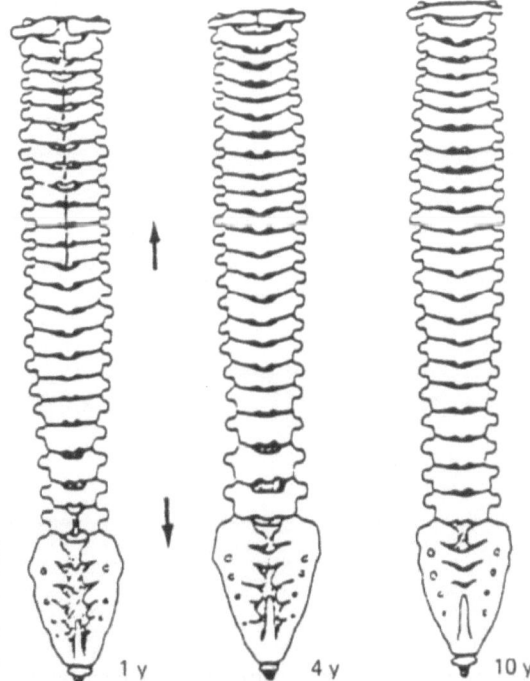

Figure 3.11. Ossification and closure of the posterior arch of the vertebra. (From Paturet G: Traité de anatomie, Volume 1, Ostéologie. Masson, Paris, 1951, p. 395.)

1 y   4 y   10 y

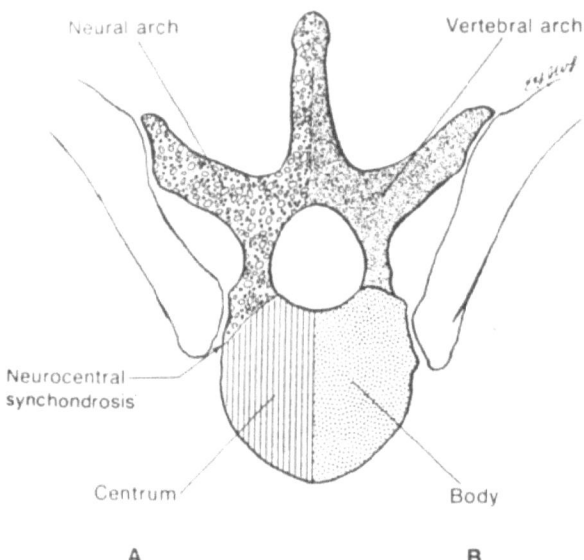

Figure 3.12. Schematic drawing of the neural arch and centrum (A), and the vertebral arch and body (B). Note that these terms are not interchangeable. It should be noted that the rib does not articulate with the centrum, but only with the neural arch. Neural arch becomes vertebral arch when there is fusion dorsally, and the centrum becomes vertebral body when there is fusion of the neuro–central synchondrosis.

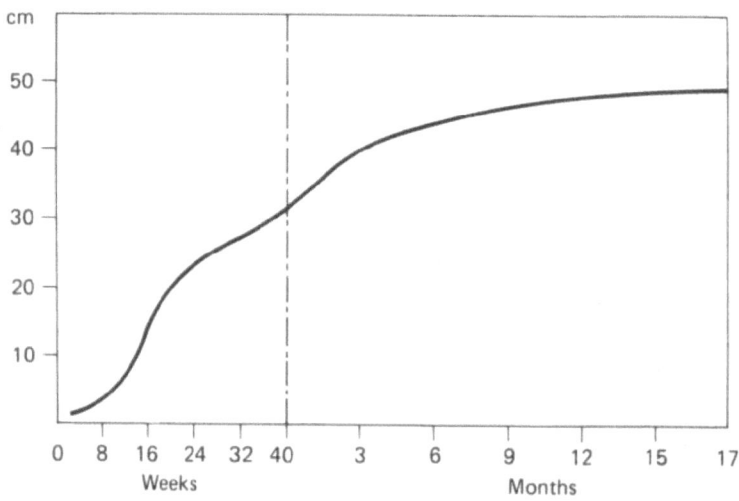

Figure 3.13. Chart of the sitting height growth during intrauterine life, and the 18 first months of extrauterine life.

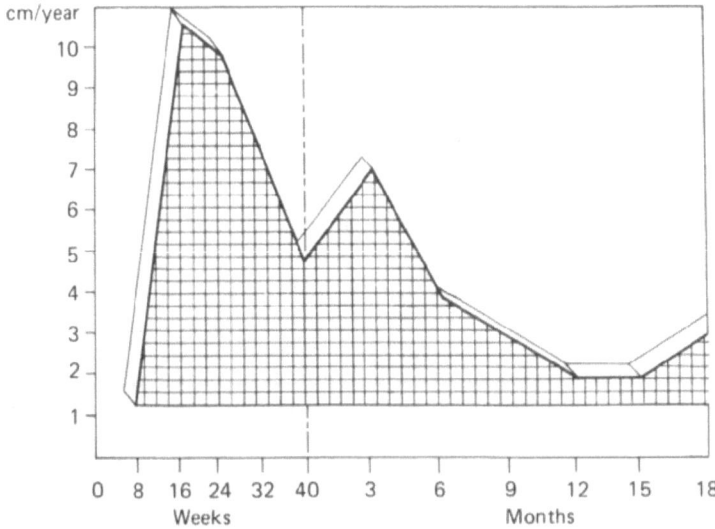

Figure 3.14. Chart of growth velocity of the sitting height during intrauterine life and the first 18 months of extrauterine life: the most significant growth occurs from the second to the sixth month in utero. A second acceleration occurs at month 3 after birth.

From age 1 to 5, neurologic maturation allows new motor attainments, particularly in the upper (drawing and so on) and lower (going upstairs and downstairs) limbs.

Thus, growth remains active during the fetal period and first 5 years of life: the sitting height goes from 35 cm to 47 cm (+12 cm) from age 0 to 1, from 47 cm to 62 cm (+15 cm) from age 1 to 5. This is a height increase of 27 cm within 5 years! The growth spurt occurring during the 5 first years of life is even more significant than the pubertal growth spurt.

From age 5 to 10, the growth of the trunk, and consequently the growth of the spine, slows down. The sitting height increases only 10 cm. The annual growth rate of the trunk is about 2 cm.

From age 10 on, the growing spine starts a new stage, characterized by puberty during which there is another remarkable growth spurt which is almost as great as that during the first 5 years of life. In fact, from age 10 to 18, the sitting height gains 20 cm in boys and 15 cm in girls. The pubertal peak starts at skeletal age 11 in girls (onset of the thumb sesamoid). It is characterized by 2 years of rapid growth during which the sitting height increases 7 cm, and by 3 years of slow growth during which the sitting height increases 5 cm.

The pubertal peak starts later in boys, at skeletal age 13. It is characterized by 2 years of rapid growth, from skeletal age 13 to 15, during which the sitting height increases 8 cm, and a slow growth, from skeletal age 15 to 18, during which the sitting height increases 5 cm.

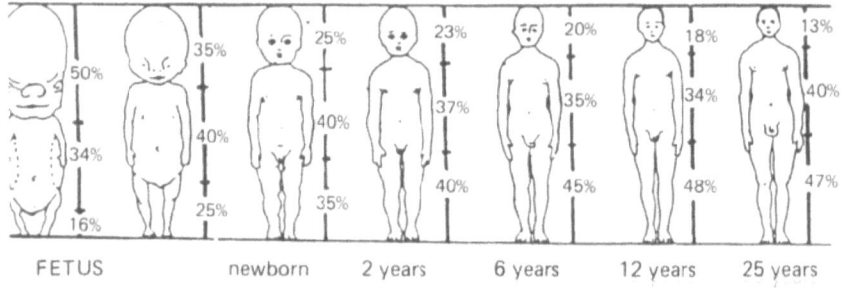

FETUS   newborn   2 years   6 years   12 years   25 years

months   5 months

Figure 3.15. A sharper study of the comparative evolution of the three segments (head, trunk, lower limbs) during growth shows that the percentage involving the head steadily decreases from fetal life to adulthood, whereas, on the other hand, the percentage of the lower limbs steadily increases. The trunk is the only segment whose percentage varies during growth with a very distinct increase at puberty, after a phase of deceleration from birth to puberty.

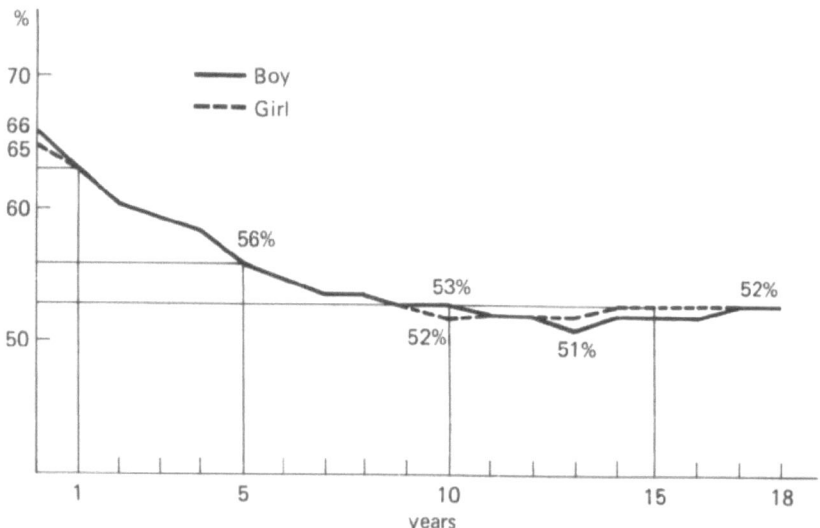

Figure 3.16. Evaluation of the "sitting height/standing height" ratio during growth: a strong deceleration occurs during the first 6 years. The stabilization at 52% occurs only at the end of puberty.

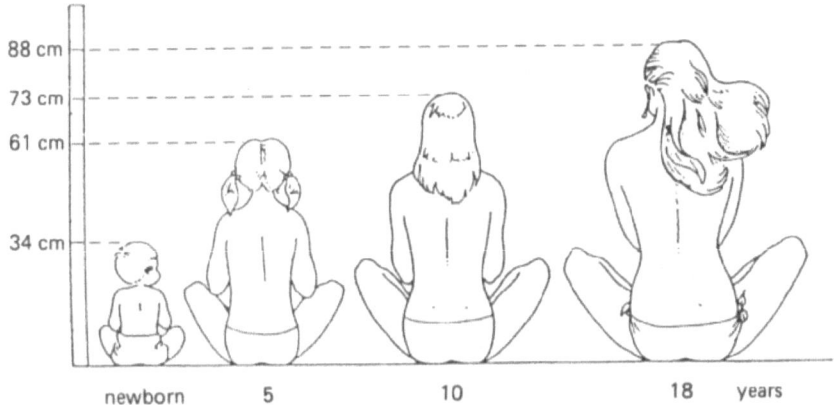

Figure 3.17. Sitting height, girls.

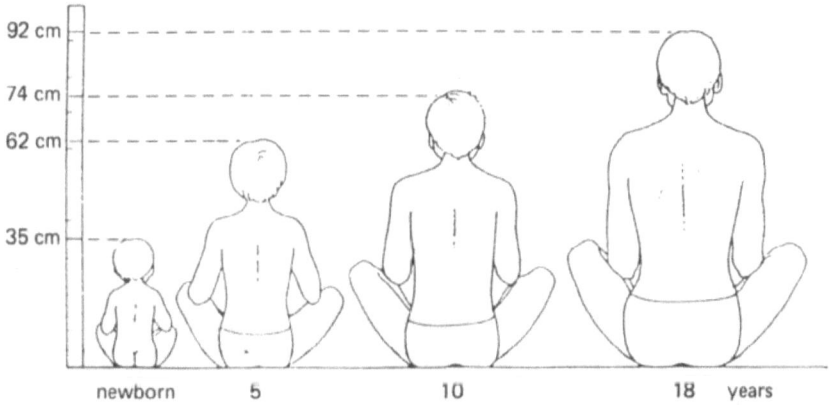

Figure 3.18. Sitting height, boys.

All these data are important because the sitting height, which represents the macrogrowth, is only the result of microgrowths occurring especially in the spine. It is important to notice that from age 10 to 17, the vertebral volume nearly doubles, and that the secondary ossification centers appear at puberty—particularly at the posterior arch level—as well as the marginal listel which "braids" the vertebral body.

Vertebral Growth

This follows an endochondral-type ossification, that is to say the typical process through membranous, cartilaginous, and osseous phases, the three blending imperceptibly one into the other, going from birth, when the vertebra is a cartilaginous mass on to complete ossification from growth cartilages. The three ossification lines proceed one toward the other, in order to fuse. The two lateral ossification lines form the posterior arch, and the one, median, ossification line the vertebral body.

Growth of the Posterior Arch

This is linked to the neural tube. Each posterior half-arch is made of a pedicle, a lamina, and an inferior articular apophysis which is bigger than the superior articular apophysis. The pars interarticularis can be clearly observed and is already ossified at birth. Nonossification of the pars interarticularis is never encountered. This notion is basic to understand the pathogenesis of spondylolisthesis, which is due to a stress fracture.

The two ossification lines approach one another posteriorly, mid-line, and fuse about age 1. The fusion starts in the thoracic area, then in the sacral area, and at the atlas and axis level at ages 2 and 4, respectively.

The formation of the posterior arch depends essentially on the medullary closure. There is a relation between the container (spinal column) and the contents (spinal cord), but we do not yet know which is the determining element. The neural tube affects the closure of the posterior arch, but it is not reciprocal: nonclosure of the posterior arch does not systematically lead to a medullary malformation. Progressively, the posterior arch and the vertebral body fuse about the fifth year of life. The fusion corresponds to a real closure of the two growth cartilages which allow the growth of the posterior arch. We can say that from age 4 on, the growth of the medullary canal is nearly completed. This concept is basic to one who plans to perform a perivertebral arthrodesis in a child. The neuro–central junction is located in the posterior zone of the vertebral body. To some extent, it contributes to the growth of the vertebral body.

Growth of the Vertebral Body

This follows a pattern similar to diaphyseal growth. In order to understand this growth, it is necessary to compare it to the growth of a long bone. In describing vertebral body growth as diaphyseal, one intends to specify that there are two growth plates, one at either extremity, which migrate toward one another, and which ossify the central part of the vertebral body. The growth of the vertebral body illustrates quite well the morphologic changes of the growth plates. At the very beginning, the vertebral body looks like a lentil, then the growth plate becomes circular, and, progressively, the vertebral body becomes rectangular: the growth cartilages are then located at the upper pole and at the lower pole of the vertebra. The upper and lower growth plates determine the length increase of the vertebra. The thickness increase of the vertebra results from the periosteum, as in the long bones.

About age 10, a listel appears at the upper and lower part of the vertebra. It is a ring which lines and braids the vertebra. This ring ossifies from the front to the

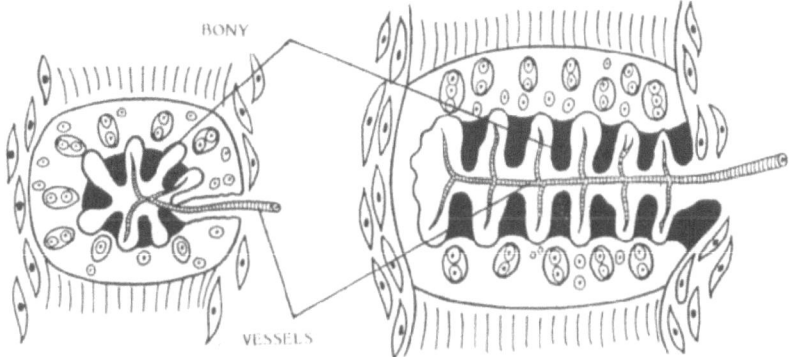

Figure 3.19. Growth by endochondral ossification of the vertebral body.

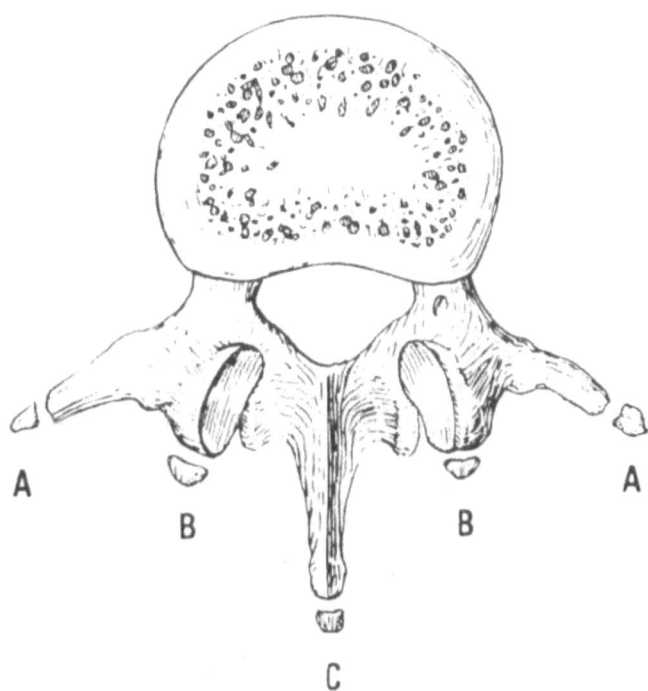

Figure 3.20. A: Transverse process. B: Mammillary process. C: Spinous process. Secondary ossification centers (apophysis) of the transverse, mammillary, and spinous processes.

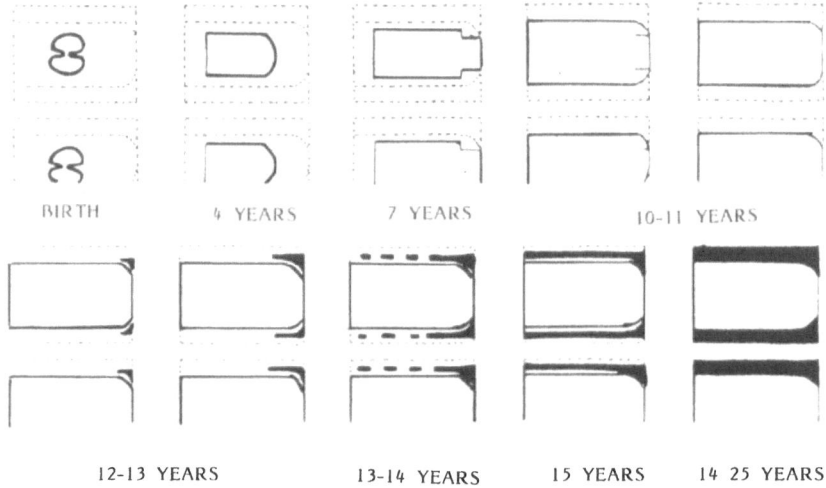

Figure 3.21. Morphology of the vertebral body. Evolution of the vertebral body from birth to the end of growth (boy). The bony centrum is first ovoid and then becomes rectangular. About age 10, a listel appears at the upper and lower part of the vertebra.

back, and fuses with the vertebral body between ages 18 and 25. Contrary to a widely held opinion, the ring is not an epiphyseal plate. It responds to the tractions of the posterior longitudinal ligament, of the prevertebral muscles, and thus behaves like an apophysis. At the same age, secondary ossification centers appear at the top of the transverse, spinal, and articular apophyses, contributing to perfect the morphology of the vertebra. They, too, as all bony processes, are under the influence of the different muscular tractions.

Winter thinks that the height of each vertebra gains about 0.07 cm per year. This assessment is useful from a mnemotechnic point of view. However, the growth of the vertebra is not linear: it is very rapid during the 5 first years of life, slackens from ages 5 to 10, to accelerate greatly during puberty.

An average thoracic vertebra, such as T7:

Age	Height	Volume
Newborn	0.6 cm	1.2 cm³
2 yrs.	1.1 cm	8.6 cm³
4 yrs.	1.3 cm	12.8 cm³
10 yrs.	1.6 cm	18.7 cm³
18 yrs.	2.2 cm	39.4 cm³

So, the vertebral height more than triples. It doubles about age 3, and reaches 50% of its final height about age 2. The vertebral volume is nearly multiplied by 8 at age 2, and by nearly 40 at the end of growth.

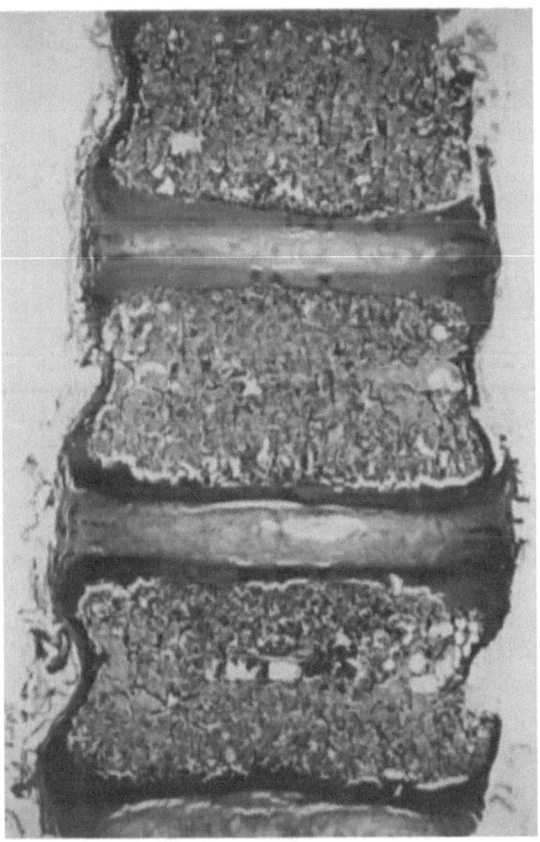

Figure 3.22. Vertebral body of lumbar vertebra at 9 years (frontal plane). Compare with Figs. 3.4 and 3.5.

An average lumbar vertebra, such as L3:

Age	Height	Volume
Newborn	0.83 cm	2.0 cm³
2 yrs.	1.6 cm	18.4 cm³
4 yrs.	2.0 cm	24.0 cm³
10 yrs.	2.4 cm	43.0 cm³
18 yrs.	3.3 cm	87.0 cm³

The height of the lumbar vertebra quadruples. It nearly reaches its final height at age 2. Its volume nearly doubles from ages 10 to 18.

These measurements are interesting as they allow one to realize that the growth notion is not only vertical and horizontal, but volumetric. This puts into relief the fact that growth is differential, and that it must be perceived as such spatially:

growth is different from the front to the back of the vertebra. In the thoracic area, the posterior elements increase more rapidly than the anterior elements. The contrary is true in the lumbar area.

These different growths result in morphologic changes. The articular apophyses, for instance, change their orientation during growth. They form a 170° angle initially, nearly an horizontal plane, to change progressively with age to a 110° angle, undergoing a 60° rotation.

Segmental Growth

The height of the spine nearly triples from birth to adulthood. The adult spine is 70 cm in the male, 65 cm in the female: cervical spine, 12 cm; thoracic spine, 28 cm; lumbar spine, 18 cm; sacrum, 12 cm.

The Cervical Spine

At birth, vertical measurement of the cervical spine is 3.7 cm, so that it grows about 9 cm to reach the adult height of 12 to 13 cm at the end of growth. The length nearly doubles at age 6; the pubertal growth spurt leads to a 3 cm gain. The cervical spine represents 22% of the C1–S1 segment, and 15 to 16% of the sitting height. The volume of the cervical spine is 9 cm³ at birth; its volume at the end of growth is about 125 cm³, that is to say that it is multiplied by approximately 15.

Cervical spine dimensions:

Age	Height
Newborn	3.7 cm
6 yrs.	7.5 cm
10 yrs.	10.0 cm
15 yrs.	13.0 cm

It is necessary to distinguish two totally different entities: (1) the upper cervical spine (C1–C2), and the lower cervical spine (C3, C4, C5, C6, C7).

The upper cervical spine, C1–C2, is characterized by its embryologic singularity. The lower part of the fourth occipital sclerotome, and the upper part of the first cervical sclerotome, form the top of the odontoid. The lower part of the first cervical sclerotome and the upper part of the second cervical sclerotome form the atlas and the base of the odontoid. The lower part of the C2 sclerotome and the upper part of the C3 sclerotome form the body of the atlas. The body of the odontoid practically represents the body of the atlas, but it fuses and inserts into the axis vertebral body.

The atlas has two lateral ossification centers, which become the lateral masses. There is a third ossification center, which is anterior, and which contributes to the formation of the posterior arch. This anterior ossification center exists at birth in 20% of the cases. Sometimes, it does not appear before age 1. It may become bifid, but this is not pathologic. The posterior ossification of the atlas

Centra   Segments or somites

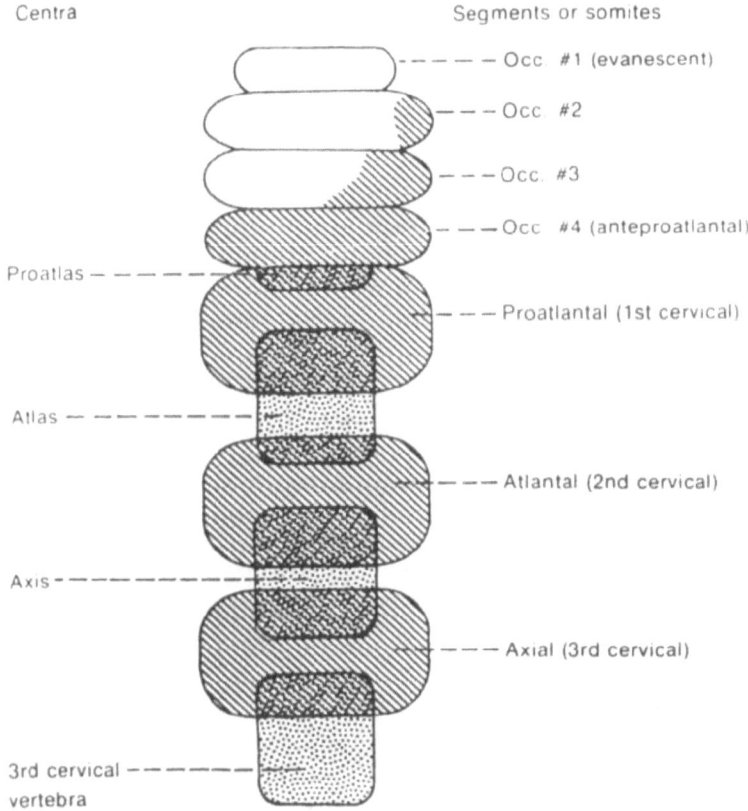

— — — — Occ. #1 (evanescent)

— — — Occ. #2

— — — Occ. #3

— — — Occ. #4 (anteproatlantal)

Proatlas — — — — —

— — — Proatlantal (1st cervical)

Atlas — — — — — — —

— — — Atlantal (2nd cervical)

Axis — — — — — — — —

— — — Axial (3rd cervical)

3rd cervical — — — — — —
vertebra

Figure 3.23. The fate of the four occipital and the upper three cervical somites. The shaded portions of occiputs 2 to 4 represent the relative contributions of the somites in the adult. (After Keith A: Human Embryology and Morphology. 6th Ed., Williams & Wilkins, Baltimore, 1948.)

may be incomplete, resulting in a pseudo-spina bifida, not to be confused with fracture lines.

The growth of the axis is even more complex. The ossification of the odontoid process appears as early as the fifth month of intrauterine life. Two longitudinal ossification centers appear, and fuse at birth. The tip of the odontoid, which does not have the same embryologic origin as the body, ossifies about age 6. This *ossiculum terminale* fuses with the rest of the body of the odontoid at age 12. Nonfusion of this secondary ossification center with the body of the odontoid results in an "os odontoideum," whose pathogenesis is not very precise (congenital or traumatic?) The body of the odontoid is separated from the body of the axis by a growth plate. However, this growth plate does not have a very elaborate structure. It fuses with the rest of the axis as early as age 6. In children, trauma of the odontoid process occurs in this growth plate, causing a "real detachment."

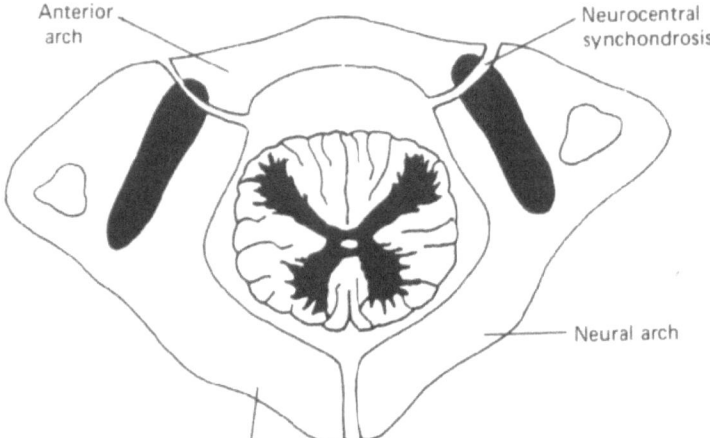

Figure 3.24. The first cervical vertebra (atlas); developmental components. The anterior arch may ossify during the last fetal months or the early postnatal months. Ossification of the neural arches begins about the seventh week of intrauterine life. The dorsal synchondrosis between the neural arches fuses about the third or fourth year of life. Fusion of the anterior arch to the lateral masses occurs by the sixth to eighth year of life.

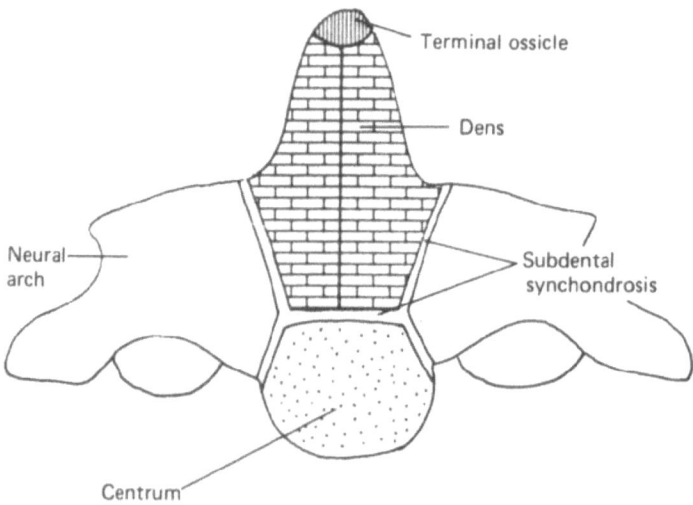

Figure 3.25. Developmental components of the second cervical vertebra (axis). A single ossification center (occasionally two) appears in the centrum in the fourth or fifth fetal month. At about the seventh month of fetal life, one ossification center appears in each neural arch, and fuses dorsally about the second or third year. The subdental and neurocentral synchondroses fuse between 4 and 7 years of age. At puberty, the inferior epiphyseal ring appears and it fuses during early life. The terminal ossicle of the dens appears at about age 2, and fuses with the dens by age 12. Two separate centers of ossification for the dens appear about the fifth or sixth prenatal months and they fuse before birth.

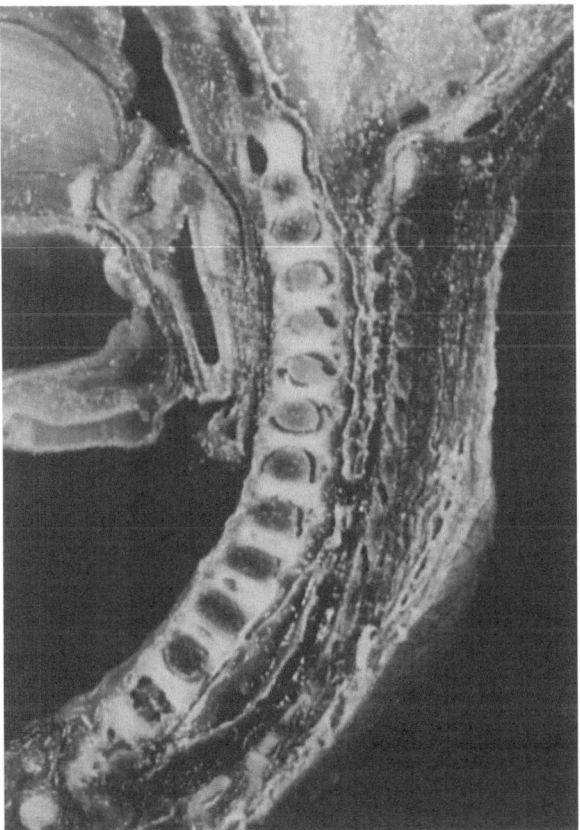

Figure 3.26. Sagittal view at birth of the cervical spine; the top of the axis is entirely cartilaginous.

The lower cervical spine – C3, C4, C5, C6, C7 – is mostly characterized by two elements: (1) The synchondrosis between the vertebral body and the arch disappears about age 6, whereas the posterior fusion of the cervical spine occurs about age 4. C2 is the last vertebra to fuse. (2) The growth plate which contributes to the growth of the posterior arch originates in the vertebral body. This growth plate contributes some 30% to the volume of the vertebral body.

The spinal (medullary) canal has been the topic of extensive radiologic studies. Significant variations exist from one person to another, but on the whole we can say that: (1) the medullary canal narrows from top to bottom, is funnel-shaped, and in the adult is large enough to permit entry of a thumb. (2) The antero-posterior diameter reaches its maximum by age 7 or 8. (3) The antero-posterior diameter is 9 mm at birth, 15 to 16 mm at age 5, and 19 mm in adulthood. An antero-posterior diameter which is less than 15 mm, at C5 level, indicates a narrow canal. (4) The transversal diameter is larger than the antero-posterior

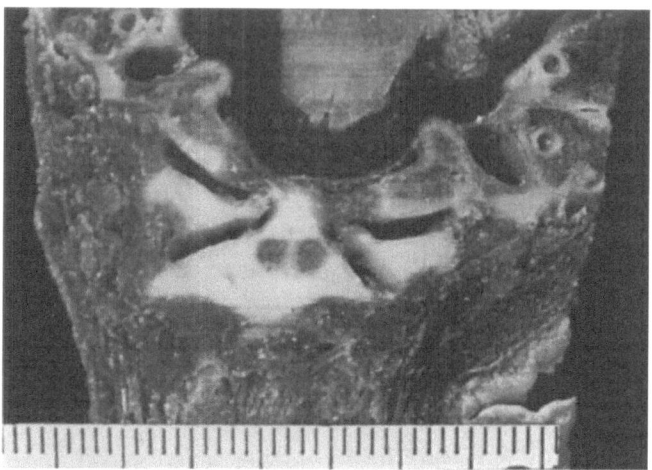

Figure 3.27. Two separate centers of ossification for the dens appear about the fifth and sixth prenatal months. On this anatomic view (frontal view) note the two ossification centers (7 months of intrauterine period).

Cervical spine

	Antero–posterior diameter	Transverse diameter	Surface
Canal	17 mm	27 mm	376 mm²
Cord	8 mm	13 mm	80 mm²

Cord	Antero–posterior	Transversal	Surface
Cervical	8 mm	13 mm	8 mm²
Thoracic	6 mm	8 mm	4 mm²

Figure 3.28. The cervical cord is comfortable in the medullary canal.

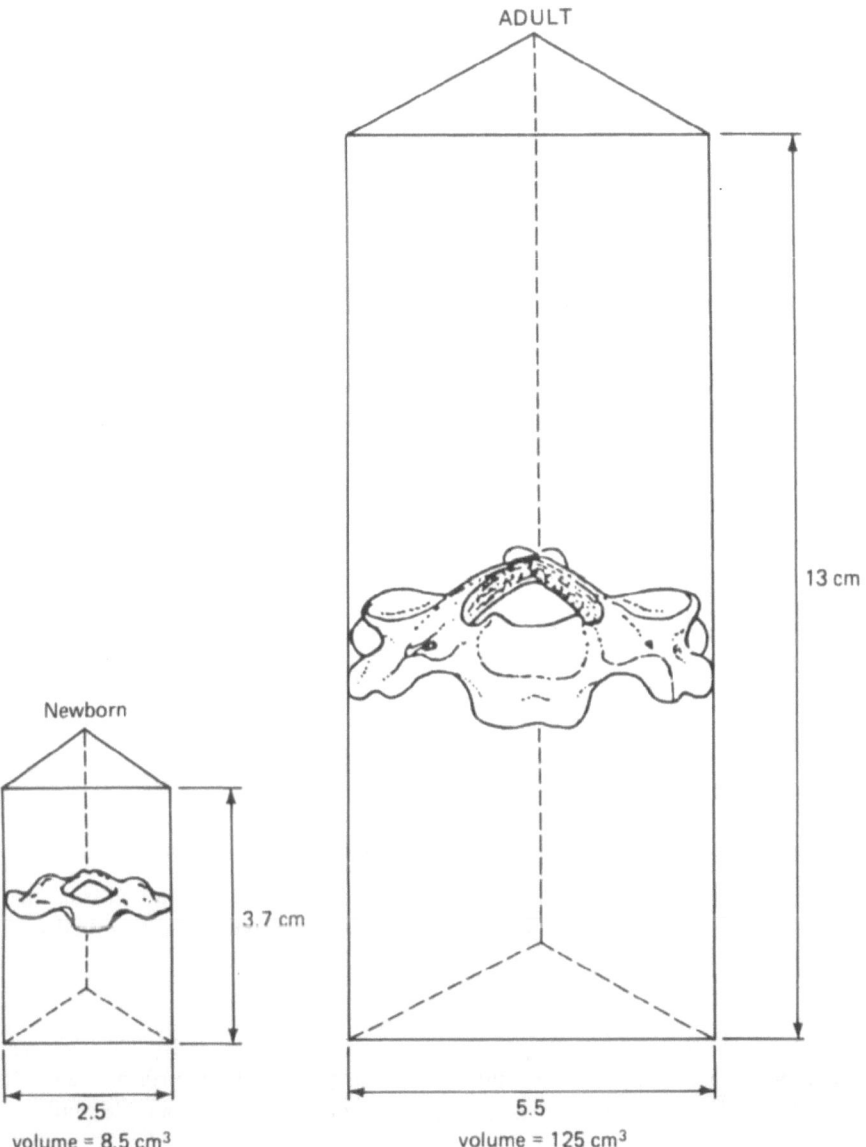

Figure 3.29. The cervical spine gains about 9 cm from birth to adulthood: it is more than three times its height at birth. The volume is multiplied by 15 within adulthood.

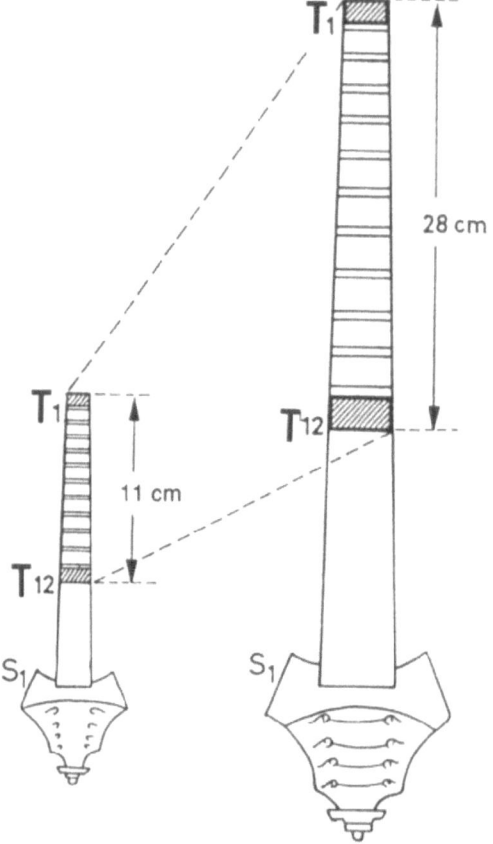

Figure 3.30. T1–T12 segment. Schematically, it is 11 cm at birth and 26 to 28 cm at the end of growth. The growth gain is thus 15 cm. So, it gains 15 cm during growth, that is to say, it is more than twice its height at birth.

diameter: 13 mm at birth, 22 mm at age 10, and 27 mm at age 16. The cervical cord has ample space in the medullary canal. In adulthood, its surface area is 80 mm², whereas the average surface area of the spinal canal is about 376 mm².

Thoracic Spine (T1–T12)

The thoracic spine is about 11 cm long at birth; at the end of growth 26 cm in girls and 28 cm in boys. Its size more than doubles from birth to the end of the growth period.

Neither in the thoracic spine does growth progress in a regular way:

Very rapid growth from age 0 to 5 (+7 cm)
Slower growth from age 5 to 10 (+4 cm)
Another growth spurt at pubertal peak (about +7 cm)

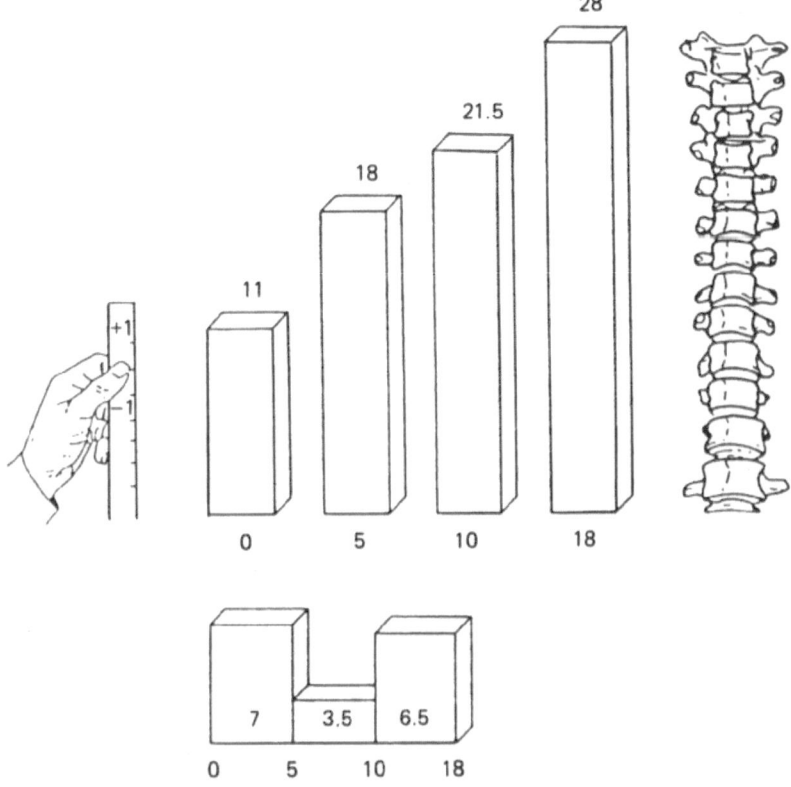

Figure 3.31. T1–T12, boy's dorsal spine. The dorsal segment in boys is slightly larger than in girls at the end of growth (28 against 26.5 cm). The dorsal segment nearly doubled at age 10. Out of all growths, the most significant is the one occurring from age 0 to 5. At age 10, in boys, 6.5 cm remain to gain on the dorsal segment (4.5 cm in girls).

The T1–T12 segment represents 30% of the sitting height, so a single thoracic vertebra represents 2.5% deficit in the sitting height. Fusion by perivertebral arthrodesis results in a 2.5% deficit in the sitting height. On the other hand, a posterior arthrodesis results in only a third of this deficit, about 0.8%. Volumetric growth, a basic notion very often ignored, goes from 22 cm³ to 249 cm³ at age 10, and reaches 504 cm³ by adulthood.

The thoracic spinal canal is narrower than either lumbar or cervical canals. The fifth finger may be introduced into this canal which attains its maximum volume by age 5.

Dimensions of T7 vertebra:

Age	Anterior/posterior diameter	Transverse diameter	Surface
Newborn	0.7 cm	0.7 cm	0.4 cm²
2 yrs.	1.4 cm	1.3 cm	1.4 cm²
10 yrs.	1.5 cm	1.5 cm	1.8 cm²
Adult	1.5 cm	1.4 cm	1.6 cm²

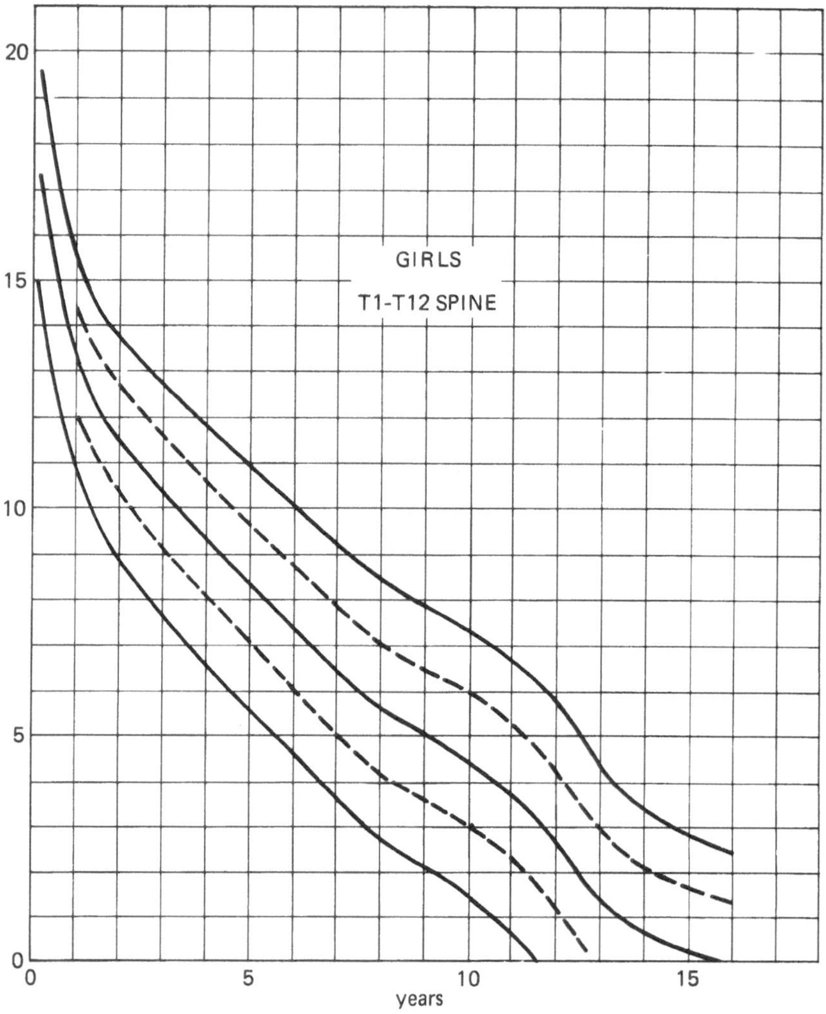

THORACIC VERTEBRA = 2.5% OF THE SITTING HEIGHT

Figure 3.32. T1–T12 spine, girls. An anterior and posterior (perivertebral) thoracic arthrodesis leads to a 30% deficit of the sitting height. A posterior thoracic arthrodesis leads to a 10% deficit of the sitting height.

First finding: there is no significant difference between the antero-posterior diameter and the transversal diameter.

Second finding: there is no very distinct variation between the medullary canal at age 2 and in adulthood.

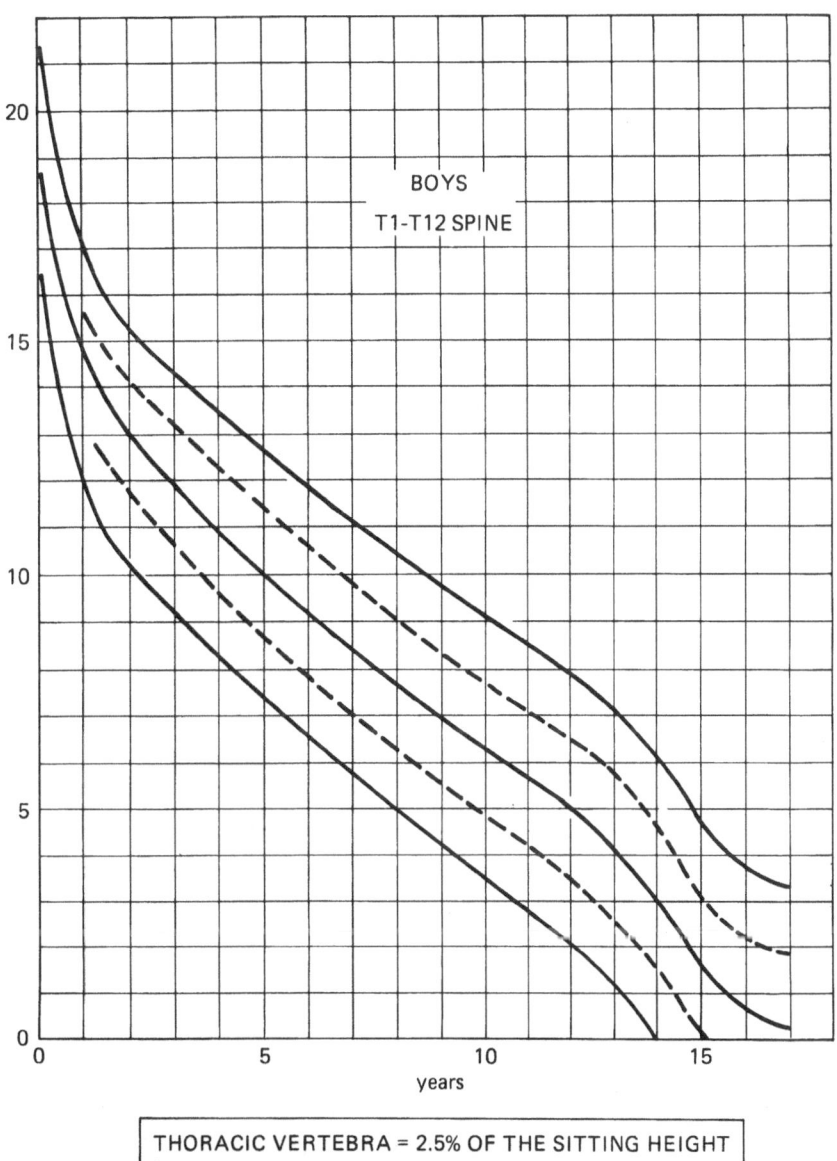

Figure 3.33. T1–T12 spine, boys. An anterior and posterior (perivertebral) thoracic arthrodesis leads to a 30% deficit of the sitting height. A posterior thoracic arthrodesis leads to a 10% deficit on the sitting height.

Third finding: The surface area of the vertebral canal increases fourfold from birth to adult life. In fact, a slight narrowing of the vertebral canal may even be

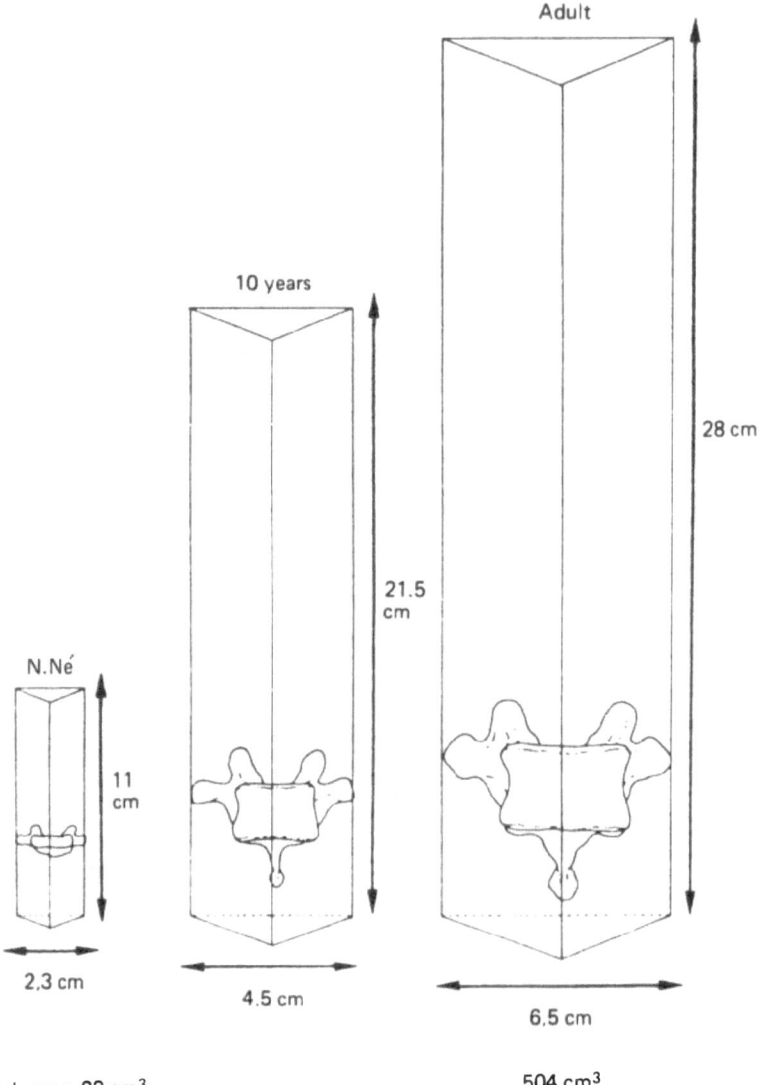

Volume = 22 cm³   504 cm³

Figure 3.34. Thoracic spine. The dorsal spine height gains about 17 cm from birth to adulthood. It doubles at age 10, and nearly triples in adulthood. But the volumetric increase is the most outstanding: the volume is 10 times greater at age 10, it is multiplied by 25 at age 20.

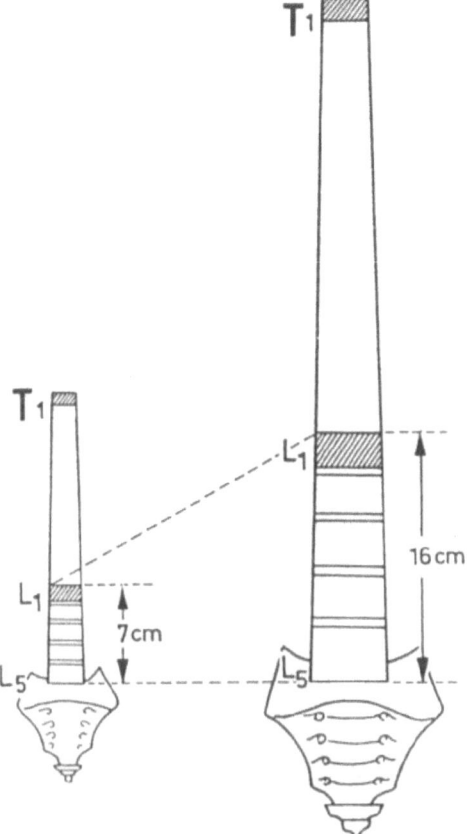

Figure 3.35. L1–L5 segment. Globally, the lumbar spine is: 7 cm at birth and 16 cm at the end of growth. Thus, it gained 9 cm. At the end of growth, the lumbar spine, as the dorsal spine, is more than twice its height at birth.

noticed in adulthood, as compared to a 10-year-old child; this is due to the thickening of the laminae by periosteal apposition. The surface area of the cord is 0.4 cm², about 25% of the medullary canal surface area.

The Lumbar Spine (L1–L5)

The L1–L5 lumbar spine is approximately 7 cm in length at birth. It grows to 16 cm in males, 15.5 cm in females. As in the thoracic spine, growth is not linear:

Rapid growth from ages 0 to 5 (+ about 3 cm)
Slow growth from ages 5 to 10 (+ about 2 cm)
Rapid growth from ages 10 to 18 (+ about 3 cm).

The lumbar spine represents 18% of the sitting height, a single lumbar vertebra 3.5% of the sitting height. Consequently, a perivertebral arthrodesis stripping all

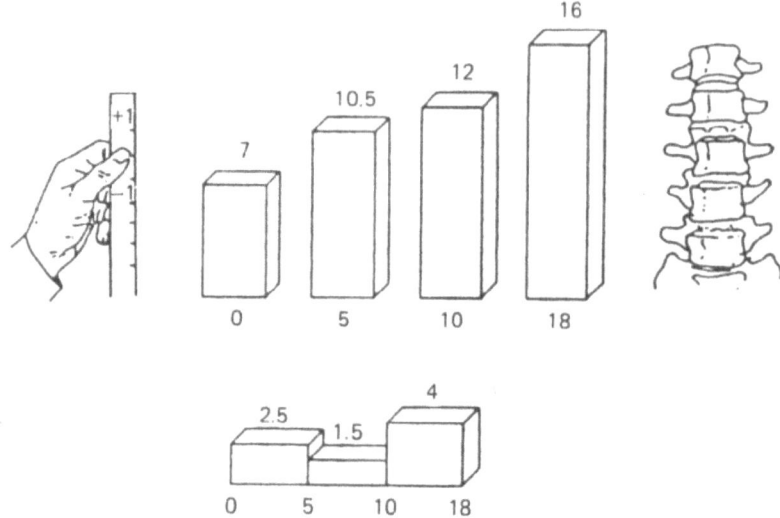

Figure 3.36. L1–L5 segment, boy's lumbar spine. At age 10, in boys, 4 cm remain to gain on the lumbar spine (3 cm in girls).

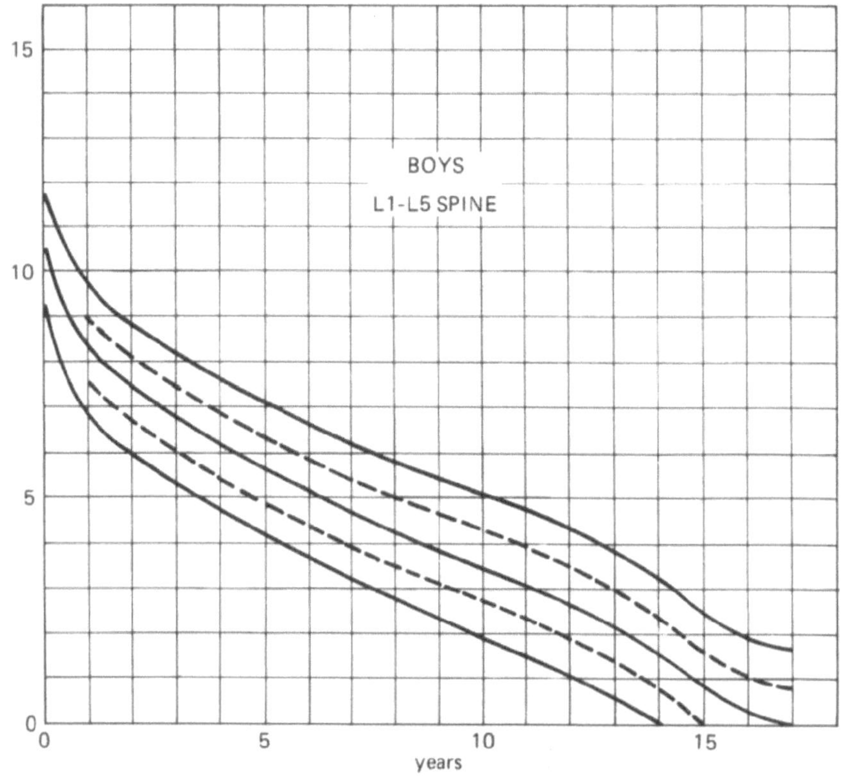

BOYS

L1–L5 SPINE

years

LUMBAR VERTEBRA = 3.5% OF THE SITTING HEIGHT

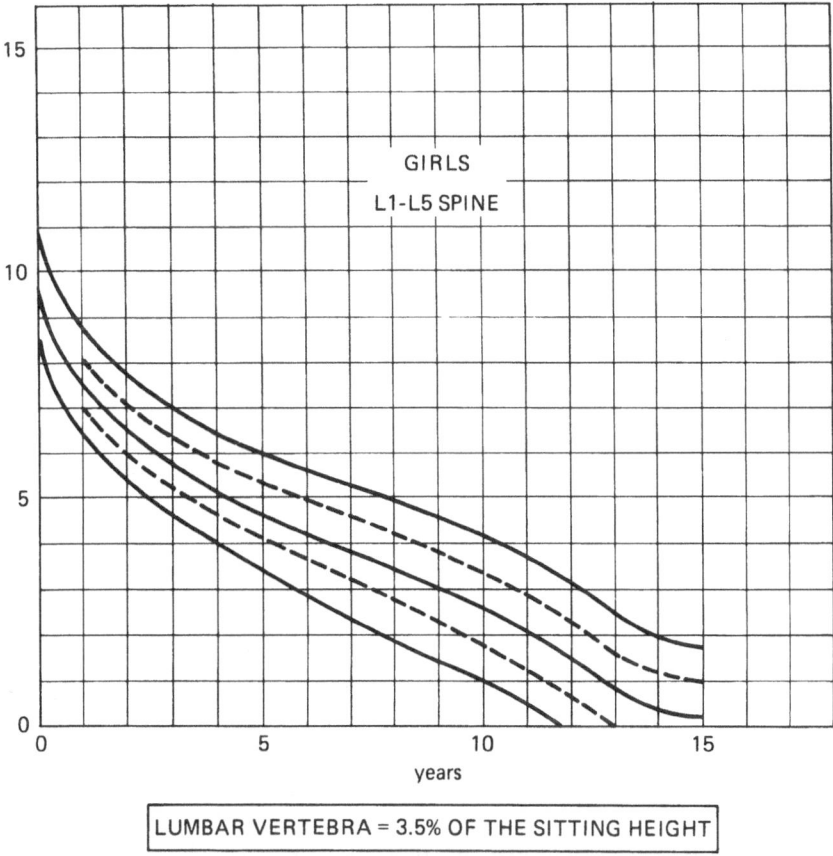

LUMBAR VERTEBRA = 3.5% OF THE SITTING HEIGHT

Figure 3.38. L1–L5 spine, girls. An anterior and posterior (perivertebral) lumbar arthrodesis leads to an 18% deficit of the sitting height. A posterior lumbar arthrodesis leads to a 6% deficit of the sitting height.

the growth cartilage from a lumbar vertebra results in a 3.5% deficit in the final sitting height. On the other hand, a posterior vertebral arthrodesis results in a deficit only one-third this great: a bit more than 1% of final sitting height. The lumbar volume is 16.5 cm³ at birth, 203 cm³ at age 10, 391 cm³ in adulthood. So, the volumetric growth is very significant. As the lumbar spine height only doubles, the volume, on the other hand, increases by a factor of 12 from birth to age 10, and by a factor of 24 from birth to adulthood. At skeletal age 10, the lumbar spine reaches 90% of its final height, but only 60% of the final volume. The

◄

Figure 3.37. L1–L5 spine, boys. An anterior and posterior (perivertebral) lumbar arthrodesis leads to an 18% deficit of the sitting height. A posterior lumbar arthrodesis leads to a 6% deficit of the sitting height.

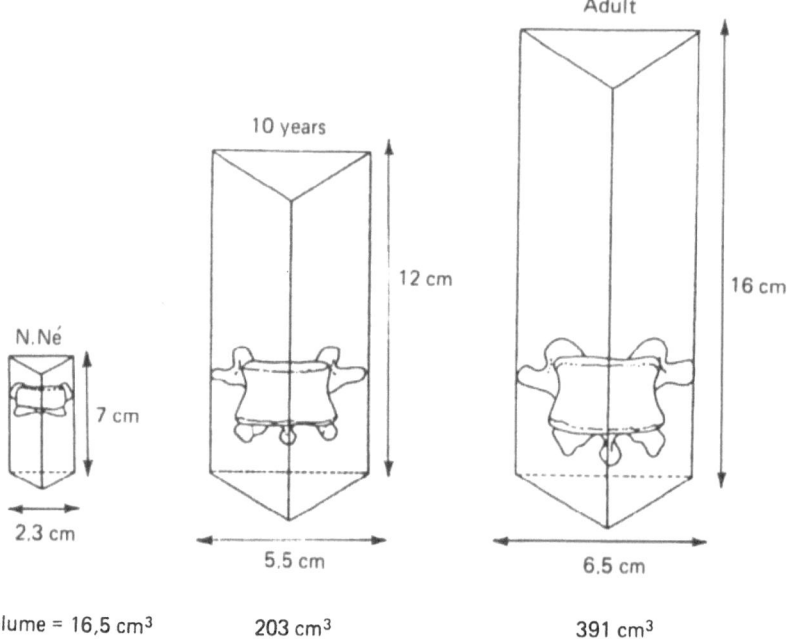

Figure 3.39. Lumbar spine. The volumetric growth is very important to consider: whereas the lumbar spine height only doubles, the volume, on the opposite, is multiplied by 24. At age 10, the lumbar spine height reaches 80%, but the volume reaches 50%. There is a difference between the height growth and the volumetric growth.

medullary canal is wider than the thoracic canal. The forefinger can be introduced. The cord stops at L1–L2.

Dimension of the L5 vertebra:

Age	Anterior/posterior diameter	Transverse diameter	Surface
Newborn	0.9 cm	0.9 cm	0.65 cm²
2 yrs.	1.4 cm	2.5 cm	2.60 cm²
10 yrs.	1.5 cm	2.3 cm	2.70 cm²
Adult	1.4 cm	2.1 cm	2.30 cm²

First finding: the transversal diameter is larger than the antero–posterior diameter.

Second finding: growth is greatest during the 2 first years of life; we even notice that the medullary canal surface tends slightly to diminish from ages 10 to 18.

Third finding: the surface area nearly quadruples from birth to adulthood.

The T1–S1 Segment

The T1–S1 segment represents a particular entity. The most frequent spinal affections (scoliosis, kyphosis) originate on this segment. It is about 19 cm at

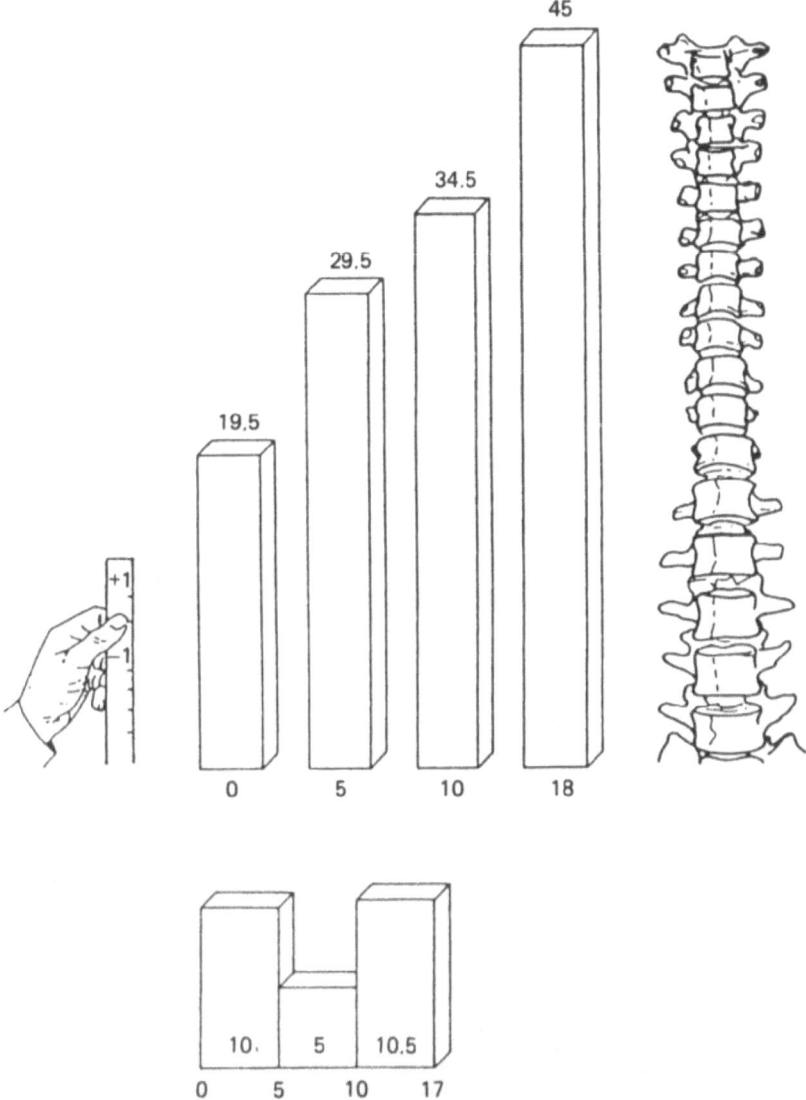

Figure 3.40. T1–S1 segment, boys. T1–S1 is about 45 cm. The overall gain is of about 25 cm during growth. From age 5 to 10, the growth velocity stunts (1 cm per year). At age 10, 10.5 cm remain to gain.

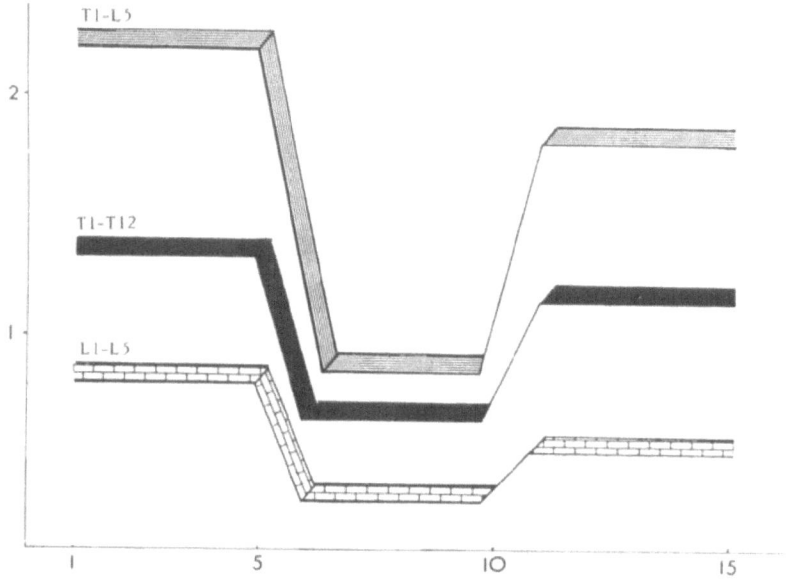

Figure 3.41. Velocity by years.

birth, and 45 cm at the end of growth in males, 42 to 43 cm in females, and represents 50% of the sitting height (exactly . . . 49%).

The Sacrum

Ossification of the sacrum is complex. There are 35 to 40 ossification centers for the sacrum which is the result of fusion of five primitive independent vertebrae.

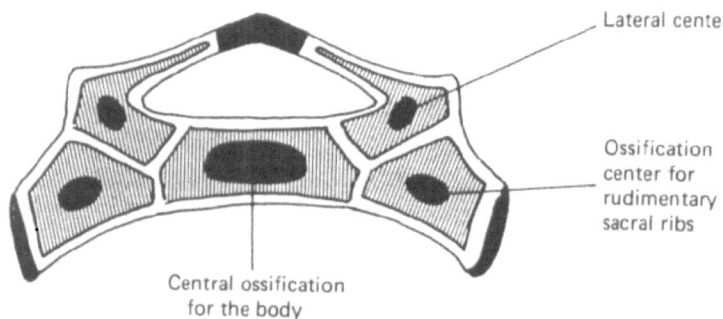

Figure 3.42. Five centers of ossification. The sacrum resembles a typical vertebra in the ossification of each of its vertebral segments. Primary centers for the centrum and each half of the vertebral arch appear between the 10th and 20th weeks. Primary centers for the costal elements appear between the sixth and eighth months of intrauterine life.

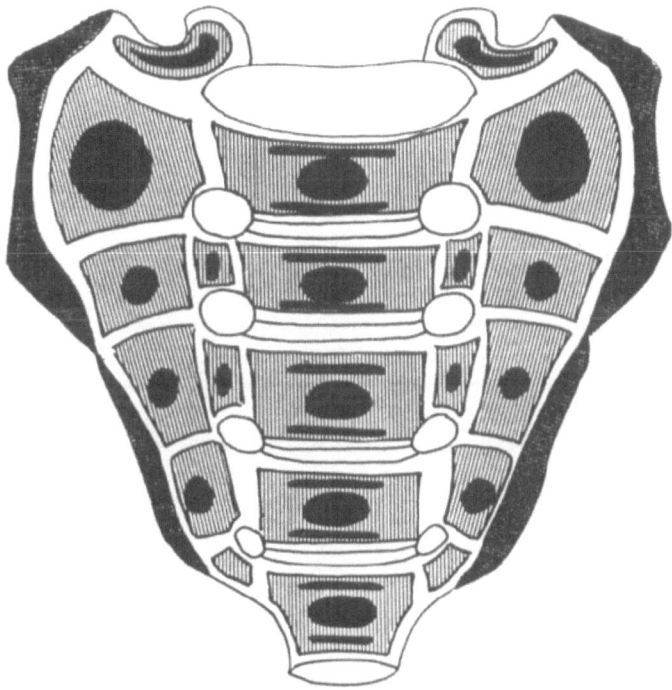

Figure 3.43. Sacral vertebrae are separated by intervertebral disks as in the other regions of the vertebral column. These disks ossify between the last two sacral vertebrae in about the 18th year. The union of sacral vertebrae then moves cranially and is completely late in the third decade.

Each sacral vertebra, like all others in the spine, has three primary centers: one median or central center for the body, and two lateral centers for the posterior arches. The centers appear in the cartilage about the fourth fetal month for the vertebral body, and about the sixth month for the lateral arches, this much later than for the thoracic or lumbar vertebra. The three upper vertebrae are characteristic in that they show, at the posterior part of the transverse apophyses, two other ossification centers corresponding to rudimentary sacral ribs. These five ossification centers, called primary, are complemented by secondary ossification centers, one of which appears at the upper part of the vertebral body, another at the lower part, and a third in the spinal apophysis. The two first ossification centers (upper and lower centers) vertebral body appear at puberty, the third at about age 18. The fusion process of the different ossification centers is the same as for the other vertebrae: the two lateral centers fuse backward in the midline, then the costal centers unite with the apophyseal mass in order to form a single element, and, lastly, this element fuses to the vertebral body.

The fusion of the different sacral elements does not occur simultaneously. Posteriorly, the posterior fusion occurs early. It starts at age 3 for the second

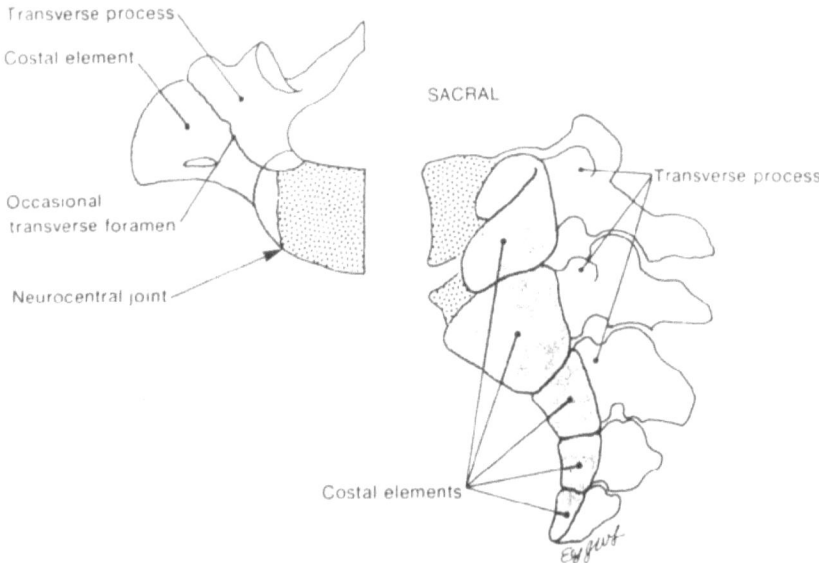

Figure 3.44. Sacral vertebrae viewed from above on the left; from side on the right. (After Romanes GS: Cunningham's Textbook of Anatomy, 10th Ed., Oxford University Press, London, 1964.)

sacral vertebra, and at age 4½ for the third vertebra. At age 7, the closure of the sacral arches is complete, and any subsequent osseous dehiscence of these arches should be considered abnormal. The normal opening of the sacral arches is observed at birth, the posterior wall being only a thin fibrous membrane.

Anteriorly, on the opposite, the fusion with the vertebral bodies with one another occurs later, about age 14. It is progressive, starting from the fifth sacral vertebra and proceeding upward to the first sacral vertebra. Thus, the fusion process is different ventrally and dorsally.

Very late, after the end of growth, four new ossification centers appear, when the sacral fusion is nearly complete. These four new ossification centers (two on each side) appear in the auricular surfaces and complete laterally the ossification of the sacrum.

The coccyx is made of four to five atrophied vertebra. As the sacrum, it is formed from the fusion of several vertebra, which are very rudimentary.

Growth of the Neural Tube: Container/Contents Ratio

The growth of the spinal cord is different from that of the vertebral column. The "container" adapts to the "contents." At the very beginning, during the embryonic period, the spine and the neural tube are synchronized in growth. The cord fills

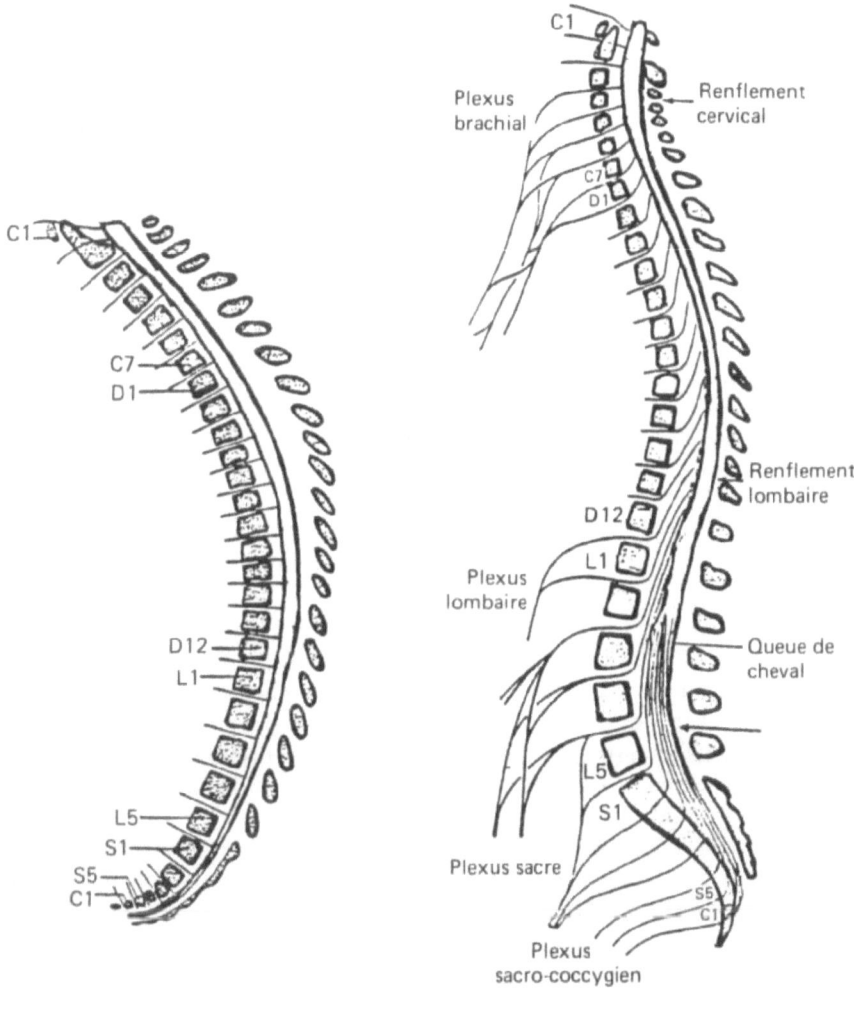

Fetus chord
before the 4th month

Adult

Figure 3.45. At the beginning, the nervous tube and the vertebral canal develop nearly parallel. The cord lies along the whole length of the canal; the spinal nerves emerge perpendicularly between the different vertebral bodies. From the fourth month on, the growth of the nervous tube slows down as that of the vertebral canal continues.

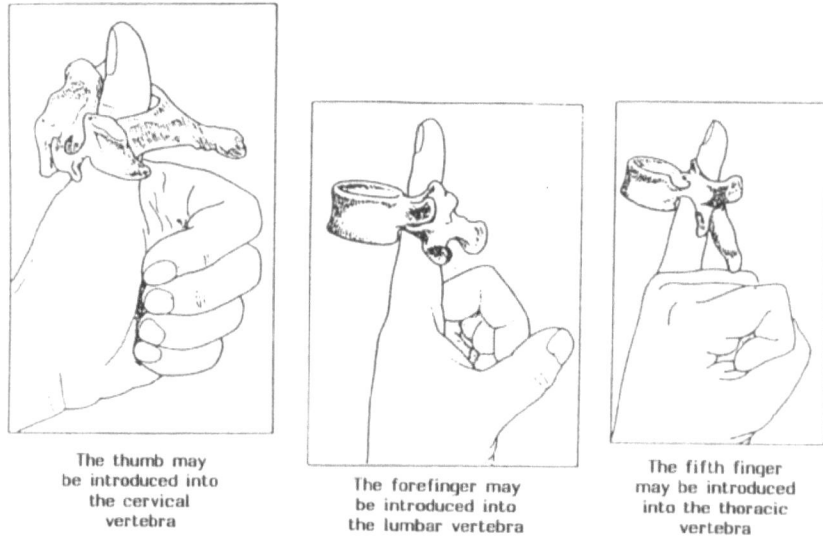

The thumb may
be introduced into
the cervical
vertebra

The forefinger may
be introduced into
the lumbar vertebra

The fifth finger
may be introduced
into the thoracic
vertebra

Figure 3.46. Container-contents ratio.

nearly the whole spinal canal. Subsequently, the spine grows faster (during the fetal period). The cord, which is initially sacral, becomes lumbar, reaching the third lumbar vertebra first and then the first or second lumbar vertebra in the second month after birth. This is its final position. The disproportionate growth between the contents (the cord) and the container (the vertebral column) occurs during the fetal period.

The Intervertebral Disc

At the end of growth, the space filled by the intervertebral discs represents about one-third to one-fourth of the body of the adjacent vertebra. In adulthood, the intervertebral disc, an avascular structure after the fourth year of life, represents 22% of the cervical spine height, 18% of the thoracic spine height, but 35% of the lumbar spine height. The height of the intervertebral disc is 4 mm at C4, 2.5 mm at T5, and 17 mm at L5. Each disc contains about 80% of water.

Pathologic Changes Secondary to Vertebral Development

Spinal pathology is pathology of the growing spine. The spine, as the femur or tibia, remains subordinated to the synchronized development of its cartilages. Abnormality of only one growth plate may affect the morphology of the whole vertebra, and the entire vertebral column. A growth disorder may affect all the

Figure 3.47. Respective percentages of bone and disc in the total height of the spine. In the cervico–dorsal spine, the discs represent about one-fourth of the total height and the vertebrae three-fourths. We notice, at the lumbar level, the importance of the discs which represent here about one-third of the height, and the vertebrae two-thirds.

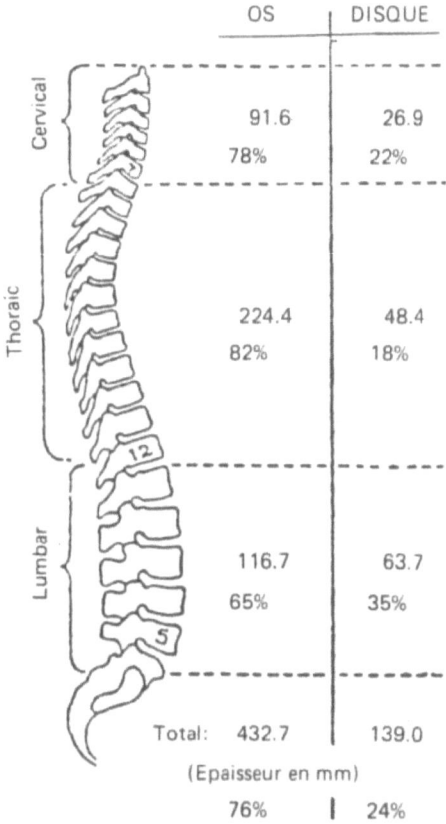

	OS	DISQUE
Cervical	91.6 78%	26.9 22%
Thoraic	224.4 82%	48.4 18%
Lumbar	116.7 65%	63.7 35%
Total:	432.7	139.0

(Epaisseur en mm)

76% | 24%

Height

Disk (mm)

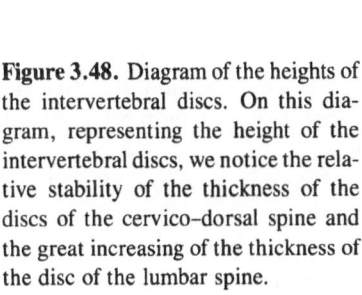

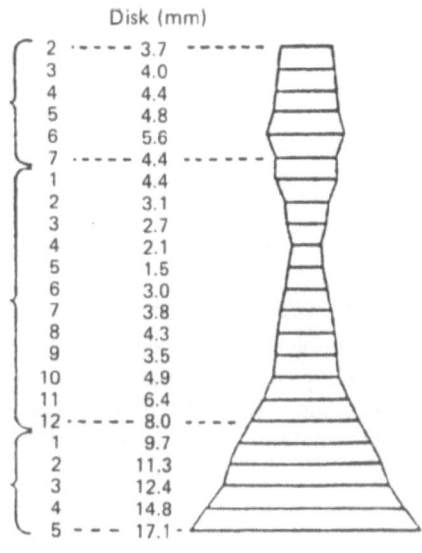

2	3.7
3	4.0
4	4.4
5	4.8
6	5.6
7	4.4
1	4.4
2	3.1
3	2.7
4	2.1
5	1.5
6	3.0
7	3.8
8	4.3
9	3.5
10	4.9
11	6.4
12	8.0
1	9.7
2	11.3
3	12.4
4	14.8
5	17.1

Figure 3.48. Diagram of the heights of the intervertebral discs. On this diagram, representing the height of the intervertebral discs, we notice the relative stability of the thickness of the discs of the cervico–dorsal spine and the great increasing of the thickness of the disc of the lumbar spine.

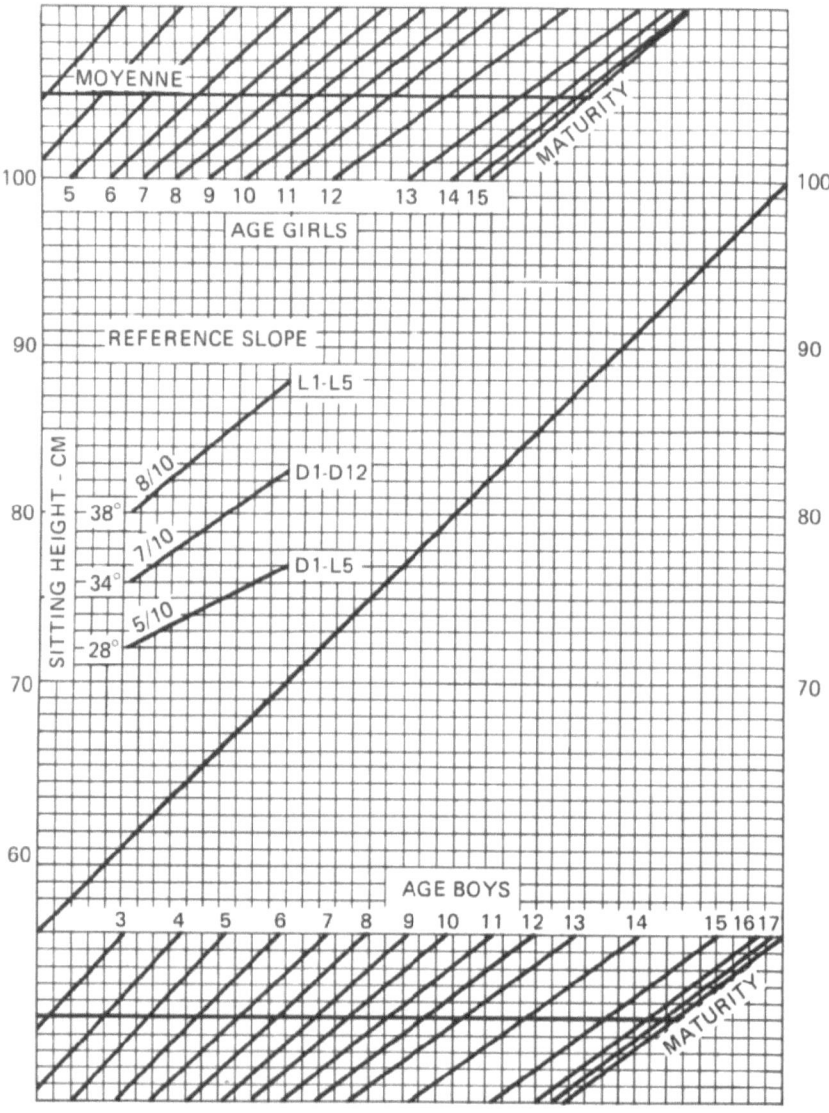

Figure 3.49. Arthrodesis chart for spine fusion.

cartilages of a same vertebra without discernment. It may be more selective and affect the posterior or anterior cartilages. In that case, it determines a growth asynchronism leading to an abnormal curvature.

Abnormalities of the posterior elements, such as one may encounter after a laminectomy, lead to kyphosis. The affection of the growth plates on one side of the vertebral body may lead to a lateral curvature (for instance, after trauma), such as stage V of Salter's classification. Scoliosis exerts a stronger pressure in

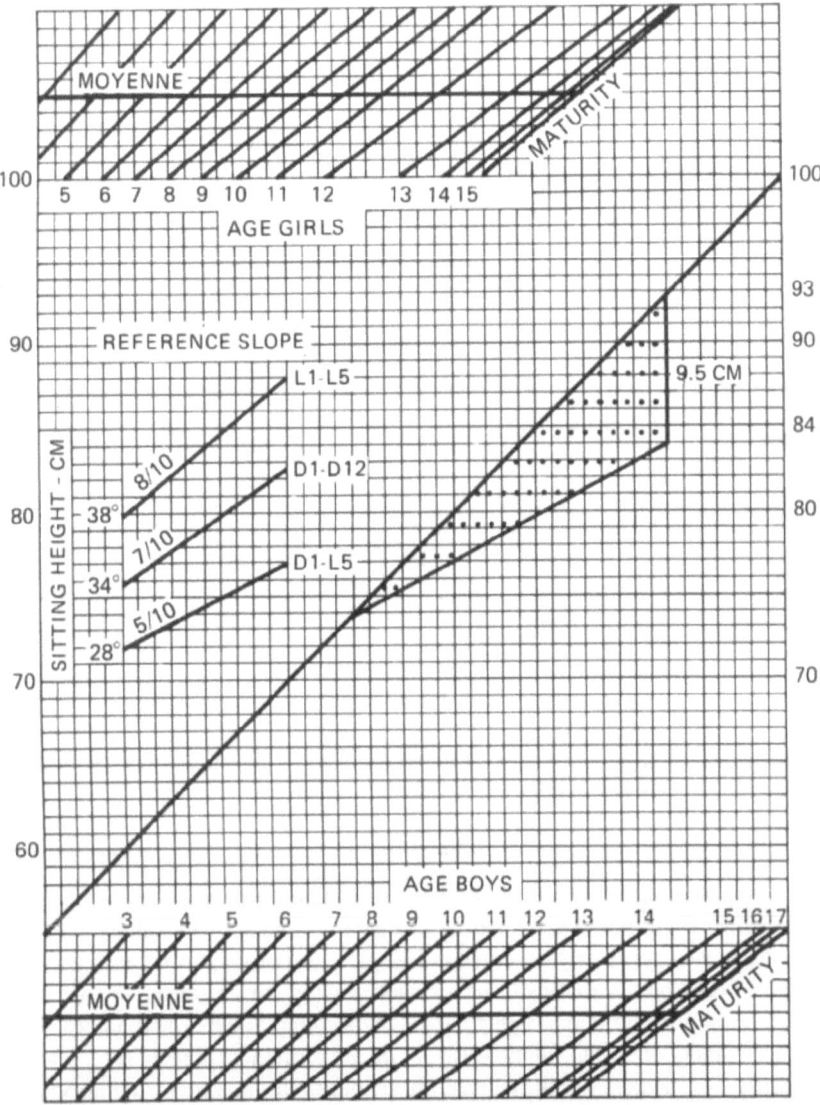

Figure 3.50. Arthrodesis chart for spine fusion. For example, a circumferential arthrodesis of T1–L5 performed at 10 years bone age leads to a deficit of sitting height of about 9 cm. For a posterior spine fusion, divide by 3.

the concave area, and a weaker pressure in the convex area. It compresses some growth plates and slackens their activity, becoming responsible for a self-maintained curvature. Kyphosis, whatever its cause, affects the anterior growth plates. It creates a difference of growth potentials favoring the benefit of the posterior arch. In Scheuermann's disease, there is a pressure excess on the

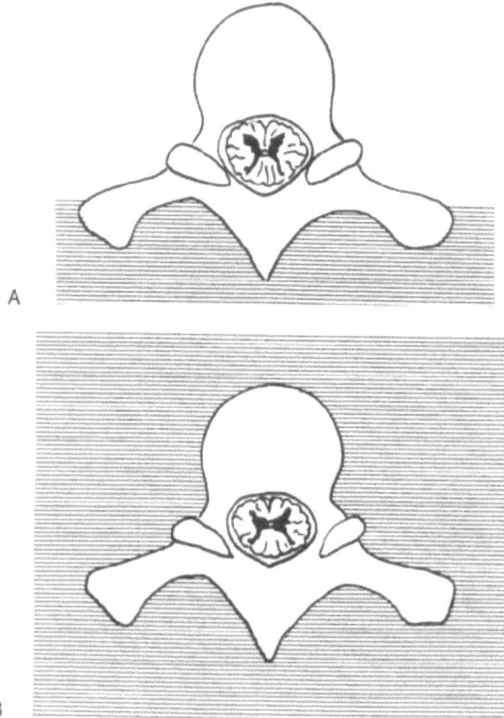

Figure 3.51. Thoracic vertebra. **A**: Posterior arthrodesis. Deficit less than 1% of sitting height. **B**: Circumferential arthrodesis. Deficit less than 3% of sitting height.

anterior part of the vertebral bodies, hence the cuneiformization. Since vertebral ossification is progressive, segmentation disorders due to a congenital malformation are not always clearly observed radiologically at birth. It is necessary to wait several years before distinguishing radiologically, for instance, the vertebral ossification disorder due to Klippel–Feil's syndrome. Since growth plates are in the vertebral bodies, the chondrodystrophies are prominent congenital anomalies identified by truncal abnormalities. In achondroplasia, the vertebral body is normal, but the spinal canal is narrow. The growth plate is the neuro–vertebral junction which is selectively affected. In Morquio's disease, the ovoid aspect of the vertebral bodies is linked to an anterior affection.

The vertebrae are sensitive to pressure forces. Thus the vertebral bodies are abnormally high in paralyzed and confined children because of the lack of pressures on the vertebral bodies. Total perivertebral arthrodesis permits one to arrest both anterior and posterior growth cartilages; it is used especially in case of paralytic spine. A total perivertebral arthrodesis of the thoracic spine leads to a 30% deficit of the sitting height, an 18% deficit of the lumbar spine, and a 15% deficit of the cervical spine. Posterior vertebral arthrodesis retards the growth of

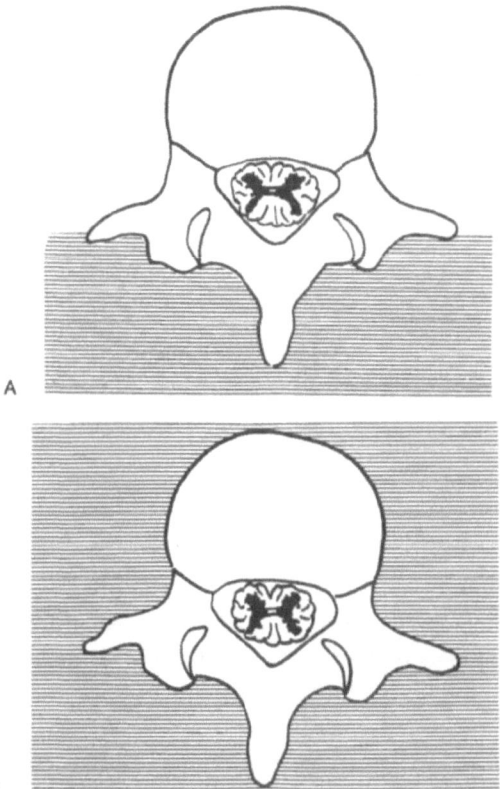

Figure 3.52. Lumbar vertebra. **A**: Posterior arthrodesis. Deficit more than 1% of sitting height. **B**: Circumferential arthrodesis. Deficit more than 3% (exactly 3.5%) of sitting height.

a vertebra by only 30%. So, its effectiveness is relative in comparison with those of perivertebral arthrodesis.

Hemi-arthrodesis is performed for congenital scoliosis. Roaf proposed it, initially, and it was used later by Winter. If performed early, before age 5, it may lead to a 15° angular correction per vertebra. Anterior and posterior hemi-arthrodesis is frequently performed in congenital scoliosis.

Posterior arthrodesis may be useful in congenital kyphosis of less than 40°. If performed early, before age 5, it may alone correct the curve. We know that a perivertebral arthrodesis of the whole thoracic spine results in an approximately 6 cm height deficit at age 10, a lumbar arthrodesis in a 3 cm height deficit.

The present state of our research shows that an early perivertebral arthrodesis, performed at age 5, does not lead to a narrow canal. Equally, a perivertebral arthrodesis at age 10, to treat, for instance, and evolutive neurologic scoliosis, will not have significant repercussions on the sitting height.

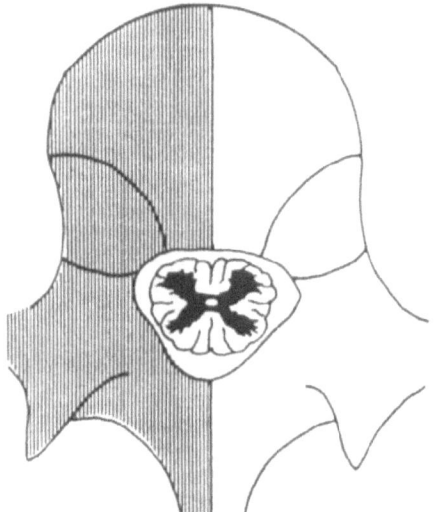

Figure 3.53. Hemiarthrodesis. (see Roaf: The treatment of progressive scoliosis by unilateral growth arrest. J.B.J.S., 1963, 45 B, 637–651 and Winter: Convex anterior and posterior hemiarthrodesis and hemiepiphysiodesis in young children with progressive congenital scoliosis. J Pediatr Orthrop 1981, 1, 361–366)

Actually, the problem with early arthrodeses, above all when they are perivertebral, concerns their volumetric dimensions. The arthrodesis locks the volumetric expansion of the vertebrae and this may have serious consequences on thoracic expansion.

Bibliography

1. Andrew T, Piggott H.: Growth arrest for progressive scoliosis. Combined anterior and posterior fusion of the convexity. J Bone Joint Surg 2:193–197, 1985.
2. Arey LB: Development of the spine and spinal cord. In: Ruge D, Wiltse LL (eds): Spinal Disorders, Diagnosis and Treatment. Lea & Febiger, Philadelphia, 1977, pp 3–13.
3. Dimeglio A, Pous JG, Bonnel F: Le cartilage de croissance. Encycl Med Chir Appareil Locomoteur. Editions Techniques, Paris. 14009 B10, 9-1983.
4. Dimeglio A: La croissance en orthopédie. Encycl Med Chir Appareil Locomoteur. Editions Techniques, Paris. 14009 A10, 3-1984.
5. Goto S, Uhthoff HK: Notochord and spinal malformations. Acta Orthop Scand 57:149–153, 1986.
6. Houston CS, Zaleski WA: The shape of the vertebral bodies and femoral necks in relation to activity. Radiology 89:59–66, 1967.
7. Jonata R: Anatomia dello schleroto umano fetale. Capelli, Bologna, 1938.
8. Lonstein JE: Spine embryology. In: Congenital Deformities of the Spine. Winter RB, Lonstein JE, Leonard AS (ed): Thieme-Stratton, New York, 1983, 1–10.
9. Lutter L: Achondroplasia: clinical manifestations and neurological significance. In: Chou SN, Seljeskog EL (eds): Spinal Deformities and Neurological Dysfunction. Raven Press, New York, 1978, pp 75–97.
10. O'Rahilly R, Benson D: The development of the vertebral column. In: Bradford DS, Hensinger RN (eds): The Pediatric Spine. Thieme, New York, 1985, pp 3–17.

11. O'Rahilly R, Meyer DB: The timing and sequence of events in the development of the human vertebral column during the embryonic period proper. Anat Embryol 157:167–176, 1979.

12. O'Rahilly R, Muller F: The early development of the hypoglossal nerve and occipital somites in staged human embryos. Am J Anat 169:237–257, 1984.

13. Parke WW: Development of the spine. In: Rothman RH, Simeone FA (eds): The Spine. WB Saunders, Philadelphia, 1975, pp 1–18.

14. Peacock A: Observations on the prenatal development of the intervertebral disc in man. J Anat 85:260, 1951.

15. Rivard C, Narbaitz R, Uithoff HK: Congenital vertebral malformations. Orthop Rev 8:135–139, 1979.

16. Roaf R: Spinal deformities. 2nd edition. Turnbridge Wells, Pitman Medical, 1980, p 337.

17. Roaf R: The treatment of progressive scoliosis by unilateral growth arrest. J Bone Joint Surg 45-B:637–651, 1963.

18. Roth M: The role of relative osteoneural growth in the gross morphogenesis of the skeleton. A hypothesis. Anat Clin 4:211–225, 1982.

19. Sauvegrain J, Nahum H, Bronstein H: Etude de la maturation osseuse du coude. Ann Radiol 5:542–550, 1962.

20. Schmorl G: The human spine in health and disease. 2nd American edition, Grune & Stratton, New York, 1971.

21. Tanaka T., Uhthoff HK: Significance of resegmentation in the pathogenesis of vertebral body malformation. Acta Orthop Scand 52:331–338, 1981.

22. Tanaka T, Uhthoff HK: The pathogenesis of congenital vertebral malformations: a study based on observations made in 11 human embryos and fetuses. Acta Orthop Scand 52:413–425, 1981.

23. Taylor JR: Growth of human intervertebral disks and vertebral bodies. J Anat 120: 49–68, 1975.

24. Tondury G: Engtwicklungsgeschichte und Fehlbildungen der Wirbelsäule. Hippokrates, Stuttgart, 1958.

25. Tsou PM: Embryology of congenital kyphosis. Clin Orthop 128:18–25, 1977.

26. Tuchmann-Duplessis H, David G, Haegel P: Illustrated human embryology, Vol. 1. Embryogenesis: Springer-Verlag, New York, 1972.

27. Winter RB: Convex anterior and posterior hemiarthrodesis and hemiepiphysiodesis in young children with progressive congenital scoliosis. J Pediatr Orthop 1:361–366, 1981.

CHAPTER 4

Neurophysiologic Basis for Diagnosis

E. Bertini, M. Di Capua, and F. Vigevano

The combination of neurophysiologic studies of motor and sensory somatic functions and kinesiologic assessment of the mechanisms of micturition is a useful approach to evaluate spinal cord damage in infants and children,[1] since spinal column lesions may occur in infants and toddlers with little or no radiographic, computed tomography (CT) scan, or myelographic evidence. Disturbances of micturition and continence, although frequent in diseases affecting the spinal cord, are difficult to confirm clinically before 3 years of age. Furthermore, it is not easy to obtain a precise clinical examination of the sensory and motor function in children before 8 to 10 years of age and, therefore, correct diagnosis of the level of spinal cord damage cannot be precise.

The neurophysiologic study of motor function may be conducted with the following diagnostic methods:

1. Electromyography (EMG) of somatic muscles to assess the level of lower motor neuron damage, considering the metameric distribution of muscles examined.

2. EMG study of muscles of the pelvic floor (bulbocavernosus, urethral, and anal) combined with study of reflex activity using manual stimuli, voluntary increased abdominal pressure, Valsalva's maneuver, coughing, sobbing, or electrical stimuli. These studies are particularly useful in lesions involving the cauda equina or the conus medullaris.

3. Kinesiologic assessment during bladder filling, observation of reflex activity during micturition, voluntary depression of reflex activity, and volitional induced or interrupted voiding. These tests are performed by means of EMG of urethral or anal sphincters in combination with cystometry, an examination that allows investigation of relationships between detrusor reflex and striated sphincter activity.

Neurophysiologic studies of sensory function are performed by means of spinal and cortical evoked potentials, obtained by stimulating electrically the peripheral sensory and/or mixed nerves, or directly the skin of the perineal area. All these diagnostic methods have been widely used in adult patients. Only in recent years have they been applied in diseases affecting the spinal cord and spinal roots in the pediatric age groups.

Our purpose is to review the most important results heretofore obtained by using these methods, demonstrating both the diagnostic usefulness and the limits of each.

Application of these methods in acquired (not hereditary) disorders of the pediatric spinal cord will also be presented.

Neurophysiologic Study of Motor Function

Basic EMG Study of Somatic Muscles

Basic EMG is most commonly performed using the standard concentric (coaxial) needle for intramuscular recording, as introduced by Adrian and Bronk.[2] Electrical potentials generated by the muscle are detected, amplified, and elaborated by a commercially available EMG apparatus. The EMG examination of skeletal muscles is performed in four steps:

1. When the needle electrode is placed in the muscle, the electrical activity associated with its insertion is evaluated (insertional activity).
2. The muscle is evaluated at rest (presence of spontaneous activity).
3. Muscle potentials evoked by isolated discharges of motor neurons are recorded with mild voluntary contraction of the muscle [single motor unit potentials (MUPs)].
4. The changes in electrical potential, as the level of muscle contraction gradually increases and eventually reaches a maximum (recruitment and interference pattern), are recorded.

It is generally necessary to sample many different areas by frequently repositioning the needle because the electrode detects muscle action potentials only from a limited area.

Selection of muscles to be studied is programmed after a previous clinical examination of the patient to establish the levels of lower motor neuron damage. This first operation requires a knowledge of the segmental innervation of somatic muscles, gained from excellent manuals available for this purpose.[3,4] Obviously, this technique is applied for limb muscles when the spinal cord damage is located at levels that have their projections from cervical (C5 to T1) and lumbosacral segments (T12 to S2). For damage of the thoracic segments, EMG of the paraspinal muscles, innervated by the posterior rami,[5] or of the abdominal muscles, innervated by the anterior rami, is indicated. As we are concerned exclusively with lesions of lower and upper motor neurons of the spinal cord, we present the EMG abnormalities for these conditions only.

In *lower motor neuron* lesions, insertional activity is generally increased because instability of the muscle membrane is enhanced during muscular denervation. A marked decrease or absence of insertional activity usually indicates a reduced number of muscle fibers, namely, in cases of fibrotic or severely atrophied muscles. Spontaneous activities at rest are also characteristic in the form of fibrillation potentials and positive sharp waves.

During a mild voluntary contraction, single MUPs appear with large amplitude, long duration, and a polyphasic morphology, indicating an increased area of residual motor units by axonal sprouting reinnervation. During maximal effort, reduced recruitment pattern with a fast firing rate of each single unit activity is found.

Increased insertional activity and the appearance of spontaneous activity in the muscle is generally evident after the first 2 weeks following denervation. These features are particularly useful in children because they do not require full collaboration of the patient. A decreased number of motor units can also be demonstrated after stimulation of the nerve corresponding to the muscle examined by means of needle or superficial skin recording electrodes. In this case a reduced amplitude of the compound muscle action potential (CMAP) appears.

In *upper motor neuron* lesions, insertional activity is normal, no spontaneous activity is detected, and single MUPs have a normal appearance. However, during maximal voluntary effort, a reduced interference pattern with slow rate firing of individual MUPs is evident.

EMG Studies in Disorders of the Spinal Cord (Excluding Inherited Diseases)

Disorders affecting the spinal cord may have their primary effect on the ventral horn. Infections, lesions from direct trauma, malformations, infiltration from tumors, radiation, and vascular insults may have an effect on the anterior horn, or motor neurons, producing an EMG pattern that can be identical with motor neuron disease. The clinical impression must then be confirmed in light of the history, physical examination, and clinical course, as well as other laboratory methods.

Poliomyelitis, fortunately, is rare today in almost all countries. The virus attacks the motor neurons preferentially. There is no segmental distribution and weakness is a matter of where and how many motor neurons lose their physiologic function. EMG in polio shows denervation and reinnervation in affected muscles.

Many other infectious and inflammatory diseases can attack the spinal cord. They usually present with a clinical picture of transverse myelitis and with evidence of upper motor neuron damage. Rarely are they selective in affecting only motor neurons; EMG examination can be of value in identifying the level of the spinal cord injury. EMG and neurographic studies, as well as clinical features of sphincter incontinence, can help in making an early differential diagnosis between transverse myelitis and Guillain–Barré syndrome.

Compression of the spinal cord and/or infiltration by both primary and secondary tumors can produce a myelopathy; however, direct metastases and primary tumors of the spinal cord are rare. EMG can detect injuries to lower motor neurons or roots.

Spina bifida with meningomyelocele is the spinal cord malformation most studied by EMG. Ingberg and Johnson[6] studied 33 infants with myelodysplasia, ranging from 1 week to 9 months of age. Conclusions can be summarized as follows: (1) EMG examination is helpful for an accurate evaluation of infants affected by lumbar meningomyelocele; (2) insertional activity is a good indicator of ultimate muscular function since stimulating the muscle mechanically with a needle electrode will evoke electrical activity in the presence of functioning or potentially functioning muscle fibers; conversely, marked fibrosis of denervated muscles may account for marked reduction in insertional activity and increased resistance to advancement of the needle electrode; (3) after surgical repair of the sac, EMG examination may show signs of reinnervation in many limb muscles; (4) muscles innervated by spinal cord levels lying between the site of major involvement and a distally involved area were relatively spared in one third of the infants. This spotty involvement is understandable in light of what was viewed at surgery (some nerves lay within the sac, some tethered to the sac lining, and others free within the CSF (cerebrospinal fluid), thus explaining the asymmetric involvement of lower limbs in some cases).

Chantraine et al.[7] published an EMG study of 53 unselected children with spina bifida aperta, ranging from 2 to 18 years of age. Generally, the weakest muscles demonstrated fibrosis with increased resistance to needle insertion, diminished insertion activity, and reduced recruitment of MUPs. Fibrillation occurred most frequently in muscles with minimal fibrosis which tested zero and poor. Subsequent EMG studies[8,9] were performed before and after surgical repair of the lumbosacral sac, to demonstrate the apparent usefulness of very early surgical repair for a better outcome of lower limb and sphincter function. One must remember that even unclosed meningomyelocele children improve somewhat during the postnatal period.

In cases with early surgical repair of the sac, postoperative EMG studies of lower limbs and sphincteric muscles demonstrated a decrease of fibrillation potentials, onset of early reinnervation polyphasic potentials, and increased amplitude and recruitment of MUPs where voluntary activity was already present before surgery.

Other series of children affected by spina bifida cystica have been published.[10-13] These authors have published control trials of immediate and delayed closure of spina bifida cystica and have searched for predictive factors by means of sensory and motor clinical evaluation only. Results seem to indicate that the clinical sensory motor evaluation is a reliable examination to assess prognosis of survival and capacity to walk. They have confirmed the usefulness of immediate closure of the neural plaque. These studies have demonstrated that EMG studies, as well as other neurophysiologic procedures, are not able to add further information to early clinical sensory–motor evaluation before and after the surgical closure of the neural plaque.

A very recent study, on the other hand, of a large series (261 meningomyeloceles)[14] has confirmed the usefulness of the sensory–motor evaluation for prognostic and functional assessment. These authors have considered electrodiagnostic tests, as well as somatic evoked responses, quite unhelpful.

EMG studies, in sum, seem more helpful during the follow-up of a child affected by meningomyelocele: (1) for the evaluation of limited muscle groups of lower limbs, when tendon transplantations are suggested by an orthopedic surgeon, and (2) to confirm or exclude involvement of the pyramidal pathways.

In traumatic lesions of the spinal cord, the EMG examination may help to localize the level of the lesion. A perinatal traumatic lesion of the cervical cord, generally provoked by a dystocic delivery,[15] can be assessed by EMG examination. This technique is helpful to perform a proper differential diagnosis between perinatal cervical cord traumatic damage, congenital cervical spinal atrophy,[16] and infantile spinal muscular atrophy (SMA type 1).

EMG Study of Muscles of the Pelvic Floor: The Reflex Activity of Urethral, Anal, and Bulbocavernosus Muscles

The perineum may be divided into the urogenital and the anal triangles. The urethra is surrounded by the external urethral sphincter quite superficially in the female (Fig. 4.1A). This sphincter, together with the deep transverse perineal muscles, forms the urogenital diaphragm and covers the whole area of the urogenital triangle. Bulbocavernosus (BC) muscle in the female surrounds the urethral meatus and introitus vaginae bilaterally. In the male the BC muscle envelopes the bulb of the urethra (Fig. 4.1B). The lateral sides of the triangle are formed by the ischiocavernosus muscles and the base by the superficial transverse perineal muscles, which also form the base of the anal triangle. The two sides of the anal triangle are formed by the gluteus maximus. The external anal sphincter is located in the central area of the anal triangle; the rest of the area is occupied by the levator ani.

These muscles are innervated by the sacral segments S2 to S4 and by the sacral plexus. Through the formation of the pudendal plexus and nerve, these roots supply the external sphincters with afferent and efferent fibers: the urethral sphincter through the perineal nerve and the anal sphincter mainly through the inferior hemorrhoidal nerve (Fig. 4.1B).

Motor activity of the sphincters maintains constant tone and responds to reflex and volitional signals. Relaxation of the sphincters is reciprocal with bladder contraction. It can normally be affected voluntarily, as will be specified below.

EMG of the external urethral sphincter is performed employing concentric needle electrodes placed medially and deeply through the perineum and behind the scrotum in the male, and lateral to the urethral meatus in the female. BC muscle is reached superficially in the midline of the perineum, behind the scrotum in the male. The anal sphincter is reached in the perianal region, in the posterior midline or on one side of this region. When possible, it is useful to study simultaneously urethral and anal sphincters because their response can sometimes be dissociated.[17,18] The EMG examination should include observation of action potentials at rest, recruitment activity during volitional contraction, and, when possible, on maximal effort.

At rest, urethral and anal sphincters almost always show continuous low-frequency activity. Amplitude of these potentials varies between 50 and 300 µV

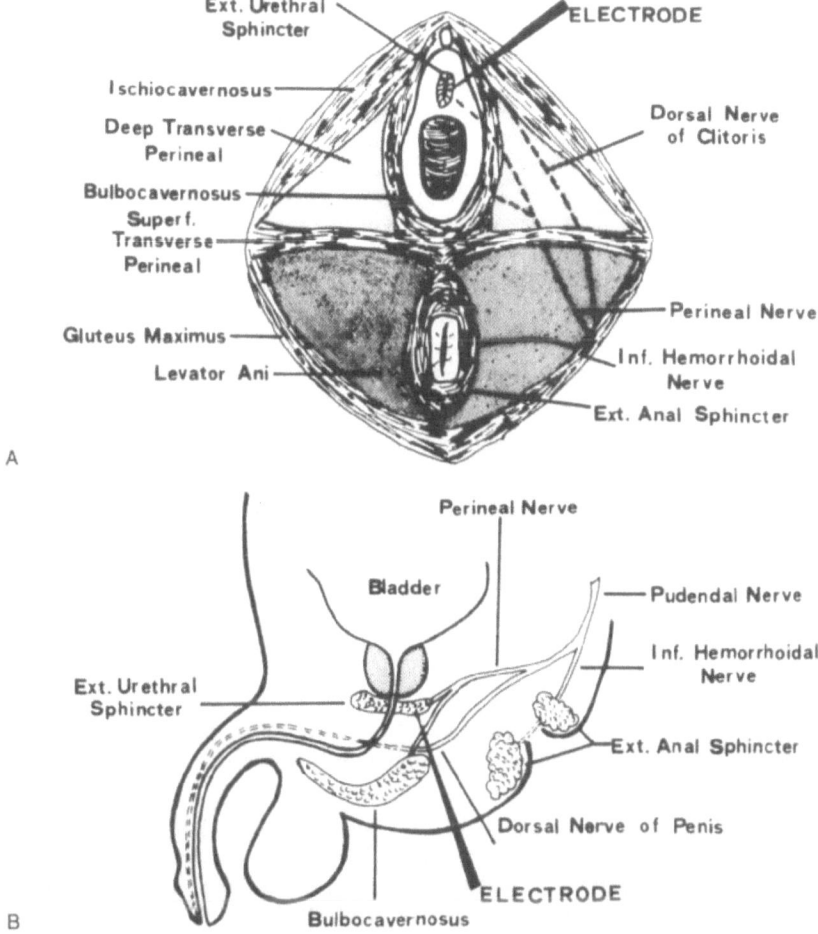

Figure 4.1. A. Female pelvic floor. Frontal view. **B.** Male pelvic floor. Lateral view. For explanation see text.

and 3 to 5 msec duration.[18] Complete relaxation of the sphincters is never detected unless the patient is simulating or performing micturition or defecation. According to Chantraine et al.,[19] the appearance of electrical silence during the resting period indicates displacement of the needle to pelvic floor muscles, which do show silence at rest. Others have noted a complete silence of sphincter muscles in healthy patients, especially in the anal sphincter, after prolonged examination.[18]

During bladder filling there is a gradual increase in motor unit activity in amplitude, number, and rate of firing in sphincter muscles (detrusor reflex); therefore, the state of the bladder should be considered during the EMG examination.

Table 4.1. Duration of MUPs in anal and urethral sphincters

	Adults		Children	
	Mean (msec)	Range (msec)	Mean (msec)	Range (msec)
Anal	5.62	2.8–11	4.58	2–9
Urethral	5.5	2–12	4.25	2–7

From Chantraine A.[19]

Volitional activity and maximal effort are difficult to obtain in children under 8 to 10 years, so spontaneous and reflex activity are the EMG parameters most often used at this age. For normal values of MUPs in urethral and anal sphincters see Table 4.1. As in skeletal muscles, 7 to 12% of polyphasics are to be considered within normal limits.

According to Waylonis,[20] in sphincter muscles children do not show the normal recruitment pattern of adults until about 70 weeks of age. Anal sphincter EMG seems particularly useful presurgically in children affected by imperforate anus, to ensure proper results.[21]

EMG of Muscles of the Pelvic Floor in Pathologic Conditions of the Spinal Cord

EMG abnormalities of pelvic floor muscles can be found in pathologic conditions involving essentially lower motor neurons of the sacral segments and roots, exclusively pyramidal pathways projecting to the lower sacral motor neurons, or in cases of mixed central and peripheral lesions.

Lower motor neuron lesions (S2 to S4 levels) are generally the result of a disorder of sacral axons due to a cauda equina syndrome or damage of the conus medullaris. Congenital malformations of the lumbosacral cord generally provoke a mixed paralysis of both central and peripheral origin.

In lower motor neuron lesions the patient cannot perceive bladder fullness or voluntarily initiate voiding as a result of loss of the sensory and/or motor limbs of the reflex arc (autonomous bladder). Peripheral paralysis of striated sphincters decreases their ability to function and explains urinary incontinence. Voiding, however, can mostly be accomplished by Crede's maneuver.

Paralysis of striated sphincters is rarely complete.

At rest: In complete early lesions there are many fibrillation potentials. In partial lesions resting activity is either diminished or normal. On bladder filling there is less activation of motor units.

On volition: Isolated or grouped MUPs discharging at a relatively high frequency appear, but never reach an interference pattern. These potentials are frequently polyphasic and of increased duration.

Upper motor neuron lesions (reflex or automatic bladder): The patient cannot perceive bladder filling or fullness and cannot voluntarily initiate voiding. Micturition is reflex and involuntary. There is often a high residual. Central paralysis is provoked by interruption of pyramidal pathways interfering with their voluntary action, though reflex activity is normal or exaggerated.

In the normal subject, micturition and defecation are controlled by the reciprocal innervation between vesical and rectal musculature, and the striated sphincters. In this condition, this reciprocal innervation is not preserved and relaxation of the sphincter during micturition may not take place (vescicourethral dyssinergia).

At rest, there may be a more marked sphincter activity than normal; activity is also increased during bladder filling. When *voiding* starts, instead of relaxation, further increase in striated sphincter activity is observed (bladder–sphincter dyssinergia). EMG can show a complete absence or a residual voluntary contraction of the sphincters and assess the extent of increased reflex activity.

Mixed central (upper motor) and peripheral (lower motor) sphincter paralysis is found mainly in malformations of the lumbosacral cord, such as spina bifida with meningomyelocele. Such spinal lesions produce not only an interruption of pyramidal tracts but also a more or less complete destruction of sacral anterior horn cells. In infants with meningomyelocele, control of sphincters is practically abolished. This type of spinal lesion produces a "mixed bladder" and all types of behavior between automatic bladder and autonomous bladder may be observed. Reflex activity may be absent when there is complete destruction of all sacral motor neurons, with evidence of spontaneous denervation. No MUPs are detected and electrical silence is present even if reflex activation is attempted. Denervation can be permanent, but it may be partially reversible.[9] In cases of total denervation, the bladder is "autonomous," incapable of contraction. It undergoes a process of retractile sclerosis of the wall. Retention of urine is the rule, as is constipation; urine may spontaneously dribble continuously or it may be made to do so if pressure is applied to the abdominal wall (Crede's maneuver). There is generally no uretheric *reflux*, as there is in cases of "automatic bladder."

After total denervation, the urethral sphincter can also become sclerosed. The EMG examination can distinguish between totally denervated sphincter with sclerotic retraction and truly increased reflex activity of the urethral sphincter. When reflex activity persists, it is reduced and, as in neurogenic atrophy, large potentials fire at high frequencies (generally over 25 cm/sec).

Functional value of the bladder in meningomyelocele seems roughly proportional to the decrease in the number of MUPs of the reflex activity recorded from the striated urethral sphincter.[22] In certain patients the presence of uretheric reflux on micturition confirms the presence of vesical contraction.[22]

Reflex Activity of the Anal and Urethral Sphincter Muscles and of the Bulbocavernosus Muscle

The demonstration of reflex contractions of the BC, periurethral striated muscle, anal sphincter, and the other perineal muscles during stimulation of the perineal nerve at the glans penis or clitoris is known as eliciting a *BC reflex*.

Motor fibers of pudendal nerves innervate most of the muscles of the pelvic floor musculature (levator ani, the paraurethral striated muscle, the superficial perineal muscles, and the anal sphincter). Innervation originates in the anterior horn cells of the sacral cord segments (S2 to S4). Their axons traverse the anterior roots. These axons follow the lateral branch of the pudendal nerve plexus to terminate in the pudendal nerves, which contain efferent and afferent fibers, and autonomic nerves from the sympathetic ganglion chain. The afferent components of the pudendal nerves supply the anterior and a portion of the posterior urethra, and the skin of the genitalia of both sexes. Stimulation of the area supplied by these sensory nerves will reflexly cause contraction of the muscles supplied by the motor fibers of the pudendal nerves.

The BC reflex is elicited clinically by pinching the glans penis or clitoris, causing reflex contraction of the pelvic floor musculature.[23,24] The absence of the BC reflex is considered to be an indicator of a neurogenic cause for bladder dysfunction. Clinically, this is often difficult to evaluate, especially in normal patients because of volitional inhibitory influences. EMG of the sphincters enhances the ability to recognize the presence of this phenomenon.

Increase of abdominal pressure, as in the Valsalva or Crede maneuvers, coughing, sobbing, and electrically evoked responses cause sudden bursts of electrical activity in both sphincters, with a complete interference EMG pattern.

Furthermore, gradual increase in electrical activity occurs with bladder filling. Voiding results in complete electrical silence; command to stop voiding results in a complete interference pattern. These reflexes and volitional responses cannot be observed in low sacral lesions or after involvement of lower thoracic and upper lumbar segments supplying the musculature affecting intraabdominal pressure. Electrically evoked reflex responses have been demonstrated to be the most useful method to assess sacral spinal cord function.

In 1967, Rushworth[25] stressed the diagnostic value of the BC reflex, reporting briefly an electrophysiologic method evoking the reflex by electrical shocks applied to the glans penis. The reflex was recorded on the BC muscles and was found to be very stable, without exhaustion. Its latency was about 35 to 40 msec in normal male subjects. Later, Dick et al.,[26] in their study of 10 normal adult men, stimulated the dorsal nerve of the penis, recording from bulbo- and ischiocavernosus muscles. Latency of responses ranged 24 to 40 msec (mean 31 msec). Eretkin and Reel[27] studied 14 normal adult male subjects. They stimulated the penis with ring electrodes and recorded responses by means of a concentric needle electrode placed in the BC muscles. At the same time, another recording electrode was placed in the anal sphincter. Mean latency was 36.1 ± 1.2 (range: 27.5 to 42.5). Only 21% of the subjects showed a response in the BC muscle. A higher (62.5%) percentage of anal responses was obtained in patients with spinal cord injury, with increased duration of the response. This was explained by the generally exaggerated polysynaptic cutaneous reflexes present in spasticity.

Siroky et al.,[28] using the same technique of Eretkin[27] for BC muscle, obtained a reflex stimulating threshold with a latency of 35 ± 2 (range 28 to 42 msec) in nine normal adult men. Latency diminished only slightly as the stimulating voltage was increased, and the reflex response did not exhaust with repetitive stimulation. When stimuli were delivered unilaterally, a contralateral and ipsilateral response was always recorded. This examination was considered useful to evaluate patients suspected to have sacral cord lesions or pudendal neuropathy.

The same authors[29] later confirmed that BC reflex had the characteristics of a cutaneous polysynaptic bilateral flexor response (as blink response). In some cases the response was composed of two well-defined components. They found that in spinal cord lesions with damage of the upper motor neuron, latency of the response was normal or sometimes shorter.

Haldemann et al.[30] studied 10 normal subjects in 1982. In doing so, they performed a new technique, using percutaneous electrodes to record responses at the BC muscle. The active electrode was positioned on the perineum, midway between the base of penis and the anus; the reference electrode was placed on the anterior-superior iliac spine; stimulation was at the base of the penis. Values ranged from 26 to 42 msec. Using the same position of recording electrodes, they also stimulated the perineum and obtained cortical and spinal "pudendal" evoked responses. In this way, using pudendal nerve stimulation they were able to demonstrate both a sacral lesion of the spinal cord and damage of the medullary sensory pathways. Other authors[31] have stressed the usefulness of recording, when possible, the BC reflex at the urethral and anal sphincter simultaneously: in pathologic cases they can be dissociated. However, this procedure has, up to now, had very few applications.

Besides BC reflex, Bradley[32] and Dick et al.[26] have introduced another reflex named "detrusor and urethral evoked response." They evoked an anal sphincter response stimulating vesical neck or wall by means of a Foley catheter with a bipolar concentric electrode. Recording of the response was performed by concentric needle electrode and by an anal plug. With this technique, they evoked a response with a latency of 50 to 80 msec; the amplitude ranged from 25 to 150 μV. Nordling[33] reported, using the same technique, values of 53 to 64 msec in normal males and 60 to 75 msec in normal females. The response was similar in amplitude and latency whether produced by stimulation of the detrusor muscle or of the posterior urethra. This "detrusor reflex" was proposed to measure the anatomic integrity of loop III[34] (see Fig. 4.2), a neural reflex pathway physiologically responsible for coordination of detrusor contraction and relaxation of periurethral striated muscle.[35] This fact is evident because the evoked anal sphincter response is most easily obtained when the bladder is empty. With the appearance of the detrusor reflex during bladder filling, attenuation of the sphincter EMG occurs. The "detrusor reflex" also permits the assessment of the function of loop IVA[34] (see Fig. 4.2). Loop IVA consists of the pyramidal tract innervation of the pudendal nucleus. In the normal individual an inhibitory synaptic potential can be generated via the pyramidal tract in the pudendal nucleus, provoking voluntary relaxation of the periurethral striated muscles.

Voluntary relaxation of the periurethral striated muscles is performed by depressing or blocking loop IVB (see Fig. 4.2). Loop IVB consists of a segmental arc whose afferent pathways originate in the spindles of sphincter muscles and

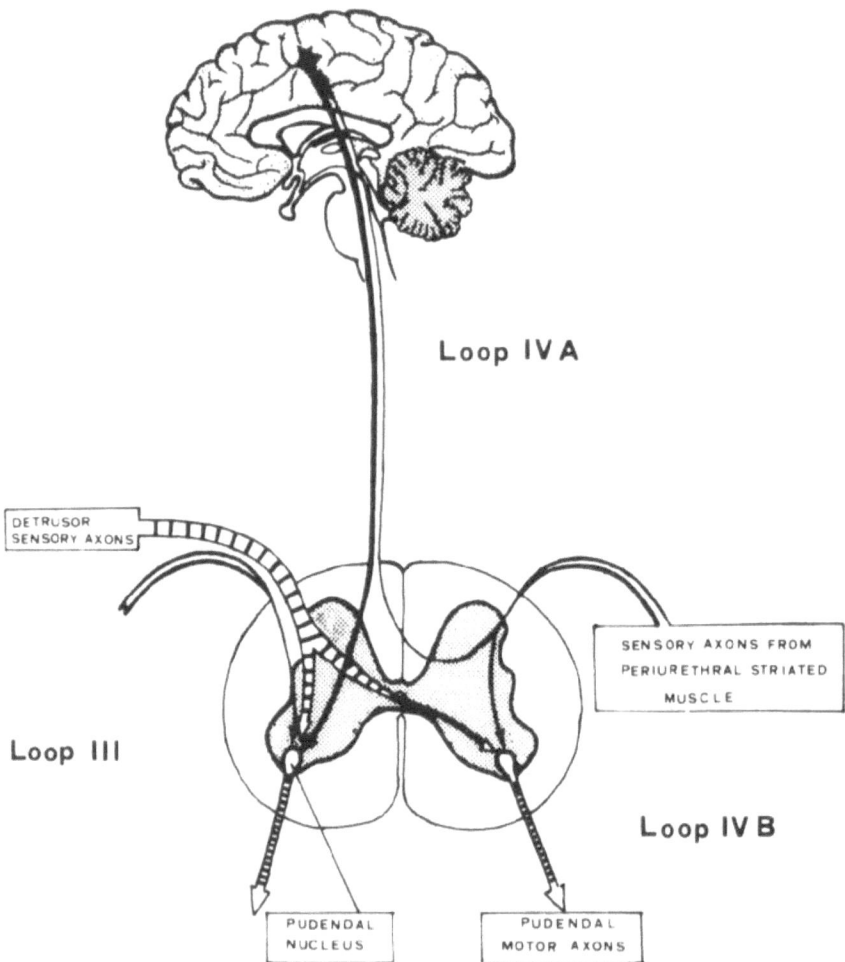

Loop IVA

DETRUSOR
SENSORY AXONS

SENSORY AXONS FROM
PERIURETHRAL STRIATED
MUSCLE

Loop III

Loop IVB

PUDENDAL
NUCLEUS

PUDENDAL
MOTOR AXONS

Figure 4.2. Schematic representation of anatomic pathways involved in reciprocal inner-vation between the vesical detrusor muscle and the urethral striated sphincter muscle. (After Bradley WE et al.[34])

terminate in the motor neurons of the pudendal nucleus.[34] At this termination, synaptic transmission may be depressed or blocked by an inhibitory signal devel-oped in loop IVA. Instructing the patient to relax perineal muscles voluntarily, the evoked anal sphincter response is attenuated by stimulation of the proximal ure-thra. Loop IVA may be interrupted by cortical and spinal cord lesions, so gener-ally no voluntary attenuation of the EMG anal response is obtained in these cases.

Another sacral reflex to be considered is the so-called *anal reflex*.[36] The reflex is elicited by stimulation of the perianal skin. The response is detected by a con-centric needle EMG electrode inserted into the superficial portion of the external anal sphincter muscle, in the midline position, posterior to the verge. Latency reported by Henry and Swash,[36] in 32 normal adults, has a mean of 8.3 msec with a range of 5 to 11.3 msec. Normal amplitudes ranged from 25 to 350 μV. This reflex has been considered a useful method to study idiopathic fecal incontinence in adult subjects. Afferent pathways of the anal reflex lie in the perianal branch of the pudendal nerves, which synapse in S2 and S3 segments of the spinal cord. Efferent pathways lie in the pudendal nerves, and arrive through the inferior hemorrhoidal nerve to the external anal sphincter muscle. Since the reflex is evoked by cutaneous stimulation, it is probably polysynaptic. When recording the latency of the anal reflex it is important, therefore, to establish the shortest possible latency with a supramaximal stimulation. In the same year Pedersen et al.[37] reported the results of anal reflex using the same technique. They studied and recorded the late components of the anal reflex in 30 normal subjects. Minimum latency was obtained around 50 msec (SD ± 10.5 msec). These authors also recorded an anal reflex stimulating the posterior tibial nerve at the lateral malleolus. The mean value of the minimum latency was 93 msec (SD ±21.1 msec). They noted that, in patients with a suprasegmental lesion, EMG response was more pronounced, concluding that perianally and peripherally elicited reflexes of the anal sphincter have many features in common with the flexor reflex of tibialis anterior elicited by the stimulation of the posterior tibial nerve at the lateral malleolus (minimum latency values of 64 msec, SD ±7.9 msec). Peripherally elicited reflex recorded from the anal reflex had a longer latency and a lower threshold than the reflex recorded from the tibialis anterior muscle. During the early stages of a spinal shock, in nine patients the anal reflex with perianal stimulation was preserved while the peripherally elicited anal reflex was not always evocable.

Pedersen et al.[38] reviewed the subject of the anal reflex after perianal electrical stimulation, studying 10 normal subjects. They were able to record early responses in all subjects. These generally had two different latencies; the first of 2 to 8 msec, the second of 13 to 18 msec. In some subjects, only the early responses were recorded. In all cases early responses had a higher threshold than the classic anal reflex, but they had a very constant latency. The classic anal reflex had a longer latency of 30 to 60 msec. Early responses were not abolished by epidural anesthesia, whereas the classic anal reflex disappeared. They concluded that early responses were not spinal reflexes but probably due to direct and antidromic impulse propagation in the efferent fibers. These considerations have been recently confirmed and demonstrated in another study.[39]

Vodusek et al.[40] tried to review the problem of "direct and reflex responses in perineal muscles" after electrical stimulation. They recorded responses in the external anal and urethral sphincters, as well as the bulbocavernosus muscles after supramaximal electrical stimulation of the penis (or clitoris), perineum, and perianal region, in 82 males and 9 females (5 to 73 years old). Their work is a first among comprehensive reviews on the subject of spinal sacral reflexes.

On perineal stimulation (penis, clitoris, lateral perineal region) reflex responses had a mean latency around 33 msec (range 26 to 40 msec), did not show exhaustion, and were evocable in all the muscles examined. These were named

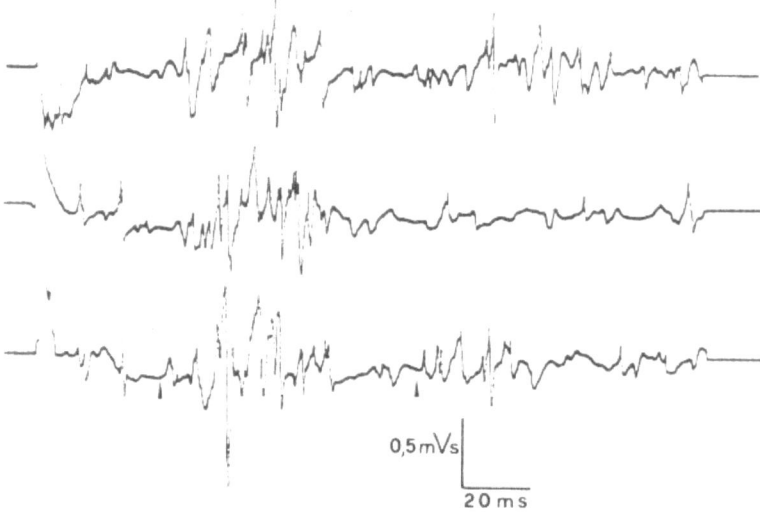

Figure 4.3. Three consecutive responses are represented with a latency around 43 msec. A second component can be observed clearly only in two responses with a latency around 112 msec. Responses are recorded at the urethral sphincter muscle and stimulation is delivered at the lateral right perineal region (stimulus intensity of 105 mAmp, 0.1 sec duration). Electromyographic examination, urodynamic evaluation, and well as the neurologic examination gave normal results. The child, S.M., 11 years old, complained of nocturnal enuresis.

R3 responses. Stimulation of the perianal region revealed exhaustion reflex responses with a mean latency of 55 msec (range 38 to 83 msec) in all muscles examined; painful stimulation was necessary in this case to have available values. These responses were named R4 responses.

These authors also obtained, in some subjects, earlier responses of 2.6 to 8 msec, called R1 responses and evocable in all muscles examined by perineal and perianal stimulation. Another group of responses, of 11.6 to 14.1 msec, called R2, were sometimes evocable in the external anal sphincter by perianal stimulation. Only R1 was interpreted to be a direct response, R2 a later and separate component of a long-duration R1 response. Early responses were evocable with strong stimulations and showed no exhaustion. They were frequently disturbed by a large stimulus artifact.

Recently, a first study of reflexes of the external urethral sphincter in children has been published.[41] Fourteen patients (ranging from 6 to 20 years) had only signs of recurrent urinary tract infections without apparent neurologic abnormalities. Another 22 patients (ranging in age from 1 month to 27 years) had suprasacral spinal cord lesions. Reflexes were evoked during urodynamic evaluation. Stimulation was applied to the penis or clitoris; the recording electrode consisted of a concentric needle inserted in the external urethral sphincter. They recorded a response with two general components. The first component ranged 20 to 45 msec in latency, with a consistent appearance, low threshold, and increasing more in magnitude than changing in latency, as strength of stimulation was increased. The second component ranged from 58 to 135, increasing in magnitude and duration with stimulus strength. Reflexes were present in about 80% of control patients. The same values were evocable in children with suprasacral cord lesions. They concluded that latency values in children were superimposable on adult values and demonstrated the analogy of these reflexes to other flexor reflexes. The reflex response of the external urethral sphincter to electrical stimulation was considered to be a useful addition to the urodynamic battery to probe the integrity of the entire reflex arc and the sacral spinal cord.

We have personally examined 14 children (seven males and seven females) who complained of enuresis or unstable bladder and had a normal neurologic examination. The age ranged from 8 to 14 years (mean 11 years). An external sphincter urethral reflex was evocable in 13 patients. Stimulations were applied to the lateral perineal region and reflexes were all evoked with a stimulus strength of 105 mAmp, 0.1 msec duration. Responses showed no exhaustion and were stable. Latencies ranged from 26 to 45 msec with a mean of 36.88 (SD ±5.87 msec). In eight cases we could distinguish a second component (Fig. 4.3). We have seen that lateral perineal stimulation was well tolerated by all children and was better accepted than stimulation of the clitoris or penis. Latency of the response was clearly abnormal in three children with tethered cord, five children with meningomyelocele, one with spastic paraplegia associated with neuropathy, and one with sacral agenesis.

Kinesiologic Assessment

This evaluation consists of EMG of urethral and anal sphincters during bladder filling, observation of reflex activity during micturition and voluntary depression of reflex activity, volitionally induced, or interrupted voiding. These tests are performed in conjunction with cystometry, allowing investigations of time relationships between detrusor reflex and striated sphincter activity. This examination should generally be performed by a skilled urologist or neurourologist. During kinesiologic assessment the study of the sacral spinal reflexes can be performed as explained above. This type of examination should always be performed when spinal cord injury is suspected because abnormalities of bladder storing and bladder emptying are frequent in this situation and can cause further urologic complications.

Cystometry is the graphic representation of changes in vesical pressure as a function of volume. Generally, this is combined with graphic representation of urinary flow rate, EMG of external urethral sphincter, and fluoroscopic visualization of the bladder and urethra during micturition (voiding cystourethrography). The combined technique of synchronous video/pressure/flow/EMG monitoring has enhanced understanding of micturition disorders and increased the possibility to study reciprocal action occurring between the bladder and

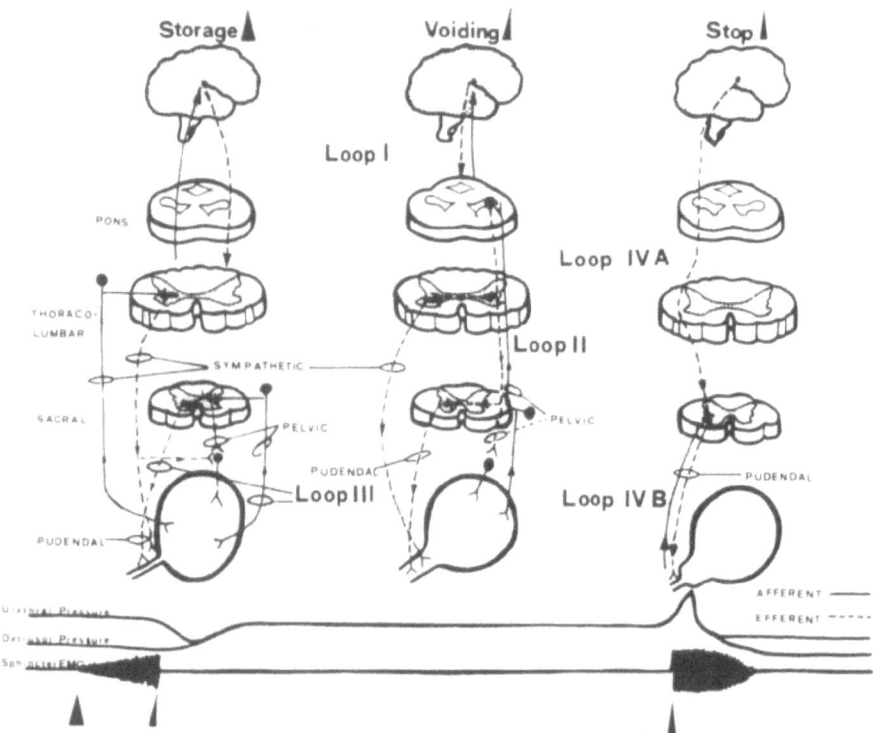

Figure 4.4. Schematic representation of anatomical pathways involved in bladder function (storage, voiding, and stop voiding). The corresponding cystourethrographic examination can be observed below and the different functional stages are indicated by different arrows. For further explanation see text. (Modified from Blaivais JG.[46])

sphincter mechanisms. For further information consultation of comprehensive manuals is suggested.[42,43]

To understand how spinal cord lesions can affect micturition, it is meaningful to synthesize neurologic pathways concerned with this complex function.

It has long been recognized that the sacral cord (S2 to S4) contains neural pathways involved in micturition reflexes. The first theory proposed by Denny-Brown and Robertson[44] suggested that the micturition reflex was nothing more than a local sacral reflex mediated entirely by the pelvic and pudendal nerves. According to this theory, bladder distension stimulates afferent fibers (from receptors of bladder mucosa and smooth muscles) of the pelvic nerve, which enter the spinal cord via the posterior roots of the second through fourth sacral segments. These fibers synapse with neurons of pelvic (intermediolateral nuclei to detrusor muscle) and pudendal nuclei (anterior horn nuclei to external urethral sphincter). The resulting efferent discharges traverse the anterior roots of the pelvic and pudendal nerves to cause detrusor contraction and striated sphincter relaxation. This reflex may be either facilitated or inhibited by suprasegmental descending pathways (Fig. 4.4).

Further studies[45] have demonstrated that local stimuli arising from the bladder cause afferent discharges in the pelvic nerve that synapse directly in a supraspinal micturition center in the pontine-mesencephalic reticular formation (nucleus tegmento-lateralis dorsalis). This pontine micturition center modulates the neural impulses in such a manner as to effect detrusor contraction and sphincter relaxation. Hald and Bradley[43] denominates loop II (see Fig. 4.4), pathways consisting of detrusor sensory afferents in the spinal cord and brain stem (nucleus tegmento-lateralis dorsalis) as well as descending pathways to the detrusor motor neurons in the sacral gray matter. This routing of detrusor sensory impulses provides an amplification of the time course of the detrusor reflex. Loop I consists of to and fro connections from nucleus tegmento-lateralis dorsalis to a specific portion of the frontal lobe. This loop provides a substrate for voluntary control of the detrusor reflex, provoking voluntary decontraction of the detrusor muscle avoiding detrusor hyperreflexia.

Loop III (see Fig. 4.4) is composed of the peripheral detrusor afferent axons and their pathways in the spinal cord, which terminates by synapsing on pudendal motor neurons. The pudendal motor neurons give rise to axons that innervate the periurethral striated muscle. Impulses in this pathway produce inhibition of pudendal motor neurons. The synchronous action of loop II and loop III provides synergic detrusor contraction and urethral external sphincter relaxation during micturition, avoiding vescico-sphincter dyssynergia.

Another reflex arc suggested by Hald and Bradley[43] is loop IV. This loop consists of two components: A and B (see Figs. 4.2 and 4.4).

Loop IVA is composed of a supraspinal, voluntary innervation of pudendal motor neurons, permitting voluntary interruption of the urinary stream. Loop IVB is composed of segmental innervation of the periurethral striated muscle, consisting of pudendal afferents of muscle spindles and pudendal motor axons to the external urethral sphincter.

As reported by Blaivais,[46] De Groot and associates have stressed the importance of the sympathetic nervous system in modulating lower urinary tract function providing bladder filling. The thoracolumbar intermediolateral cell column receives afferent discharges from receptors in the bladder wall. Efferent impulses (hypogastric nerves) result in contraction of the internal sphincter, helping to maintain continence. Other efferent sympathetic pathways synapse on postganglionic parasympathetic neurons, resulting in inhibition of detrusor contraction.

Blaivais,[46] in a detailed urodynamic and neurologic evaluation of 550 patients, has reviewed the neurophysiologic pathways involved in micturition. They differ somewhat from the theories of Bradley. His assumptions can be summarized as follows. Voiding can be described in terms of three major and different neurophysiologic and anatomic pathways (Fig. 4.4). During storage, bladder distension results in afferent pelvic nerve discharges that through the pudendal nerve reach the pudendal nucleus, impulses that result in contraction of the external urethral sphincter. Simultaneously, afferent sympathetic discharges traverse hypogastric nerves. After synapse in sympathetic thoracolumbar nuclei, efferent discharges cause: (1) inhibition of transmission at the preganglionic parasympathetic neuron, which inhibits detrusor contraction and (2) increased tone at bladder neck. Urodynamic findings are characterized by an urethral pressure that is greater than the detrusor pressure, accompanied by concomitant bursts of electrical activity in the external urethral sphincter.

During voiding, afferent pelvic nerve discharges ascend in spinal cord and synapse with the pontine micturition center. Descending efferent pathways cause: (1) inhibition of pudendal firing and relaxation of external urethral sphincter, (2) inhibition of sympathetic firing which opens the bladder neck and permits postganglionic transmission, and (3) pelvic parasympathetic firing which causes detrusor contraction.

During micturition it is possible to stop voluntarily the urinary stream. Descending corticospinal pathways originating from the motor cortex synapse in the pudendal nucleus, resulting in contraction of the external urethral sphincter.

Spinal cord injuries always cause a neurourologic disorder. Following the classification of Krane and Siroky,[42] we can divide neurogenic bladder into two main categories: with detrusor hyperreflexia and with detrusor areflexia.

Detrusor hyperreflexia can be associated with coordinated urethral sphincter, dyssynergia of the external urethral sphincter, or dyssynergia at the level of the proximal smooth muscle sphincter. Detrusor areflexia can be associated with coordinated urethral sphincters, nonrelaxing striated sphincter, external urethral sphincter denervation, or nonrelaxation of the smooth muscle sphincter.

Neurophysiologic Study of Sensory Function

Somatosensory Evoked Potentials in Pediatric Spinal Cord Pathology

Somatosensory evoked potentials (SEPs) are useful to evaluate the integrity of the nervous system at different levels, from the periphery to the cerebral cortex. They provide information on sensory fibers of larger diameter in the peripheral nervous system, the dorsal columns, brain stem lemniscal pathways, and thalamocortical projections of the central nervous system.

Stimulation of sensory and/or mixed nerves produces low-amplitude evoked potentials, recorded by means of superficial electrodes at different spinal levels and from the scalp. Summation of these evoked potentials with the method of averaging has improved the signal-to-noise ratio. The use of SEPs in children is relatively recent. Only a few studies are available with regard to maturation. Furthermore, methodologies and results obtained are, at the moment, too variable to propose standardized values.

SEPs from Upper Extremity Stimulation

Stimulation of the second or third finger, or of the median nerve at the wrist, produces the appearance, in healthy adults, of a negative wave called N1 or N20

Table 4.2. Mean latencies (msec) of SEPs from birth to 12 months of age; left median nerve stimulation at the wrist

Age	Erb's point-Fz	CII-Fz	C'4-Fz
Birth	6.2 ± 0.7	9.4 ± 0.4	24.3 ± 2.1[a]
2 months	5.6 ± 0.5	8.7 ± 0.7	20.2 ± 1.6[a]
4 months	5.6 ± 0.3	8.3 ± 0.5	19.1 ± 1.3[a]
6 months	5.6 ± 0.6	8.3 ± 0.4	17.4 ± 1.1[a]
8 months	5.3 ± 0.6	8.1 ± 0.6	17.2 ± 1.7[u]
10 months	5.5 ± 0.7	8.1 ± 0.8	17.3 ± 0.9[a]
12 months	5.8 ± 0.8	8.1 ± 0.7	16.7 ± 0.8[a]

Modified from Willis J. et al.[52]
[a] N1 peak latency.

(in relation to the mean latency of the peak around 20 msec). The recording is contralateral, from the parietal cortex. In the child this early negative component goes through progressive changes. Only around the age of 8 years does it reach the typical pattern found in adults.[47,48] This wave reflects the activity of the thalamocortical fibers and the cortex. Recording from Erb's point, cervical spinal cord, and from the scalp, against a noncephalic reference, four potentials of brief latencies around 9, 11, 13, and 14 msec appear, presenting different polarities (N or P) in relation to the different locations of the recording electrodes. The suggested generators of these waves could be, respectively, the brachial plexus, dorsal columns, nucleus caudatus, and medial lemniscus.[49-51] Using the measurement of the distance from the stimulating electrode to Erb's point, it is possible to determine the peripheral nerve conduction velocity. The interpeak latencies from Erb's point to the spine, and from the spine to the scalp, permit one to determine the central conduction times.

Willis et al.[52] reported a study of normal infants in the first year of life. They observed that the latency of Erb's point potential remained stable throughout this age, whereas the latencies of the cervical, spine, and scalp potentials decreased with maturation (Table 4.2).

SEPs to Lower Extremity Stimulation

By stimulation of the common peroneal nerve at the ankle, evoked potentials over both the spine and the scalp are elicitable, using surface electrodes. In adults, the earlier and most stable positive scalp potentials are obtained at about 27 msec and 37 msec of latency, stimulating, respectively, the common peroneal nerve and the posterior tibial nerve. In bipolar leads, spinal evoked responses consist of an initially positive triphasic potential. This is greatest in amplitude and duration, most complex in configuration from leads placed over the lower thoracic spine. Conversely, leads over rostral cord segments produce a response that is small and poorly defined. The presumed neural generators of the spinal SEPs are the roots of the cauda equina, the intramedullary continuations of dorsal root fibers, and the afferent pathways of the dorsal columns from leads positioned

Table 4.3. Mean and standard deviation for spinal conduction velocities (m/sec) in six age categories

Age	Stim. –L3	T12–T6	T6–C7	L3–C7
0–1 month	34.36 ± 3.29	17.14 ± 3.82	43.00 ± 5.24	27.00 ± 3.42
1–12 months	42.00 ± 6.12	25.71 ± 3.50	53.56 ± 10.63	39.15 ± 4.75
13–36 months	56.36 ± 6.08	33.56 ± 4.01	64.93 ± 11.54	50.33 ± 4.95
3–6 years	59.25 ± 5.85	37.00 ± 3.32	70.67 ± 16.07	58.33 ± 6.17
6–10 years	62.86 ± 4.26	45.60 ± 4.67	84.93 ± 8.03	66.56 ± 4.55
10–30 years	65.74 ± 3.77	49.60 ± 4.19	88.74 ± 6.45	67.91 ± 3.85

Modified from Cracco J.B. et al.[53]

over the lumbar spine, the lower thoracic spine, and the rostral spinal cord, respectively. The onset of the first negative component, recording over L3, T12, T6, and C7, is used as the indicator of the spinal latency. Using the onset latencies of the spine SEPs and the peak latency of the scalp component, and measuring the distances between the point of stimulation and spine/scalp recording electrodes, the different conduction velocities can be determined.

Peripheral conduction velocity, from the stimulating electrode at the knee to L3, is around 65 m/sec in normal adults. Spine-to-spine conduction velocity (L3 to C7, T12 to T6, and T6 to C7) are respectively around 70 m/sec, 50 m/sec, and 85 m/sec.[53] These conduction velocity values in the newborn are about 50% of the adult values. They increase with age (Table 4.3). Peripheral conduction velocities reach adult values by the third year, whereas not until the fifth year are spinal cord velocities within the adult range. This is related to the different rate of maturation between the peripheral system and the afferent central pathways.

Cracco et al.[54] also measured, in normal adults, the conduction velocities between the spinal responses, with leads over L3, T12, T6, and C7, and cortical responses; values were respectively: 39.7 ± 1.4 msec, 36.6 ± 1.8 msec, 33.5 ± 1.3 msec, 22.9 ± 1.0 msec.

Spine–scalp conduction velocities are shorter than intraspinal velocities. This is probably related to synaptic slowing through the brain stem.

Clinical Applications of SEPs (Excluding Inherited Diseases)

In adult patients with traumatic spinal cord lesions above C6 to C7, clinically considered to be complete, neither median nor peroneal nerve evoked potentials can be recorded. Conversely, in complete cord lesions at the C6 to C7 level or below, evoked responses were recorded stimulating the median nerve but not after stimulation of the peroneal nerve. Patients with incomplete lesions of the cervical cord generally showed abnormal wave forms and prolonged latencies. Patients with clinical improvement frequently showed normal potentials.[55]

In children with meningomyelocele, a good correlation between the neurologic status and the spinal evoked potentials has been suggested.[56] A clinically complete lesion of the spinal cord produced normal evoked potentials in the leads

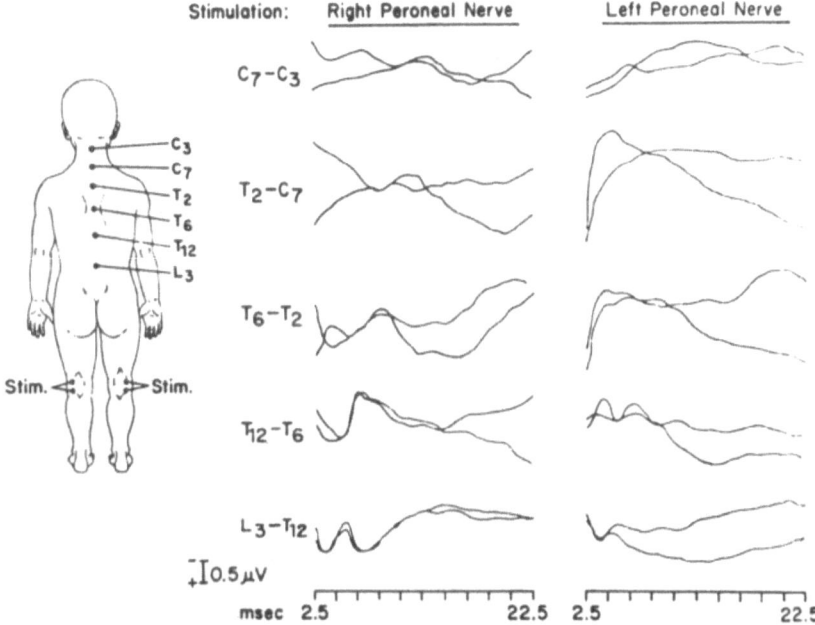

Figure 4.5. Spinal evoked potentials obtained from a 6-month-old infant who presented a clinically asymmetric defect from a lumbosacral meningomyelocele. The stimulation of the left (paralyzed) leg produced small potentials only over the cauda equina and caudal spinal cord, whereas normal responses were recorded at all levels by stimulation of the relatively normal right leg. (From Cracco RQ et al.[59])

below it and the absence of response rostral to the lesion. Some children with meningomyelocele showed a positive potential in the leads immediately rostral to the lesion. This potential progressively decreased in amplitude in rostral leads but did not change in latency.[57] It can be considered as a nonpropagated volume-conducted potential, experimentally demonstrated in spinal cord transection, so-called "killed-end effect."[58] Infants with mild defects showed no abnormal potentials in leads rostral to the lesion. Furthermore, Cracco et al.[59] obtained normal spinal potentials, stimulating the normal leg in infants with a clinically asymmetric defect (Fig. 4.5). The same authors have also noticed, with leads over the lumbar spinous processes, evoked responses normally recorded over the lower thoracic spine, in a few patients with either meningomyelocele or occult dysraphism. This suggested caudal displacement of the spinal cord, later confirmed by myelography.

Other authors[60] have observed reduced conduction velocities from the spine (L3, T12, T6) to the cortex in children with atlanto-axial subluxation, intramedullary astrocytoma, transverse myelitis, and cervical cord trauma. SEPs have been shown to be a useful tool in the diagnosis of birth-related spinal cord injuries.[61]

Intraoperative Spinal Cord Monitoring

Spinal and cortical SEPs have been used for monitoring afferent ascending spinal transmission in a variety of neurosurgic, orthopedic, and vascular conditions. It has been observed experimentally that cortical SEPs are attenuated or abolished by ischemia before spinal SEPs. Conversely, they are both affected to a similar degree and with the same time course following spinal cord manipulation.[62] This suggests the usefulness of simultaneous recording of both spinal and cortical SEPs.

During operations using Harrington rod applications, only minimal changes of the spinal SEPs, epidurally recorded at the upper thoracic or cervical spinal levels, have been observed. Amplitudes did not fall over 50% except in one case in whom the responses disappeared after distraction, in which case the patient suffered a transient postoperative spasticity.[63]

Whittle et al.[64] utilized the intraoperative monitoring of SEPs during surgery for congenital malformations of the spinal axis, such as the tethered cord syndrome, in an attempt to minimize iatrogenic morbidity to the sacral spinal cord and roots. These authors considered that monitoring of spinal SEPs is a suboptimal method to assess neural integrity of S3 to S4 roots during surgery, because these roots are not activated by tibial and peroneal nerve stimulation. Furthermore, the signal evoked at the lumbar region is essentially a "conus" potential representing the potential field generated in the dorsal horns of the spinal segments from L4 to S3. In this situation, a lesion of one or two sacral roots could provoke only insignificant changes of the spinal SEPs at the lumbar region. To avoid this problem, they suggest the simultaneous recording of spinal evoked potentials together with a method of assessing anal or vesical function.[65]

References

1. Light KJ, Faganel J, Roth DR, Dimitrijevic MR: Meningomyelocele: a clinical, urodynamic and neurophysiological evaluation. J Urol 131:717–721, 1984.
2. Adrian ED, Bronk DW: The discharge of impulses in motor nerve fibers. Part 2. The frequency of discharge in reflex and voluntary contractions. J Physiol (Lond) 67:119, 1929.
3. Delagi EF, Perotto A: Anatomic Guide for the Electromyographer, 2nd Edit. Charles C Thomas, Springfield, Illinois, 1980.
4. Kendall FP, McCrear E: Muscles: Testing and Function, 3rd Edit. Williams & Wilkins, Baltimore, 1983.
5. Johnson EW: Practical Electromyography. Williams & Wilkins, Baltimore, 1980.
6. Ingberg HO, Johnson EW: Electromyographic evaluation of infants with lumbar meningomyelocele. Arch Phys Med Rehabil 44:86–92, 1963.
7. Chantraine A, Lloyd K, Swinyard CA: An electromyographic study of children with spina bifida manifesta. Dev Med Child Neurol 6:7–17, 1964.
8. Chantraine A, Stevenvaert A, Timmermans L: Electromyographic study before and after operation in spina bifida with myelomeningocele. A preliminary report. Dev Med Child Neurol (Suppl) 13:136–137, 1967.

9. Chantraine A, Stevenvaert A, Carlier G, Bonnal J: Evolution electromyographique du bilan pré et postopératoire du spina bifida avec troubles neurologiques. Acta Paediatr Belg 22:127–140, 1968.

10. Sharrard WJW, Zachary RB, Lorber J, Bruce AM: A controlled trial of immediate and delayed closure of spina bifida cystica. Arch Dis Child 38:18–22, 1963.

11. Hunt G, Lewin W, Gleave J, Gairdner D: Predictive factors in open myelomeningocele with special reference to sensory level. Br Med J 4:197–201, 1973.

12. Lorber J: Early results of selective treatment of spina bifida cystica. Br Med J 4:201–204, 1973.

13. Sharrard WJW: Assessment of the myelomeningocele in children. In: Laurin RL (ed): Myelomeningocele. Grune & Stratton, New York, 1977, pp 389–419.

14. Simpson D, Corney A, Creswell J: Myelomeningoceles: Validity of early postnatal assessment. J Pediatr Neurosci 1:187–202, 1985.

15. Jellinger K, Schingshackl A: Birth injury of the spinal cord: report of two necropsy cases with several weeks survival. Neuropaediatrie 4:111, 1973.

16. Darwish H, Sarnat H, Archer C, Brownel K, Kotagal S: Congenital cervical spinal atrophy. Muscle Nerve 4:106–110, 1981.

17. Vereeken RL, Verduyn H: The electrical activity of the paraurethral and perineal muscles in normal and pathological conditions. Br J Urol 42:457–463, 1970.

18. Di Benedetto M: Electromyography and Nerve Conduction in Neuro-Urology. American Association of Electromyography and Electrodiagnosis, Minimonograph No. 4, 1977.

19. Chantraine A: EMG examination of the anal and urethral sphincters. In: Desmedt JE (ed): New Developments in Electromyography and Clinical Neurophysiology, Vol 2. Karger, Basel, 1973, pp 421–432.

20. Waylonis WG, Aseff JN: Anal sphincter electromyography in the first two years of life. Arch Phys Med Rehabil 54:525–527, 1973.

21. Archibald KC, Goldsmith EI: Spincteric electromyography. Arch Phys Med Rehabil 48:387–392, 1967.

22. Jesel M, Isch-Treussard C, Isch F: Electromyography of striated muscles of anal and urethral sphincters. In: Desmedt JE (ed): New Developments in Electromyography and Clinical Neurophysiology, Vol. 2. Karger, Basel, 1973, pp 406–420.

23. Bors E, French JD: Management of paroxysmal hypertension following injuries to cervical and upper thoracic segments of spinal cord: AMA Arch Surg 64:803–812, 1952.

24. Lapides J, Bobbit JM: Diagnostic value of bulbocavernosus reflex. JAMA 162:971–972, 1956.

25. Rushworth G: Diagnostic value of the electromyographic study of reflex activity in man. In: Widen L (ed): Recent Advances in Clinical Neurophysiology, Suppl 25 to Electroencephalography and Neurophysiology. Elsevier, Amsterdam, 1967, pp. 65–73.

26. Dick HC, Bradley WE, Scott FB, Timm GW: Pudendal sexual reflexes and electrophysiologic investigations. J Urol 3:376–379, 1974.

27. Eretkin C, Reel F: Bulbocavernosus reflex in normal bladder and/or impotence. J Neurol Sci 28:1–15, 1976.

28. Siroky M, Sax SD, Krane RJ: Sacral signal tracing: the electrophysiology of the bulbocavernosus reflex. J Urol 122:661–664, 1979.

29. Krane JK, Siroky MB: Studies on sacral evoked potentials. J Urol 124:872–876, 1980.

30. Haldemann S, Bradley WE, Bhatia N: Evoked responses from the pudendal nerve. J Urol 128:974–980, 1982.

31. Opsomer RJ, Wese FX, Knoops P, Van Cangh PJ: Etude de l'arc réflex sacré par potentiels évoqués moteurs. Résultats préliminaires. Acta Urol Belg 51:325–333, 1983.

32. Bradley WE: Urethral electromyography. J Urol 108:563–564, 1972.

33. Nordling J, Andersen JI, Walter S, Meyhoff HH, Hald T, and Gammelgaard PA: Evoked response of the bulbocavernosus reflex. Eur Urol 5:36–38, 1979.

34. Bradley WE, Timm GW, Rockwold GL, Scott FB: Detrusor and urethral electromyography. J Urol 114:891–894, 1975.

35. Bradley WE, Timm GW, Scott FB: Innervation of the detrusor muscle and urethra. Urol Clin N Am 1:3, 1974.

36. Henry MM, Swash M: Assessment of pelvic floor disorders and incontinence by electrophysiological recording of the anal reflex. Lancet i:1290–1291, 1978.

37. Pedersen E, Harring H, Klemar B, Torring J: Human anal reflexes. J Neurol Neurosurg Psychiatry 41:813–818, 1978.

38. Pedersen E, Klemar B, Schroder HD, Törring J: Anal Sphincter Responses After Perianal Electrical Stimulation. Neurol Neurosurg Psychiatry 45:770–773, 1982.

39. De Grandis D, Audisio R, Aiello I, Serra G, Morsiani E: Response of external anal sphincter to electrical stimulation of the perineal skin. Riv Ital EEG Neurofisiol Clin 6:43–51, 1983.

40. Vodusek DB, Janko M, Lokar J: Direct and reflex responses in perineal muscles on electrical stimulation. J Neurol Neurosurg Psychiatry 46:67–71, 1983.

41. Hallet M, Bauer S, Khoshbin S, Dyro F: Reflexes of the external urethral sphincter in children. Arch Neurol 41:942–945, 1984.

42. Krane J, Siroky MB: Clinical Neuro-Urology. Little Brown & Company, Boston, 1979.

43. Hald T, Bradley WE: The Urinary Bladder. Neurology and Dynamics. Williams & Wilkins, Baltimore, 1982.

44. Denny-Brown D, Robertson EG: On the physiology of micturition. Brain 56:149, 1933.

45. Bradley WE, Conway CJ: Bladder representation in the pontine-mesencephalic reticular formation. Exp Neurol 16:237–249, 1966.

46. Blaivais JG: The neurophysiology of micturition: A clinical study of 550 patients. J Urol 127:958–963, 1982.

47. Hrbek A, Karlberg P, Olsson T: Development of visual and somatosensory evoked responses in pre-term newborn infants. Electroencephalogr Clin Neurophysiol 34:225–232, 1973.

48. Desmedt JE, Brunko E, Debecker J: Maturation of the somatosensory evoked potentials in normal infants and children, with special reference to the early N1 component. Electroencephalogr Clin Neurophysiol 40:43–58, 1976.

49. Desmedt JE, Cheron G: Central somatosensory conduction in man: neural generators and interpeak latencies of the far field components recorded from neck and right or left scalp and earlobes. Electroencephalogr Clin Neurophysiol 50:382–403, 1980.

50. Cracco RQ, Cracco JB: Somatosensory evoked potentials in man: far-field potentials. Electroencephalogr Clin Neurophysiol 41:460–466, 1976.

51. Anziska B, Cracco RQ, Cook AW, Feld EW: Somatosensory far-field potentials: studies in normal subjects and patients with multiple sclerosis. Electroencephalogr Clin Neurophysiol 45:602–610, 1978.

52. Willis J, Seales D, Frazier E: Short latency somatosensory evoked potentials in infants. Electroencephalogr Clin Neurophysiol 59:366–373, 1984.
53. Cracco JB, Cracco RQ, Stolove R: Spinal evoked potential in man: a maturational study. Electroencephalogr Clin Neurophysiol 46:58–64, 1979.
54. Cracco RQ, Anziska BJ, Cracco JB, Vas GA, Rossini PM, Maccabee PJ: Short-latency somatosensory evoked potentials to median and peroneal nerve stimulation: studies in normal subjects and patients with neurologic disease. Ann NY Acad Sci 388:412–425, 1982.
55. Perot PL Jr: The clinical use of somatosensory evoked potentials in spinal cord injury. Clin Neurosurg 20:367–381, 1973.
56. Cracco JB, Cracco RQ, Graziani LJ: Spinal evoked response in infants with myelodysplasia. Neurology 24:359–360, 1974.
57. Cracco JB, Cracco RQ: Spinal somatosensory evoked potentials: maturational and clinical studies. Ann NY Acad Sci 388:526–537, 1982.
58. Cracco RQ, Evans BE: Spinal evoked potential in the cat: effects of asphyxia, strychnine, cord section and compression. Electroencephalogr Clin Neurophysiol 44:187–201, 1978.
59. Cracco RQ, Cracco JB, Sarnowski R, Vogel HB: Spinal evoked potentials. In: Desmedt JE (ed): Clinical Uses of Cerebral, Brainstem, and Spinal Somatosensory Evoked Potentials. Karger, Basel and New York, 1980.
60. Schiff JA, Cracco RQ, Rossini PM, Cracco JB: Spine and scalp somatosensory evoked potentials in normal subjects and patients with spinal cord disease: evaluation of afferent transmission. Electroencephalogr Clin Neurophysiol 59:374–387, 1984.
61. Bell HJ, Dykstra DD: Somatosensory evoked potentials as an adjunct to diagnosis of neonatal spinal cord injury. J Pediatr 106:298–301, 1985.
62. Larson SJ, Wahs PR, Sances JA, et al: Evoked potentials in experimental myelopathy. Spine 5:299–302, 1980.
63. Jones SJ: Clinical applications of short latency somatosensory evoked potentials. Ann NY Acad Sci 388:369–387, 1982.
64. Whittle IR, Johnston IH, Besser M: Intraoperative monitoring of spinal somatosensory evoked potentials during surgery for tethered cord syndrome. Riv Neurosci Pediatr (J Pediatr Neurosci) 1:178–186, 1985.
65. Badr G, Carlsonn CA, Fall M, Friberg S, Lindstrom L, Ohlsson B: Cortical evoked potentials following stimulation of the urinary bladder in man. Electroencephalogr Clin Neurophysiol 54:494–498, 1982.

CHAPTER 5

Embryologic and Developmental Dynamics of the Dysraphic State

Massimo Caldarelli and David G. McLone

The term dysraphic state describes a number of congenital anomalies characterized by a disturbance in the formation of the neural tube and/or its coverings. Dysraphic states may involve the whole craniospinal axis or single portions of it (brain, spinal cord). In view of the specific interest of this chapter, we will restrict our analysis to spinal dysraphism, which may present under several clinical manifestations (Table 5.1).

For a better understanding of this complex matter, some initial considerations must be brought to mind concerning the timing of and the main events leading to neural tube formation.[1-6] Present knowledge of early human nervous system development is based on a great number of anatomic observations deriving from large collections of embryos and fetuses[3-14] or from single specimens. On the other hand, neither an in vivo nor an in vitro study exists dealing with human neurodevelopment. This is the reason for which experimental studies performed on animal embryos have been largely utilized to elucidate and, possibly, understand fully the dynamic process of neurodevelopment in humans (Fig. 5.1). After the pioneering studies of Streeter,[11-14] the embryonic period (first 8 postovulatory weeks) was divided into 23 "Carnegie Stages," formerly "Horizons." Besides the presence of specific anatomic patterns, the main criteria that attribute an embryo to a particular embryologic stage are the approximate gestational age and the crown–rump (C–R) length.[4,9,10] Accurate timing of normal development of an early human embryo is essential when trying to refer developmental anomalies to specific embryologic events (Table 5.2).

Development of the Human Nervous System

By Carnegie Stage 7 (0.4 mm C–R; 16 days) a cellular process which extends rostrally starting from Hensen's node is recognizable: the notochord which is believed to play a role as inducer of the neural plaque. The neural plaque region may be recognized above it, surrounded by the non-neural ectoderm.[15] The first evidence of the future nervous system, in the appearance of a shallow neural groove, is evident, however, only during the subsequent Carnegie Stage 8 (1 to

Table 5.1. Clinical manifestations of spinal dysraphism

Myeloschisis: The neural plaque remains exposed without any covering.

Myelomeningocele: Ectopic spinal cord lying outside the spinal canal, due to accumulation of cerebrospinal fluid beyond the dysraphic neural tissue, which maintains the aspect of the primitive neural plaque.

Meningocele: Mere protrusion of the meninges (dura mater and arachnoid) through a defect of the spinal arches, but still covered by intact skin.

Spina bifida occulta: Simple skeletal defect characterized by the normal position of the spinal cord and meninges within the spinal canal.

1.5 mm C–R; 18 days); at this time the neural folds are represented more in the rostral than in the caudal area.[16] The neural groove deepens and the neural folds become more evident during Carnegie Stage 9 (1.5 to 2.5 mm C–R; 20 days) which marks the beginning of the "neurulation." Major segmentations of the future brain may be identified at this stage, as the rhomboencephalon is more prominent. Mesencephalic flexure appears and caudal eminence is actively proliferating.[17] During Carnegie Stage 10 (2 to 3.5 mm C–R; 22 days; 4 to 12 pairs of somites) some new features become apparent, such as the optic sulcus.[18] The neural folds approximate and eventually fuse in an area opposite somites 2 to 7, which corresponds to the future upper cervical-rhomboencephalic level.[15,19] Telencephalon and diencephalon become more distinguishable and the "spinal" neural plaque greatly lengthens. By Carnegie Stage 11 (2.5 to 4.5 mm C–R; 24 days; 13 to 20 pairs of somites)[10,15] the neural plaque closure continues both rostrad and caudad, in a fashion that has been compared to a zip-fastner, although it has been demonstrated that the closure may take place at several levels independently. This process leads to the identification of two slits, at the rostral and caudal ends of the fusing neural tube, which are called "neuropores" (anterior and posterior). The rostral end is the first to seal (when 20 pairs of somites are identifiable). Although this closure is dependent mainly upon progressive fusion of the rhomboencephalic, mesencephalic, and prosencephalic folds, some fusion also proceeds in the opposite direction, starting at the level of the chiasmatic plate.[20] The final site of fusion of the anterior neuropore (the so-called *situs neuroporicus*) corresponds to the future commissural plate. At this time the only communication between the neuroectoderm and the amniotic fluid is through the posterior neuropore (Fig. 5.1).

Carnegie Stage 12 (3.5 mm C–R; 28 days; 30 or more pairs of somites) is characterized mainly by the closure of the posterior neuropore, which occurs when 25 pairs of somites are identifiable.[11,15] The final site of fusion of the neural folds is presumably at the future mid-lumbar level. When the posterior neuropore closes, no contact between the neuroectoderm and the amniotic fluid persists. This notion is of practical importance in relation to the α-fetoprotein presence in the amniotic fluid. By this stage the neural tube begins to fill with a protein-rich fluid, which is interpreted as a product of transudation of the

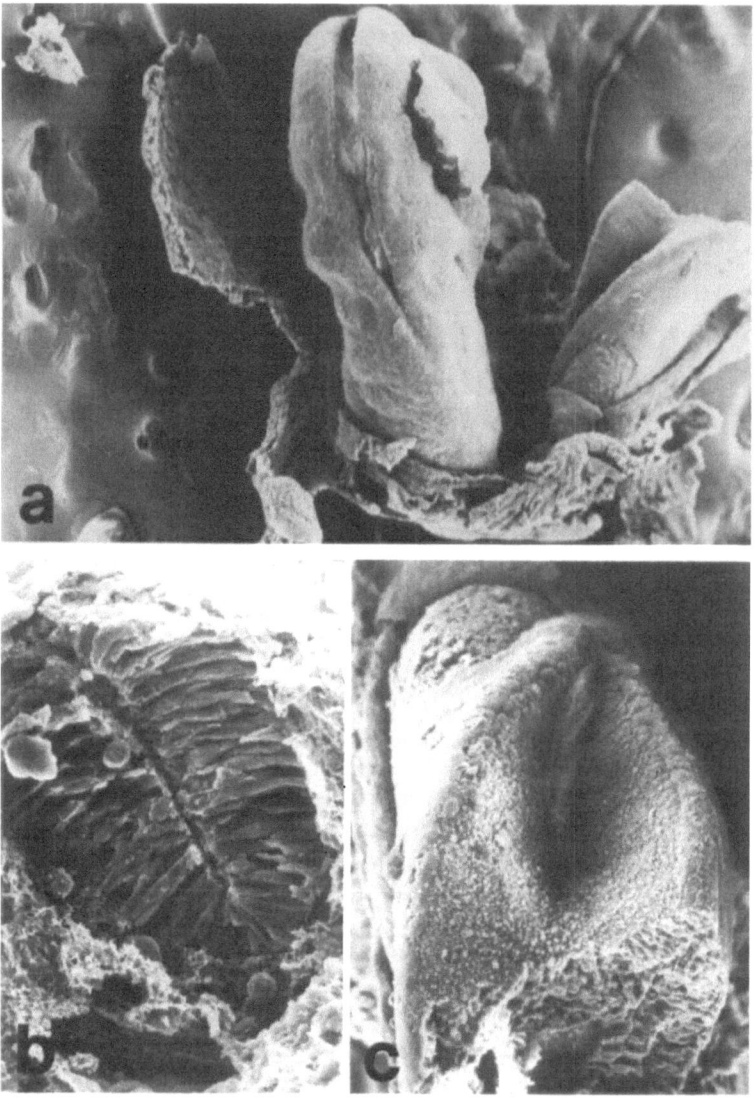

Figure 5.1. Scanning microphotograph representing a "neurulating" C57 mouse embryo (**a**); note the still open neural groove in the cephalic region. A fracture section in the mid-thoracic region (**b**) shows a normally closed neural tube; that in the tail region (**c**) shows the approximating neural folds.

Table 5.2. Outline of the main events connected with early neural tube formation, during the embryonic period proper

Carnegie Stage	C–R length	Approximate gestational age	Main events correlated with neurulation
7	0.4 mm	16	Hensen's node and notochord identifiable
8	1–1.5 mm	18	Neural folds and shallow neural grove apparent
9	1.5–2.5 mm	20	Neural groove deepens; mesencephalic flexure apparent; 1 to 3 pairs of somites
10	2–3.5 mm	22	Neural folds begin to fuse at the level of 2nd to 7th somite; 4 to 12 pairs of somites
11	2.5–4.5 mm	24	Rostral neuropore closes; neural tube formation proceeds; 13 to 20 pairs of somites
12	3–5 mm	26	Thinning of the roof of 4th ventricle; caudal neuropore closes; 21 to 29 pairs of somites
13	4–6 mm	28	Cervical flexure apparent; appearance of first occipito-spinal nerves and ganglia; 30 or more pairs of somites
14	5–7 mm	32	Pontine flexure evident; almost all spinal nerves and ganglia formed; appearance of cerebral vesicles

ependymal cells.[3,4,21,22] When the choroid plexus of the IVth ventricle appears, during Stage 15, cerebrospinal fluid (CSF) filtration begins in a specific region of the rhombic roof anterior to the choroid plexus anlage, which is referred to as Weed's *area membranacea superior*, and the central canal of the neural tube becomes filled with a fluid that has a reduced protein content. Further filtration causes distension of the neural tube, which corresponds to a physiologic, transitory phase of embryonal hydrocephalus and hydromyelia, and determines a secondary thinning in the roof of the hindbrain, the so-called Weed's *area membranacea inferior* (Carnegie Stages 18 to 20).[21–25] Finally, this area becomes increasingly permeable and leads to the outflow of the primitive CSF from within the neural tube, and this opens up the intercellular space of the "meninx primitiva"[26] to form the subarachnoid space and to start CSF circulation. Concomitantly, the central canal of the neural tube becomes slit-like and the subarachnoid space develops (Carnegie Stages 21 to 23). This sequence of events has been criticized by one of us,[27–29] who observed the development of the subarachnoid space from a preexisting "mesenchymal extracellular space," which was independent of the CSF circulation. Some authors[24,25,30] sustained the same point of view and argued that the development of the rhomboencephalic foramina is an active process, independent of CSF filtration.

The sequence of events that begins with the appearance of the neural plaque and finishes with the closure of the posterior neuropore is called neurulation ("primary" neurulation). As soon as the superficial ectoderm separates from the underlying neural ectoderm (the actual "neural tube"), it fuses in the midline. Mesenchymal cells migrate between the superficial ectoderm and the neural tube. This gives rise to the posterior vertebral arches and to the paraspinal muscles. The precise timing and interrelationship of the different stages of neurulation is fundamental to ensure a normal development of the nervous system and its surrounding structures.

When neurulation is completed, the caudalmost part of the spinal cord and vertebral segments still needs to be formed; in fact, only 25 neural and vertebral segments may be recognized at this time. The successive lengthening of the spinal cord depends on transformations of the "caudal eminence,"[3,4,6] an undifferentiated cell mass into which the notochord and the caudal end of the neural tube blend. This process approximately spans the period from Carnegie Stage 13 to 20. It is referred to as "secondary neurulation" and is not well known in humans. Observations on experimental animals[3,31-38] may suggest its nature. By Carnegie Stages 13 to 14, the initially undifferentiated mesenchymal cells within the caudal cell mass, which is now completely covered by ectoderm, begin to undergo a morphologic differentiation which results in their appearance as ependymal-like cells; these are radially oriented around some vacuoles, which also appear in this developmental phase. This morphologic event has been called the "rosette formation."[3,37,38] Progressive cell differentiation concentrically involves the other cellular layers around the primitive "rosettes" which, on the other hand, tend to differentiate into neural cells. Concomitantly the vacuoles, initially separated from each other, begin to coalesce to form a cavity that eventually makes contact with the preexisting spinal canal. In this way the primitive neural tube has further elongated beyond the area of closure of the posterior neuropore.

The third and last phase of neural tube formation begins during Carnegie Stages 18 to 20; it overlaps with the second one, and continues throughout the fetal period and also after birth. The "canalization" leads to the formation of an excessive number of spinal and vertebral segments; this last phase is characterized by the regression of the most caudal segments and, for this reason, it has been called by Streeter[39] "retrogressive differentiation," a term that emphasizes the genetic determination of the process. The final result of this third phase is the formation of the filum terminale, conus medullaris, and ventriculus terminalis,[4,36,40] as well as the ascent of the caudal end of the spinal cord up to the first lumbar vertebra throughout the gestational period.

Neurulation is accompanied by modifications in the surrounding mesenchymal tissue that lead to the formation of the musculoskeletal covering of the neural tube. The notochord represents the earliest evidence of the spinal axis. Somites, which develop from the paraxial mesoderm, give rise to the vertebrae and spinal muscles. Vertebral development passes through three subsequent phases.[2,3,6] First, membrane formation occurs (Carnegie Stages 10 to 16), during which vertebral segmentation takes place. Each somite is divided into a rostral and a caudal half by a "sclerotomic fissure": then each caudal half fuses with the rostral half of the adjacent somite. The membrane becomes stratified late in embryonic life but fusion occurs only after the end of fetal life. Membrane formation is followed by chondrification (Carnegie Stages 17 to 23). The third phase of vertebral development (ossification) occurs after birth. One can see that the closure of the spinal cord follows that of the neural tube after a long interval.

Mechanisms of Neural Tube Closure

Neurulation is the most well-known phase of neurodevelopment; nevertheless, controversy still exists concerning the forces that cause the neural plaque to fold and, eventually, to fuse into a neural tube. One point of view emphasizes the medial migration of the non-neural ectoderm lateral to the neural plaque, as the force promoting neural infolding.[41,42] This hypothesis is no longer supported by experimental evidence which, on the contrary, suggests that forces within the neural folds, or the neural plaque itself, act to perform the closure of the neural tube. The experimental observation of medial migration of the mesoderm under an excised neural plaque indicates that this phenomenon may contribute to the medial displacement of the neural folds, although neurulation cannot be reduced to this action alone.[43-45] This type of observation, as well as others such as, for instance, turning the neural plaque upside down[44] (which succeeds in achieving a normal neurulation with only a mild degree of retardation) further support the hypothesis that the neural tube formation is mainly dependent on forces intrinsic to the neural plaque.

As far as the very nature of these forces is concerned, many investigators have been attracted by the cytoskeletal components of neuroectodermal cells, such as microfilaments and microtubules.[45-48] Microtubules are correlated with cell elongation and, more precisely, paraxial microtubules are presumed to bring about cell elongation by displacing cytoplasm toward the extending base of the cell.[47] Experimental disruption of these cytoskeletal components with colchicine causes the cells of the neural anlage, which were elongated prior to treatment, to lose their elongated shape, and cells that would otherwise elongate to fail to do so.[1,45,49]

Microfilaments are inserted on the desmosomes and, thus, can flow across the cell to the next desmosome, linking the entire superficial portion of the neural ectoderm. They are regarded as having a contractile role in several systems.[45,50] They increase in number in the apical region of the neuroepithelial cells as neurulation proceeds,[51] and it has been assumed that they play a role in the constriction of the apex of each cell. Experimentally induced disruption of these microfilaments with cytochalasin B[45,52] in the neurulating embryo causes those cells, the apices of which were constricted prior to treatment, to lose their apical constriction.

Contractile protein filaments such as actin have been demonstrated on the lateral surface area and within the neural groove, which suggests that their contraction may be responsible for the first contact between the approaching neural folds.[53] These actin filaments are highly concentrated in the "luminal" portion of the neuroepithelial cells and may be attached to the plasma membrane.[54] To test the role of these actin filaments, experiments have been performed on the neurulating mammalian embryo,[48,55-58] cultured in vitro, in which the calcium ion concentration was altered by adding papaverine to the culture medium: after 24 hours of such treatment the majority of the embryos revealed neural tube closure defects. These defects could be reversed by adding ionophore, a substance capable of increasing the calcium ion concentration, to the culture medium.

The combined action of these cytoskeletal components and contractile proteins located within the superficial margin of neuroectodermal cells is responsible for the actual contraction and bringing together of the neural folds; progressive flexion finally brings the neural folds into contact. Besides this combined action, investigators' attention has recently been attracted to the complex molecules present on the cell coat or in extracellular matrix of the neurulating neural ectoderm.[59-65] These molecules which are, chemically, complex carbohydrates such as proteoglycans, glycoproteins, and glycosaminoglycans, have been accounted for intervening in processes like cellular adhesiveness,[59,66-68] intercellular recognition,[66,77] and morphologic differentiation.[68-70] Information relating to the presence of complex carbohydrates on the cell surface of the developing neuroectoderm was first derived from histochemical and scanning or electron microscope studies.[71-74] These studies permitted the appreciation of differences in the glycosaminoglycan composition of the neural folds, and gave rise to discussion regarding their specific role in neurulation by using chemical compounds such as concanavalin A,[75] which bind to the apical surface of the closing neuroectoderm and alter the surface membrane activity, thus interrupting the process of neurulation.

In several developing systems (limb, trunk, neural crest) hyaluronic acid accumulates in the stage of cell migration, while during cell differentiation chondroitin sulfate synthesis overrides the hyaluronic acid synthesis; further differentiation is characterized by the enzymatic removal of hyaluronic acid (which is essential for a normal differentiation), and sulfated glycosaminoglycan synthesis predominates.[68-70,76] Complex carbohydrates play an essential physiologic role in the permeability and hydration of the extracellular matrix, thus acting on cell migration. The complex carbohydrates' interaction with fibronectin and collagen is regarded as playing an important role in the deposition of the extracellular matrix, as well as in the regulation of the interaction between cells and their molecular environment.[59,66,77,78]

As far as the process of neurulation is concerned, complex carbohydrates account for the making of a "bridge" between the opposing neural folds. They could intervene as the final passage, after the initial joining of the neural folds brought about by actin filaments[53] and cytoskeletal elements.[45,47,49,50,52] Ultrastructural and electron microscopy studies[38,79-83] document the presence of morphologic changes such as vesicles and filopodia ("blebs") in the area of presumptive fusion along the apical neural folds. The presence of hyaluronic acid on the neuroepithelial cells during neurulation would prevent cell adhesion[69] by covering the cell surface receptors; its absence would allow for inappropriate cellular interaction which might result in neural tube (NT) defects. The possibility of inducing NT defects through hyaluronidase[84] seems to support this hypothesis. On the other hand, an excess of hyaluronic acid in the medium may also result in NT defects. Glycoconjugates also serve as recognition sites on the plasma membrane and regulate normal histogenesis and brain differentiation.[85,86] Thus, the presence of these molecules on the surface of axon tracts in the embryo may be the signal that enables specific neurons to make contact with those specific axon tracts.[87]

To ascertain the precise role of such macromolecules in neurulation, experiments were carried out in which teratogenic substances were used specifically to interfere with the metabolism of glycoconjugates. Tunicamycin is able to inhibit neurulation in an embryo culture. This antibiotic, besides other teratogenic effects, has the capacity to inhibit the asparagine-linked glycoprotein assembly and protein synthesis in general.[88,89] From a morphologic point of view, tunicamycin administration to the culture medium determines marked cellular alterations in the neuroepithelium and alterations in brain development, the result of which is obvious when considering that glycoproteins bearing asparagine-linked oligosaccharides are major plasma membrane components.

As a conclusion to this section, one can see that the more sophisticated the methods of analysis are, the deeper the analysis is to be focused on the primitive components of the system. Indeed, the dynamic interpretations of neural development in the early sixties, in terms of cell migration, have been subsequently replaced by the evidence of the role of the cellular cytoskeleton. More recently, actin filaments and surface macromolecules have been demonstrated as playing a major role in the process of neurulation. Further knowledge about these ultrastructural and biochemical components of neuroepithelial cells will certainly give further insight into our understanding of human neurulation.

Pathogenesis of Neural Tube Closure Defects

The origin of NT closure defects has long been debated. From a historical point of view Morgagni[90] first described, in 1761, the association of spina bifida and hydrocephalus, and hypothesized that the former anomaly was the cause of the latter, an embryonal hydrocephalus and hydromyelia ("hidrops cerebri and medullaris") being the causative factor of the "blow-out" of the already closed spinal cord. This interesting observation may be considered the origin of the theory of "reopening" which still exists nowadays. Likewise, from a historical point of view Lebedeff[91] in 1881 and, later on, von Recklinghausen[92] in 1886 first suggested that the influence of a genetic or environmental factor might interfere with the neurulating embryo, thus leading to a primary NT closure defect, i.e., lack of closure of the neural folds. Also this theory represents the origin of an alternative point of view on the occurrence of NT closure defects, which is at present the most accepted. Two main interpretations of neural tube closure defects are still under debate, and may be summarized as follows: (1) the neural

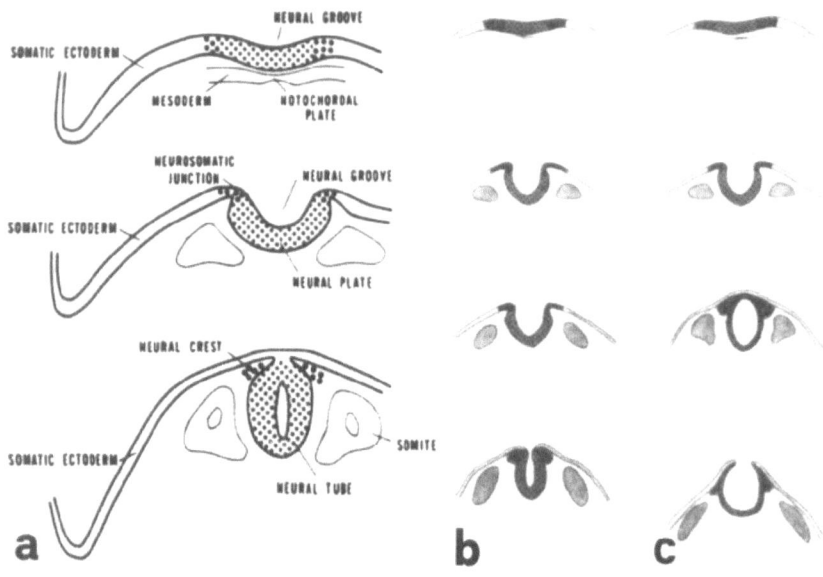

Figure 5.2. Schematic drawing of normal (**a**) and abnormal (**b,c**) neurulation; the two theories of "primary nonclosure" (b) and of "secondary re-opening" (c) of the neural tube are presented.

folds normally make contact and fuse and then "reopen" either because of increased intraluminal pressure (within the closed neural tube) or because of a primary defect in the neuroepithelium; (2) the neural tube never closes because of a primary defect intrinsic to the neuroepithelium or underlying mesoderm (Fig. 5.2).

The reopening of the neural tube, first suggested by Morgagni[90] and later on by Cleland,[93] has been recently restated by Gardner.[21-23] This author emphasized that the phase of embryonal hydrocephalus and hydromyelia may account for the blow-out of the neural tube at sites of weakness, namely the last sites to close, i.e., the regions of the anterior and posterior neuropores. Padget[94,95] suggested the occurrence of a "neuroschisis" in the dorsal neuroepithelium, followed by the formation of a "neuroschistic bleb" which might finally rupture through the overlying ectoderm. Certain observations, however, seem to restrict the applicability of this theory. In fact pathological observations of dysraphic fetuses[96] have disclosed normal IVth ventricles and subarachnoid spaces concomitant with a lumbar myelomeningocele; myeloschisis has been documented in earlier developmental stages before CSF begins to flow;[97] there is a normal permeability of the roof of the IVth ventricle and there is no particular incidence of neural tube defects or hydrocephalus in species such as the dog, in which the Magendie foramen is normally absent.[98]

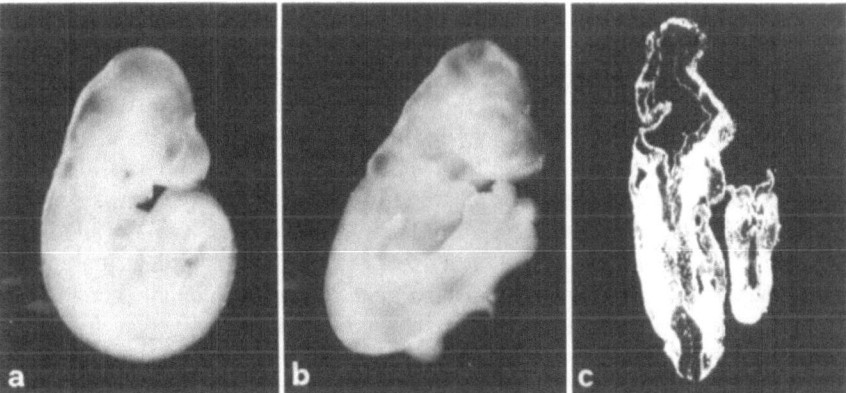

Figure 5.3. a: Normal ten-day C57 mouse embryo. **b**: Ten-day C57 mouse embryo after maternal treatment with vitamin A, showing a neural tube closure defect in the tail region. **c**: Section of the same embryo as in (b) representing the association of a dilation of the ventricular system and a fusion defect of the neural tube.

Although contrasting evidence, this theory of "secondary" neural tube closure defects has been recently reproposed as the result of experimentally induced neural tube closure defects in the mouse embryo.[89,99] These experiments utilized the administration of vitamin A to the pregnant mouse[67,79,100-102] at the time of presumed neural tube closure (Fig. 5.3). The resulting anomalies were a large number of hydrocephalic embryos (well known effect of hypervitaminosis A), and dysraphic embryos in which the embryonal hydrocephalus had been replaced by a depression in the rhombic roof, suggesting an escape of the primitive CSF through the neural tube defect. Although univocal interpretation of such results is not allowed, the possibility of a causal relationship between the two events, i.e., a "reopening" of an already closed neural tube seems likely. In terms of biochemistry, vitamin A promotes an increase in the glycosylation of the cell surface in many tissues and decreases the synthesis of glycosaminoglycans,[103] and thus may have a teratologic effect by acting on primitive CSF dynamics.

The theory of a defective closure of the neural tube, first propounded by Lebedeff[91] and von Recklinghausen,[92] assumes a "primary defect" of neurulation as its causative factor. This primary defect has been attributed to an abnormal orientation of the cells of the neural folds[104] and, more recently, to the interference of external factors on either the actine distribution[53] or cytoskeletal components[45,47,50,52,58,79] or else the cell surface material* of neurulating neuro-epithelial cells. Just recently, an alteration in the complex carbohydrates of the cell surface brought about by Trypan Blue administration to pregnant rats has

---

*Refs. 72, 74, 76, 88, 89, 99, 102, 105, 106.

been propounded as the causative factor of both neural tube closure defects, and mesodermal abnormalities (such as the shallow posterior cranial fossa) as well as the hydrocephalus often associated with spinal dysraphism.[105,106]

Some experimental data suggest that the "nonclosure" might also depend on a "primary mesodermal insufficiency" due to a reduction in the number of paraxial mesodermal cells,[107,108] although the contrasting evidence of the possibility of normal closure of an isolated neural plaque would deny this hypothesis.

Another point of view advocates the causative role of "nonclosure" to an "overgrowth" of the neural tissue[109] at the site of presumed fusion of the neural folds. This phenomenon, attributed to a disturbed mesodermal–neural interaction,[97] is actually only apparent, since neither the counts of the number of cell nuclei[104] nor autoradiographic studies[110] performed on the largely everted and protudent neural folds of myeloschistic embryos, produced statistically valid differences between normal and abnormal specimens.

Pathologic Development of the Spinal Cord and Morphology of Spinal Dysraphic State

In a normal sequencing of embryologic events, neural tube closure is expected to be followed by skin closure as well as by the induction of meningeal coverings on the spinal cord and, subsequently, by the formation of the posterior vertebral arches and paraspinal muscles. However it may be produced, spinal dysraphism results in a disorganization at the site of neural tube closure (in particular, the posterior neuropore), the affects of which may vary in depth, length, and tissue differentiation; in other words, a disorganization of the posterior neuropore results in a myeloschisis or myelomeningocele (according to whether or not CSF accumulates behind the dysplastic neural tissue). These malformations are accompanied by concomitant macroscopic anomalies (such as the kinking of the medulla, the dilatation of the central canal of the spinal cord, the alterations in the vertebral column) as well as by microscopic abnormalities in neural tissue organization (heterotopia, microgyria).

Any attempt to classify spinal dysraphism must take into consideration whether or not the lesion is covered by skin; this differentiation is based on the assumption that if there is skin covering, the lesion occurred in a later phase of neurodevelopment, namely after the closure of the posterior neuropore and the separation of the neural tube from the primitive ectoderm.[3,4,111] *Myeloschisis and myelomeningocele*[1,3,5,6] belong to the first type of malformation and they probably originate between Carnegie Stages 10 and 12 (but, according to the theory of "reopening" of the neural tube, this should happen at a later stage). In both anomalies, the abnormal spinal cord maintains in its dorsal aspect (the "ependymal" surface of the neural plaque) the appearance of the open neural plaque crossed downwards by a shallow groove. This is representative of the primitive neural groove, which continues rostrally along the central canal of the spinal cord, from which some CSF leaks independent of any rupture of the arachnoid membranes. Sometimes the neural plaque is completely disorganized and severely dysplasic, thus suggesting having undergone intrauterine infarction. This observation seems to support the idea that meningomyelocele is a "progressive intrauterine disease."[112] The ventral aspect of the open neural plaque (its "arachnoidal" surface) represents the entire outside of the would-be-normal spinal cord and both dorsal and ventral roots emerge from there. It has been seen experimentally that a myeloschisis can be commuted into meningomyelocele, depending on a CSF accumulation ventrally to the neural plaque, and such a possibility has been assumed to occur also in humans. Meningomyelocele is thus characterized by the presence of an arachnoid sac underlying the open neural plaque, and crossed by nerve roots running to the exit foramina. The underlying vertebral bodies are flattened and widened; their pedicules are evereted and lie almost horizontally, and laminae are hypoplastic. The paraspinal muscles, which are significantly reduced owing to the lack of innervation, are similarly everted and lie anteriorly rather than posteriorly, thus acting as flexors rather than as extensors of the spine. Collateral alterations such as hydromyelia or diastematomyelia, rostral (or caudal) to the lesion, may also coexist,[113] as well as concomitant anomalies of mesodermic derivates such as lipoma or vascular abnormalities.

Among the malformations arising during a later phase of embryonic development, namely between Carnegie Stages 16 and 23, *meningocele* is the most common. Meningocele is characterized by a dorsal (or, much more rarely ventral) protrusion of the meningeal sac (arachnoid and dura mater) through a defect of the bony wall of the spine. The spinal cord, although it may be abnormal, lies completely within the spinal canal. Nerve roots generally emerge in a normal fashion, even if some aberrant nerve roots are included within the herniated sac. Almost invariably it is associated with a lipoma.[114,115] In the case of *spina bifida occulta* the defect is merely situated in one or more posterior vertebral arches, but the spinal cord and meninges are normal, even though some aberrant nerve roots fibrous bands, or adhesions may be found.[116]

Conclusions

Data available to date suggest that neurulation is the result of the combined action of intra and extracellular morphological and biochemical events which are under the direction of the genome. These events are strictly correlated and a precise time sequence is fundamental in order to avoid any error which might interfere with the normal neurulation process, thus leading to neural tube closure defects. Cytoskeletal components of neuroepithelia are of the utmost importance, allowing the initial bringing together of neural folds. Complex carbohydrates on the cell surface and within the extracellular matrix also account for a correct sequence of events, which leads to the neural tube formation, as they are responsible for cell-to-cell adhesiveness and initial contact, as well as for cell recognition and migration (which are just as important for normal neurodevelopment). Data available from experimental teratology would suggest a "primary" neural tube closure defect, although some evidence still gives rise to discussion regarding the possibility of a "secondary" neural tube closure defect.

References

1. Di Rocco C, Caldarelli M: Mielomeningocele. Casa del Libro, Roma, 1983.
2. Langman J: Medical embryology. Williams & Wilkins, Baltimore, 1969.
3. Lemire RJ, Loeser JD, Leech RW, Alvord EC: Normal and abnormal development of the human nervous system. Harper & Row, Hagerstown, 1975.
4. Lemire RJ, Warkany J: Normal development of the central nervous system: correlations with selected malformations. In: Pediatric Neurosurgery. Grune & Stratton, New York, 1982, pp. 1–22.
5. Warkany J: Congenital malformations. Year Book Medical Publishers, Chicago, 1971.
6. Witschi E: Development of vertebrates. WB Saunders, Philadelphia, 1956.
7. O'Rahilly R: Developmental stages in human embryos, including a survey of the Carnegie Collection. Part A: embryos of the first three weeks (stages 1 to 9). Carnegie Institute, Washington, 1973.
8. O'Rahilly R: Early human development and the chief sources of information on staged human embryos. Eur J Obstet Gynec Reprod Biol 9:273–280, 1979.
9. O'Rahilly R, Gardner E: The time and sequence of events in the development of the human nervous system during the embryonic period proper. Z Anat Entwickl Gesch 134:1–12, 1971.
10. O'Rahilly R, Müller F: The normal and abnormal development of the nervous system in the early human embryo. Riv Neurosc Ped (J Pediatr Neurosci) 2:89–94, 1986.
11. Streeter GL: Developmental horizons in human embryos. Description of age group XI, 13 to 20 somites, and age group XII, 21 to 29 somites. Contr Embryol Carneg Instn 30:211–245, 1942.
12. Streeter GL: Developmental horizons in human embryos. Description of age group XIII, embryos about 4 or 5 millimeters long, and age group XIV, period of indentation of the lens vesicle. Contr Embryol Carneg Instn 31:27–63, 1945.
13. Streeter GL: Developmental horizons in human embryos. Description of age groups XV, XVI, XVII, XVIII, being the third issue of a survey of the Carnegie Collection. Contr Embryol Carneg Instn 32:133–203, 1948.
14. Streeter GL: Developmental horizons in human embryos. Description of age groups XIX, XX, XXI, XXII, and XXIII, being the fifth issue of a survey of the Carnegie Collection. Contr Embryol Carneg Instn 34:165–196, 1951.
15. O'Rahilly R, Gardner E: The initial development of the human brain. Acta Anat 104:123–133, 1979.
16. O'Rahilly R, Müller F: The first appearance of the human nervous system at stage 8. Anat Embryol 163:1–13, 1981.
17. Müller F, O'Rahilly R: The first appearance of the major divisions of the human brain at stage 9. Anat Embryol 168:419–432, 1983.
18. Müller F, O'Rahilly R: The first appearance of the neural tube and optic primordium in the human embryo at stage 10. Anat Embryol 172:157–169, 1985.

19. Heuser CH, Corner GW: Developmental horizons in human embryos. Description of age group X, 4 to 12 somites. Contrib Embryol 36:29–39, 1957.
20. Müller F, O'Rahilly R: Cerebral dysraphia (future anencephaly) in a human twin embryo at stage 13. Teratology 30:167–177, 1984.
21. Gardner WJ: The dysraphic states: from syringomyelia to anencephaly. Excerpta Medica, Amsterdam, 1973.
22. Gardner WJ: Etiology and pathogenesis of the development of myelomeningocele. In: McLaurin RL (ed): Myelomeningocele. Grune & Stratton, New York, 1977, pp. 3–30.
23. Gardner WJ: Rupture of the neural tube: the cause of myelomeningocele. Arch Neurol 4:1–7, 1961.
24. Osaka K, Handa H, Matsumoto S, Yasuda M: Development of cerebrospinal fluid pathways in the normal and abnormal human embryos. Child's Brain 6:26–38, 1980.
25. Osaka K, Oi S: Embryological concepts for head injury in the newborn and infant. In: Raimondi AJ, Choux M, Di Rocco C (eds): Head Injuries in the Newborn and Infant. Springer-Verlag, New York, 1986, pp. 19–31.
26. Weed LH: The development of the cerebrospinal spaces in pig and in man. Contr Embryol Carneg Instn 5:1–116, 1917.
27. McLone DG: The subarachnoid space: a review. Child Brain 6:113–120, 1980.
28. McLone DG: The cerebrospinal fluid pathways: structure and development. In: Raimondi AJ, Choux M, Di Rocco C (eds): Head Injuries in the Newborn and Infant. Springer-Verlag, New York, 1986, pp. 33–51.
29. McLone DG, Bondareff W: Developmental morphology of the subarachnoid space and continuous structures in the mouse. Am J Anat 1421:2173–2193, 1975.
30. Brocklehurst G: The pathogenesis of spina bifida: a study of the relationship between observation, hypothesis, and surgical incentive. Dev Med Child Neurol 13:147–163, 1971.
31. Bolli P: Sekundare Lumenbildungen im Neuralrohr und Ruckenmark menschlicher Embryonen. Acta Anat 64:48–81, 1966.
32. Dryden RJ: Spina bifida in chick embryos: ultrastructure of open neural defects in the transitional region between primary and secondary modes of neural tube formation. In Persaud TVN (ed): Advances in the Study of Birth Defects, Vol. 4. MTP Press, Lancaster, 1980, pp. 75–100.
33. Hughes AF,, Freeman RB: Comparative remarks on the development of the tail cord among higher vertebrates. J Embryol Exp Morphol 32:335–363, 1974.
34. Jelínek R, Seichert V, Klika E: Mechanism of morphogenesis of caudal neural tube in the chick embryo. Folia Morphol (Praha) 17:355–367, 1969.
35. Klika E, Jelínek R: The structure of the end and tail bud of the chick embryo. Folia Morphol (Praha) 17:29–40, 1969.
36. Lemire RJ: Variations in development of the caudal neural tube in human embryos. Teratology 2:361–370, 1969.
37. Schoenwolf GC: Histological and ultrastructural studies of secondary neurulation in mouse embryos. Am J Anat 169:361–376, 1984.
38. Schoenwolf GC, Kelley RO: Characterization of intercellular junctions in the caudal portion of the developing neural tube of the chick embryo. Am J Anat 158:29–41, 1980.
39. Streeter GL: Factors involved in the formation of the filum terminale. Am J Anat 25:1–11, 1919.

40. Kernohan JW: The ventriculus terminalis: its growth and development. J Comp Neurol 38:107–125, 1925.

41. Gillette R: Cell number and cell size in the ectoderm during neurulation (*Ambystoma maculatum*). J Exp Zool 96:201–222, 1944.

42. Schroeder TE: Neurulation in *Xenopus laevis*. An analysis and model based upon light and electron microscopy. J Embryol Exp Morphol 23:427–462, 1970.

43. Davis SO: Photochemical spectral analysis of neural tube formation. Biol Bull 87:73–95, 1944.

44. Jacobson CO: Cell migration in the neural plate and the process of neurulation in the axolotl larva. Zool Bidr Uppsala 35:433–449, 1962.

45. Karfunkel P: The mechanisms of neural tube formation. Int Rev Cytol 38:245–271, 1974.

46. Burnside B: Microtubules and microfilaments in amphibian neurulation. Am Zool 13:989–1006, 1973.

47. Karfunkel P: The activity of microtubules and microfilaments in the chick. J Exp Zool 181:289–302, 1972.

48. O'Shea KS: The cytoskeleton in neurulation: role of cations. In: Harrison RJ (ed): Progress in Anatomy, Vol. 1. Cambridge University Press, New York, 1981, pp. 35–60.

49. Ferm VH: Colchicine teratogenesis in hamster embryos. Proc Soc Exp Biol Med 122:775–778, 1963.

50. Jacob M: Microfilament organization and cell movement. Trends Neurosci 5:369–373, 1982.

51. Baker PC, Schroeder TE: Cytoplasmic filaments and morphogenetic movement in the amphibian neural tube. Dev Biol 15:432–450, 1967.

52. Linville G, Shepard T: Neural tube closure defects caused by cytochalasin B. Nature 236:246–247, 1972.

53. Sadler TW, Greenberg D, Coughlin P, Lessard JL: Actin distribution patterns in the mouse neural tube during neurulation. Science 215:172–174, 1982.

54. Pollard TD: Cytoplasmic contractile proteins. J Cell Biol 91:156s–165s, 1981.

55. Lee NY, Nagele RG: Neural tube closure defects caused by papaverine in explanted early chick embryos. Teratology 20:321–332, 1979.

56. O'Shea KS: Calcium and neural tube closure defects: an in vitro study. In: Birth Defects: Original Article Series, Vol. 18. March of Dimes Birth Defects Foundation, 1982, pp. 95–106.

57. Smedley MJ, Stanisstreet M: Calcium and neurulation in mammalian embryos. J Embryol Exp Morphol 89:1–14, 1985.

58. Stanisstreet M, Jumah H: Calcium, microfilaments and morphogenesis. Life Sci 33:1433–1441, 1983.

59. Brauer PR, Bolender DL, Markwald RR: The distribution and spatial organization of the extracellular matrix encountered by mesencephalic neural crest cells. Anat Rec 211:57–68, 1985.

60. Edelman GM: Cell-adhesion molecules: a molecular basis for animal form. Sci Am 250:118–129, 1984.

61. Hay ED: Extracellular matrix. J Cell Biol 91:205s–223s, 1981.

62. Hay ED: Collagen and embryonic development. In: Hay ED (ed): Cell Biology of Extracellular Matrix. Plenum Press, New York, 1983, pp. 379–409.

63. Heifetz A, Lennarz WJ, Libbus B, Hsu Y: Synthesis of glycoconjugates during the development of mouse embryos in vitro. Dev Biol 80:398–408, 1980.

64. Jacobson AG: Morphogenesis of the neural plate and tube. In: Connelly TG, Brinkley LL, Carlson BM (eds): Morphogenesis and Pattern Formation. Raven Press, New York, 1981, pp. 233–263.
65. Reddi AH: Extracellular matrix and development. In: Piez KA, Reddi AH (eds): Extracellular Matrix Biochemistry. Elsevier, New York, 1984, pp. 375–412.
66. Culp LA: Fibronectin and proteoglycans as determinants of cell substratum adhesion. J Supramol Struct 11:401–427, 1979.
67. Thorogood P, Smith L, Nicol A, McGinty R, Garrod D: Effects of vitamin A on the behaviour of migratory neural crest cells in vitro. J Cell Sci 57:331–350, 1982.
68. Toole BP: Glycosaminoglycans in morphogenesis. In: Hay ED (ed): Cell Biology of Extracellular Matrix. Plenum Press, New York, 1981, pp. 259–294.
69. Toole BP: Hyaluronate and hyaluronidase in morphogenesis and differentiation. Am Zool 13:1061–1065, 1973.
70. Underhill CB, Toole BP: Binding of hyaluronate to the surface of cultured cells. J Cell Biol 82:475–484, 1979.
71. Mak L: Ultrastructural studies on amphibian neural fold fusion. Dev Biol 65:435–446, 1978.
72. Moran D, Rice RW: An ultrastructural examination of the role of cell membrane surface coat material during neurulation. J Cell Biol 64:172–181, 1975.
73. O'Shea KS, Kaufman MH: Phospholipase C-induced neural tube defects in the mouse embryo. Experientia 36:1217–1219, 1980.
74. Sadler TW: Distribution of surface coat material on fusing neural folds of mouse embryos during neurulation. Anat Rec 191:345–350, 1978.
75. Lee NY: Inhibition of neurulation and interkinetic nuclear migration by Concanavalin A in explanted early chick embryos. Dev Biol 48:392–399, 1976.
76. Pintar JE: Distribution and synthesis of glycosaminoglycans during quail neural crest morphogenesis. Dev Biol 67:444–464, 1978.
77. Rollins BJ, Cathcart MK, Culp LA: Fibronectin-proteoglycan binding as the molecular basis for fibroblast adhesion to extracellular matrices. In: Horowitz MI (ed): The Glycoconjugates. Academic Press, New York, 1982, pp. 289–329.
78. Yamada KM, Hayashi M, Akiyama SK: Structure and function of fibronectin. In: Hawkes S, Wang JL (eds): Extracellular Matrix. Academic Press, New York, 1982, pp. 25–34.
79. Geelen JAG, Langman J, Lowdon JD: The influence of excess vitamin A on neural tube closure in the mouse embryo. Anat Embryol 159:223–234, 1980.
80. Jacobson AG, Tam PPL: Cephalic neurulation in the mouse embryo analyzed by SEM and morphometry. Anat Rec 203:375–396, 1982.
81. Schoenwolf GC: Observation on closure of the neuropores in the chick embryo. Am J Anat 155:445–466, 1979.
82. Waterman RE: SEM observations of surface alterations associated with neural tube closure in the mouse and hamster. Anat Rec 183:95–98, 1975.
83. Waterman RE: Topographical changes along the neural fold associated with neurulation in the hamster and mouse. Am J Anat 146:151–172, 1976.
84. Schoenwolf GC, Fisher M: Analysis of the effects of Streptomyces hyaluronidase on formation of the neural tube. J Embryol Exp Morphol 73:1–15, 1983.
85. Cotman CW, Lasher RS, Mena EE, Erickson PF: Synapse glycoproteins. In: Coates PW, Markwald RP, Kenny AD (eds): Neurology and Neurobiology, Vol. 6. Alan R. Liss, New York, 1983, pp. 19–39.

86. Margolis RK, Margolis RU: Structure and distribution of glycoproteins and glycosaminoglycans. In: Margolis RU, Margolis RK (eds): Complex Carbohydrates of Nervous Tissue. Plenum Press, New York, 1979, pp. 45–73.

87. McKay RDG, Hockfield S, Johanson J, Thompson I, Frederikson R: Surface molecules identify groups of growing axons. Science 222:788–794, 1983.

88. Atienza-Samols SB, Razon Pine P, Sherman MI: Effects of tunicamycin upon glycoprotein synthesis and development of early mouse embryo. Dev Biol 79:19–32, 1980.

89. McLone DG, Suwa J, Collins JA, Poznanski S, Knepper PA: Neurulation: biochemical and morphological studies on primary and secondary neural tube defects. Concepts Pediatr Neurosurg 4:15–29, 1983.

90. Morgagni GB: De sedibus et causis morborum per anatomen indagatis, Vol. 1, Epist XII. Venice, 1761.

91. Lebedeff A: Ueber die Enstehung der Anencephalie und Spina bifida bei Vogeln und Menschen. Virchow Arch Path Anat 86:263, 1881.

92. Recklinghausen von F: Untersuchungen uber die Spina Bifida. II: uber die Art und die Entsehung der Spina Bifida, ihre Beziehung zur Ruckernmarks und Darmspalte. Virchow Arch Path Anat 105:296–330, 1886.

93. Cleland J: Contribution to the study of spina bifida, encephalocele, and anencephalus. J Anat Physiol 17:257–291, 1883.

94. Padget DH: Spina bifida and embryonic neuroschisis. A causal relationship; definition of postnatal confirmations involving a bifid spine. Johns Hopkins Med J 128:233–252, 1968.

95. Padget DH: Neuroschisis and human embryonic maldevelopment: new evidence on anencephaly, spina bifida and diverse mammalian defects. J Neuropathol Exp Neurol 29:192–216, 1970.

96. Osaka K, Matsumoto S, Tanimura T: Myeloschisis in early human embryos. Child's Brain 4:347–359, 1978.

97. Källén B: Early embryogenesis of the central nervous system with special reference to closure defects. Dev Med Child Neurol 10 (Suppl 16):44–53, 1968.

98. Cohen LA: Absence of a foramen of Magendie in the dog, cat, rabbit, and goat. Arch Neurol 16:524–528, 1967.

99. Caldarelli M, McLone DG, Collins JA, Suwa J, Knepper PA: Vitamin A induced neural tube defects in the mouse. Concepts Pediatr Neurosurg 6:161–171, 1985.

100. Cohlan SQ: Congenital anomalies in the rat produced by excessive intake of vitamin A during pregnancy. Pediatrics 13:556–567, 1954.

101. Langman J, Welch GW: Effect of vitamin A on development of the central nervous system. J Comp Neurol 128:1–16, 1966.

102. Peters PWJ, Dormans JAMA, Geelen JAG: Light microscopic and ultrastructural observations in advanced stages of induced anencephaly and spina bifida. Teratology 19:183–196, 1979.

103. Lindahl U, Höök M: Glycosaminoglycans and their binding to biological macromolecules. Annu Rev Biochem 47:385–417, 1978.

104. Dekaban AS, Bartelmez GW: Complete dysraphism in a 14 somite human embryo. Am J Anat 115:27–42, 1964.

105. Di Rocco C, Rende M: Neural tube defects. Some remarks on the possible role of glycosaminoglycans in the genesis of the dysraphic state, the anomaly in the configuration of the posterior cranial fossa, and hydrocephalus. Child's Nerv Syst 3:334–341, 1987.

106. Di Rocco C, Rende M: Congenital hydrocephalus and mucopolysaccharides. Riv Neurosc Ped (J Pediatr Neurosci) 1:61–67, 1985.
107. Marin-Padilla M, Ferm VH: Somite necrosis and developmental malformations induced by vitamin A in golden hamster. J Embryol Exp Morphol 13:1–8, 1965.
108. Marin-Padilla M: Notochordal-basichondrocranium relationships: abnormalities in experimental axial skeletal (dysraphic) disorders. J Embryol Exp Morphol 53:15–38, 1979.
109. Patten BM: Overgrowth of neural tube in young human embryos. Anat Rec 113:381–393, 1952.
110. Lendon RG: An autoradiographic study of induced myelomeningocele. Dev Med Child Neurol 14:(Suppl 27):80–85, 1972.
111. Lemire RJ, Shepard TH, Alvord EC Jr: Caudal myeloschisis (lumbosacral spina bifida cystica) in a five millimeter (horizon XIV) human embryo. Anat Rec 152: 9–16, 1965.
112. Epstein F, Marlin A, Hochwald G, Ransohoff J: Myelomeningocele: a progressive intrauterine disease. In: McLaurin RL (ed): Myelomeningocele. Grune & Stratton, New York, 1977, pp. 171–178.
113. Emery JL, Lendon RG: Lipomas of the cauda equina related to neurospinal dysraphism. Dev Med Child Neurol 20 (Suppl):62–70, 1969.
114. James CCM, Lassman LP: Spinal dysraphism: spina bifida occulta. Appleton-Century-Crofts, New York, 1972.
115. McLone DG, Mutluer S, Naidich TP: Lipomeningoceles of the conus medullaris. Concepts Pediatr Neurosurg 3:170–177, 1982.
116. Lassman LP, James CCM: Lumbosacral lipomas: critical survey of 26 cases submitted to laminectomy. J Neurol Neurosurg Psychiatry 30:174–181, 1967.

CHAPTER 6

Epidemiology and Clues to the Etiology of Neural Tube Defects

Rita P.M. Luciano and Francesco Velardi

Since the pioneering studies of Record and McKeown[1] published in 1949 an increasing number of epidemiologic surveys have been conducted to gather information on the etiology of neural tube defects (NTD). This accounts for the evolution from the puzzled attitude of the past to the present plans for primary prevention. Although a definitive answer to the interlacing thread of questions and apparent contradictions arising from different sources is far from available, some evidence is now clearly discernible, indicating clues to further knowledge and indications for interventional programs.

The most outstanding landmarks in our understanding of the etiology of NTD may be summarized as follows:

1. NTD are etiologically and epidemiologically related, except for cases presenting in association with other malformations or in which the defect is part of a known syndrome.
2. Genetic factors have been recognized to act in combination with environmental influences.
3. Different environmental influences, presumably acting through a common pathogenetic mechanism, seem to be able to produce a dysraphic alteration with a variable efficacy depending on a genetically determined threshold.
4. A significant decline in the prevalence of NTD has been widely reported for the last decade.

Etiologic and Epidemiologic Homogeneity/Heterogeneity of NTD

Evidence that different phenotypical manifestations of a dysraphic state, such as meningocele, meningomyelocele, encephalocele, anencephaly, and craniorachischisis, are to be considered as an etiologically related group derives from epidemiologic and family studies, as well as experimental models. In fact, figures collected in different countries indicate a concordance in the high or low risk of occurrence for different types of NTD (Table 6.1) as well as parallel secular

Table 6.1. Concordance in the High or Low Risk of Occurrence for Spina Bifida and Anencephaly in Different Countries

Place of Survey	Spina Bifida	Anencephaly	
Lagos[2]	0.2	0.8	Low incidence
Hiroshima and Nagasaki[3]	0.3	0.6	
Australia[4]	1.11	0.91	Intermediate incidence
Boston[5]	1.26	0.98	
South Wales[6]	4.13	3.54	High incidence
Belfast[7]	4.5	4.2	

trends. Moreover a coherent tendency is apparent when other epidemiologic variables are considered.[8] Accordingly, it is evident from family studies that the risk of occurrence in siblings is not limited to the same defect, but involves any of the possible dysraphic conditions, even if it is more likely to be manifested with the same phenotypic feature (Table 6.2). On the other hand, experimental models clearly outline that a teratogenic agent able to affect neural tube closure may cause any of the various expressions of a dysraphic state, depending on the specific sequential closure step that was occurring at the time of its administration.[12] However, whereas the different alterations of neural tube closure are considered to be an homogeneous group when presenting in isolation, in recent studies a new differentiation has become apparent for those cases in which the defect is found in combination with other nonrelated congenital anomalies.[13-16] This separation, first of all, refers to well-classified complex syndromes that include NTD,[13] with a specific genetic (disease due to a single mutant gene or a chromosomal abnormality) or nongenetic (such as the syndrome of amnios rupture sequence or oculoauriculovertebral dysplasia) etiology (Table 6.3).

These anomalies, however, account for only a very small percentage of NTD, and although a chromosomal abnormality was found in 40% of abortuses with

Table 6.2. Types of Neural Tube Defects Observed in Sibs of Index Patient

	Anencephalus	Spina bifida
South Wales[9]		
Anencephalus	16	13
Spina bifida	20	32
Liverpool[10]		
Anencephalus	26	20
Spina bifida	13	11
Southhampton[11]		
Anencephalus	2	0
Spina bifida	1	6

Table 6.3. Recognized Syndromes Including a Neural Tube Defect

Genetic syndromes
  Meckel
  Median cleft-face
  Robert's
  Anterior sacral meningomyelocele and anal stenosis
  Trisomy-13
  Trisomy-18
  Triploidy
  Other abnormalities as umbalanced translocation and ring
    chromosome

Nongenetic syndromes
  Syndrome of the amnios rupture sequence
  Oculoauriculovertebral dysplasia

central nervous system defects that were miscarried at the embryonic stage, it is seldom observed in conceptuses reaching term.[17] More recently, besides these well-identified syndromes, an etiologic heterogeneity has also been proposed for the mere association of NTD with other unrelated congenital anomalies. In fact, when considered separately, they were demonstrated to show epidemiologic patterns unlike those of the isolated NTD.[14,15]

Among the associated anomalies, an increased incidence has been reported for oral cleft,[16] omphalocele, and diaphragmatic hernia;[18] this combination was suggested to be interpretable as a "generalized weakness" of the midline, due to its "poorly buffered" morphogenetic properties.[19] The recently reported high risk for NTD among sibs of children with tracheoesophageal dysraphism could be interpreted in this light, but this finding has not been consistently reported.[20]

Genetic Factors

Results from epidemiologic surveys reveal various incidence rates of NTD in different populations and recurrence of the disease in affected families. The following analyses are helpful in elucidating the specific effects of genetic versus environmental factors: (1) sex ratio; (2) geographic variations and ethnic studies among native and immigrant populations; and (3) family aggregation (models of recurrence in relatives, importance of parental consanguineity, twin studies).

Sex Ratio

It is common knowledge that NTD affect females more frequently than males.[8,21] However, no satisfactory explanation for this difference is available to date.

The most striking statistics concern anencephaly. The male/female ratio has been observed to be as low as 0.40 in the British Isles (although this is subject to wide regional variations), becoming 1:1 in the oriental countries. The sex ratio for spina bifida is lower, but more stable in various populations, with levels ranging between 0.6 and 0.9 in most surveys.[22] Actually, females are, in general, more severely affected than males, and it has been recently reported[23] that they represent a higher percentage of stillborn among NTD cases. On the other hand, no sex difference was found by Creasy and Alberman[17] examining aborted fetuses affected by neural tube malformations. Nevertheless, no clear evidence is available to date for the hypothesis proposed by Burn and Gibbens,[24] who claimed that an X-linked protection from miscarriage may account for the reported female prevalence, nor for James' suggestion that female embryos, showing a "delayed" development at the initial stages, are more likely to be affected by teratogens.[8] Support is also lacking for Knox's hypothesis based on the fetus–fetus interaction model.[25]

Geographic and Ethnic Variations

Areas of high, intermediate, and low incidence have been identified (Fig. 6.1). Racial variations might explain the wide range from the highest rates recorded among Irish, British, Sikhs, and Egyptians of Alexandria, through to the lowest

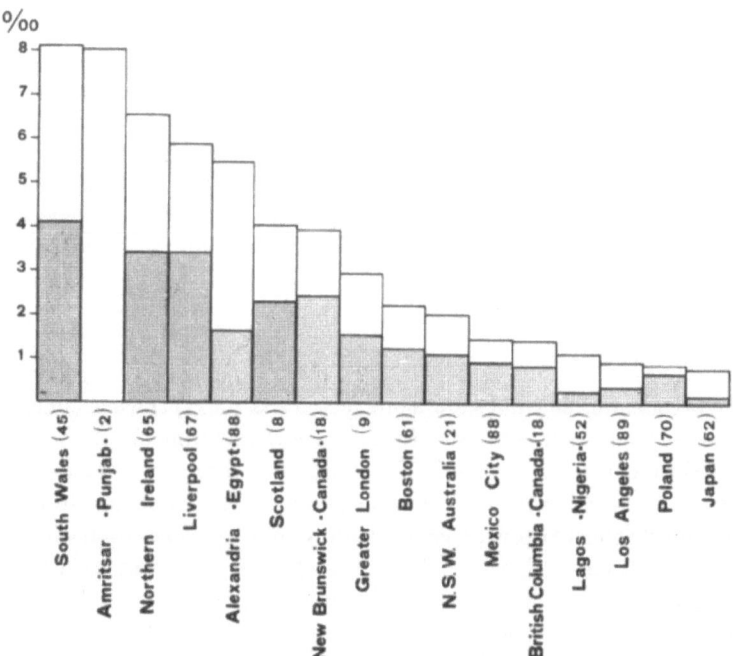

Figure 6.1. Incidence of neural tube defects in different series. The shaded areas indicate the incidence of spina bifida.

occurrence risk among Midland Europe, Negro, and Far Eastern populations with an intermediate rate recorded in the USA and Canada. The two latter display a characteristic downward trend from east to west.[21,26] However, locally acting environmental factors might be a determinant as well. Studies dealing with the incidence among ethnic groups after migration could clarify whether geographic or racial influences are involved. However the possibility of cultural differences, handed down through tradition and maintained for several generations (even far away from the country of origin) must be taken into account, as well as a possible socioeconomic gradient among ethnic groups. When the prevalence of NTD among migrant populations is considered, birth ranks intermediate between the place of origin and residence are often found. White Australians show a lower incidence rate than the British; white Australians of English descendant display a higher rate relative to native Australians, whereas those of non-English (European) descent show a lower incidence. Japanese individuals living in Hawaii show an increased risk of NTD, from the low level present in their country of origin toward the higher level of their new place of residence. Couples of Irish ancestry born in Boston have rates intermediate between Bostonians of other ethnic origin and first-generation immigrants from Ireland. In Israel, a country with a low birth frequency for NTD, the higher incidence documented among the offspring of mothers immigrating from other Middle-Eastern countries is no longer observed in the next generation, when the parents are born in Israel.[4,5,21,27] Since an inter-ethnic mating is unlikely to account for such a rapid variation, environmental factors must be considered. However, a high incidence is present among Sikhs, even those living outside of India,[28] whereas the disease is rare among Ashkenazim Jews, regardless of the rate found in the country they settled in.[29] Moreover, the constantly low occurrence of dysraphic states among Negro populations, wherever analyzed, despite centuries of separation from their places of origin, strongly suggests an underlying genetic protection.[9] In light of all this, a combined effect of genetic factors and geographic, cultural, and socioeconomic differences determining individual life styles can be outlined as the most likely source of variations.

Family Aggregation

Siblings of an affected child show an increased risk for NTD when compared to the general population. The rate of recurrence ranges from about 1% to nearly 10% in different series. A similar figure has been observed in the offspring of affected parents (either the mother or the father).[21] These findings strongly support the involvement of genetic factors in the etiology of NTD, even when taking into account that a family shares, besides the genetic patrimony, environmental characteristics, such as life style and socioeconomic status.

When considering the possible inheritance model involved in family aggregation, one can appreciate that, in all epidemiologic surveys, the proportion of affected siblings and offspring is far from the 25% expected for recessive inheritance. Also, a dominant inheritance is not likely, even assuming a very low penetrance. This pattern, however, has been recently proposed by Fineman et al.[30] on the basis of their finding of a high frequency of spina bifida occulta or other related vertebral and external anomalies in relatives of affected children. An X-linked recessive inheritance has been described only in two families.[29,31] On the other hand, the birth of affected children in families where the father is affected rules out the possibility of a cytoplasmic transmission. However, the importance of genetic influences in the occurrence of NTD is, furthermore, stressed by the increased risk recorded in the offspring of consanguineous marriages. In fact, in Alexandria, Egypt, where an exceptionally high rate of marriages between cousins is encountered (30%) an NTD incidence of 14.2 per thousand births was recorded from consanguineous marriages, whereas among nonconsanguineous couples the rate was 5.7 per thousand births.[32]

On the contrary, concordance rates of monozygotic (MZ) versus dizygotic (DZ) twins (another important feature often utilized by geneticists to ascertain whether genetic factors are a determinant in the etiology of the disease), far from helping to draw definitive conclusions, add some new puzzling questions to be answered. As all twins share the same intrauterine environment but only MZ twins share the same genetic patrimony, a genetically determined condition has to be more likely to recur in MZ than in DZ twins. Initial studies failed to demonstrate a concordance for NTD in twins, either MZ or DZ, higher than in sibs. As a high percentage of miscarriages has been estimated in embryos with a neural tube malformation, it was suggested that when both twins are affected the mother is more likely to miscarry, whereas the presence of a normal co-twin prevents the miscarriage of the affected one, thus accounting for the deficit of concordantly affected twins at term. This being the case, a higher percentage of concordantly affected twins should be obtained when fetal deaths are included in the study. Accordingly, data collected by Janerich and Piper,[33] as well as by Windham et al.,[23] based on both live-birth and fetal-death certificates, show an occurrence of 8.8% and 5.3%, respectively, among same sex twins, who are mostly MZ, whereas no concordant pair was observed among opposite-sex twins, who are necessarily DZ twins. Similarly, in the Elwood and Elwood review,[21] the concordance rate was 7.6% for same-sex pairs and only 2.8% for opposite-sex pairs. Windham and Sever[23,34] found a larger proportion of twins, either concordantly or discordantly affected, among infants with NTD than among the general population. Thus, they suggested a common etiologic factor for the twinning process and neural tube malformations. This was related to previous hypotheses proposing that developmental delay[35] or an alteration of the developmental clock[36] may cause a greater susceptibility to malformations in multiple pregnancies. This also holds in James' contention that an early insult might cause both duplication and morphologic alterations.[37]

On the other hand, Janerich[33] invoked a polygenic model, modified by environmental factors, to explain the increasing recurrence risk for NTD recorded among half-sibs, full-sibs, and MZ twins. In fact, once recognized that inheritance factors are likely to play a role, but also excluded the classic genetic patterns of transmission, a polygenic model was considered. In 1969 Edwards[38] described a multifactorial model according to which there is a critical threshold, determined by the presence of a certain number of predisposing genes. In this view, embryos possessing predisposing genetic factors beyond this threshold are prone to develop the disease when exposed to environmental conditions that are able to act as a trigger. The number of genes determining the genetic threshold is encountered at the highest frequency, that is about half-way between the index patient and the general population, among first-degree relatives, sharing half of their genetic patrimony with the affected patient, and at levels progressively closer to the overall rate when higher degree relatives are considered. Accordingly, when two affected births have occurred in the same family, the expected occurrence rate is furthermore increased. As far as the absolute rate of recurrence in affected families is concerned, the greatest level, as may be expected, is reached in high-risk countries. However, due to the slope of the normal curve, the lower the incidence for a given geographic area, the greater the increment of the risk for relatives.[9] These features, predicted by the multifactorial model, have been verified in family studies.[22] For this reason, notwithstanding some imprecise correspondence between expected versus observed figures (i.e., the lack of a higher sibship risk related to affected males), this model is at present considered the most able to fit the current data.

Environmental Factors

Environmental influences are concordantly claimed to justify the puzzling epidemiologic patterns of dysraphic states. These must be taken into account when interpreting the heterogeneous geographic distribution and the observed seasonal and secular variations in the frequency of affected births. Moreover, since nongenetic factors affecting the intrauterine environment must concur with genetic factors to explain the family recurrence model, maternal circumstances, such as socioeconomic status, age, parity, metabolic disorders, and unbalanced dietary intake, must also be considered. Finally, the teratogenic effects of exposure to chemical, physical, and infectious agents have to be analyzed. So far, the great number of chemical, epidemiologic, and experimental studies pointing to the significance of any of the various environmental factors indicates that multiple causes, rather than a single one, may be able to trigger an altered closure of the neural tube when acting on a genetically predisposed embryo. A common pathogenetic mechanism may be speculated. It is noteworthy that environmental factors may differ in importance with respect to genetic factors when low- or high-risk areas are considered.[34,39] A causative agent, playing a role in determining a local rate, may not have the same importance everywhere. On the other hand the interference of unselected biases should also be considered.

Geographic Factors

As discussed above, the different birth rates across countries may be justified on a racial basis in terms of predisposing genetic characteristics, life style, and socioeconomic standards only to a certain degree. Moreover, environmental rather than genetic factors are more likely to act in determining local variations within the same country. This has been observed in France, Scotland, and Wales.[6] Thus, geographic variables such as climate, water supply, geologic structure, radioactivity, and population density have been tested. Analyzing the differences among small areas in the South Wales region, Laurence et al.[6] did not find any correlation between these variables and the occurrence of the disease, except for some evidence of an urban–rural gradient. This latter finding, confirmed by Field,[4] was not observed in other studies.[21,27,37,40] Other analyses dealing with background radioactivity[41,42] failed to demonstrate any positive correlation with the incidence of NTD, even though radiation damage is extremely significant in experimental models. Climate variables do not seem to be consistently related to NTD occurrence, although a relationship with rainfall or average temperature has been reported occasionally.[4,21,43]

Correlation between content of various oligoelements (calcium, magnesium, chromium, zinc, copper, cadmium, lead, mercury, and molybdenum) in water and occurrence of NTD has been investigated by many authors since Penrose, in 1957,[44] excited interest in the possible concurrence of the softness of local drinking water and the variation of NTD across the British Isles. These studies failed to yield definitive evidence, mostly because these surveys, realized across populations or in different time periods, were not supported by a case-control analysis within each population. The only oligoelement for which some significant correlation with NTD was shown was zinc. Zinc deficiency has been reported in the high prevalence areas of the Middle East.[27] In addition, a statistically significant relationship between zinc content in the mother's drinking water, serum, and red cells and NTD in her offspring was found in a case-control study by St. Leger et al.,[45] although the biologic significance of this result was argued by the authors themselves. More recently Dorsch et al.[46] carried out a study in rural South Australia, where the place of residence during pregnancy was considered in matching case-control pairs. A significantly higher incidence of anencephaly and spina bifida was found in the offspring of mothers who drank primarily ground or bore water, relative to children of mothers who consumed only rainwater. The most striking difference was the higher content of nitrates in bore and ground water. This finding is consistent with experimental studies, and with the significant correlation documented by Knox[47] between anencephalic births and the mother's intake of nitrate-cured meats.

Seasonal Variations and Secular Trends

The efforts to find a seasonal variation in the occurrence of NTD are justified by the support it could offer for the etiologic role of some environmental influences, i.e., dietary, viral, climatic, and so on. Unfortunately, the relationship between season and NTD occurrence varies with a complicated pattern according to the years and places of survey, as well as the defect considered.[21,22] Moreover, seasonal variations of all births must be taken into account. Misinterpretations may occur when times of conception are estimated, using birth dates regardless of the duration of pregnancy. In fact, Smithells et al.[48] found a significant excess of affected infants among winter births relative to summer births, but no seasonality when conceptions were analyzed, because of different rates of premature delivery throughout the year.

Spring seems to be the highest risk period for conception of affected fetuses in several surveys from England, Hungary (in respect to spina bifida but not anencephaly), and some regions of Canada (only for anencephaly).[21,49] This is not consistent with the reported fall prevalence in a Quebec study[50] or with the summer peak in Australia (December, January, February),[4] whereas no seasonal variation has been found elsewhere.[21,22,41,51,52] In a recent study from the United Kingdom,[53] the seasonal peaks for NTD were in phase with an embryo's increased susceptibility to anencephaly in May and June and to spina bifida in July. A local difference in environmental factors, acting in different seasons, might account for these heterogeneous findings. Moreover, the tendency of seasonal variations to show up in high-risk areas and to disappear where the defects are not common has been pointed out.[51,53] It might suggest a preponderant importance of environmental factors in countries with high frequency. In some cases a known local seasonal prevalence was no longer identified in years of high incidence,[53] possibly due to a new emerging factor being more relevant in that period.

The incidence of NTD is known to have widely varied during the last century (Fig. 6.2), showing long-term trends in which the prevalence rose from baseline or from a previous trough level toward a peak incidence, eventually falling again to the original or even lower level. In several surveys,[22,56,58] the shape of the incidence slope seems to define some kind of "epidemics," usually not concurrently observed in different countries. We are not able, at the moment, to understand completely the ultimate meaning of secular trends, as we are not aware of the actual etiology of the malformation. The attempt to propose likely candidates for the "epidemic" waves could have provided clues for the causation of NTD but, unfortunately, although suggestive correlations have been hypothesized, they have not been adequately documented.

One of the most striking "epidemics" is that described between 1920 and 1944 in the northeastern United States, which showed, during the quinquennium 1930 to 1934, a peak rate twice as high as in the years before 1920 and after 1944. The linking with the great economic depression of 1929 proposed by McMahon[56] was highly suggestive, and it fitted well with the reported association between low socioeconomic status and occurrence of NTD. However, the lack of a precise temporal correspondence leaves some residual questions.

A drop in the general welfare might be, again, a clue for interpreting the "epidemic" that occurred in Berlin during and shortly after the Second World War, although a wider diffusion of the phenomenon should have been observed. Actually, in such a troubled period it is really hard to extract a causative factor and, in spite of careful analyses, no definite etiologic explanation could be offered.[58]

In view of the experimentally demonstrated efficacy of viral infections and febrile episodes in determining NTD, an attempt has been made to link influenza

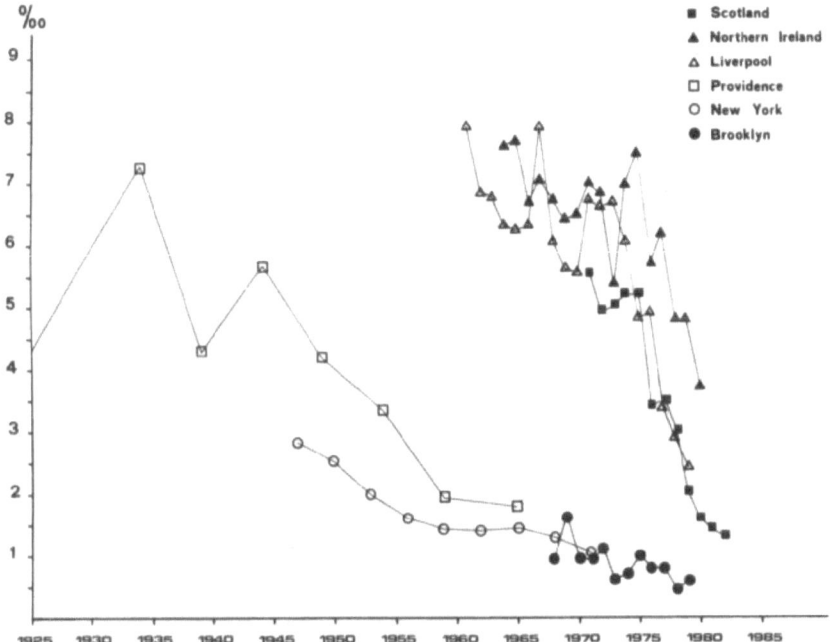

Figure 6.2. Time-trends of neural tube defects in Scotland,[54] Northern Ireland,[7] Liverpool,[55] Providence,[56] New York,[57] Brooklyn, New York.[57]

outbreaks with the epidemic increase of the malformation. However, no rise in the incidence of NTD was found after three different influenza epidemics across 1960.[59] It has also been suggested that the peak increments in secular trends are not related to the years of birth of the affected children but to the age ranks of their mothers, suggesting that the causative factor should have acted in women of a particular generation.[22,57] This hypothesis is far from being proved.

Maternal Circumstances: Socioeconomic Status and Life Style

A correlation between NTD and social class has been investigated on the rationale that possible environmental risk factors, such as unsafe working conditions, infections due to overcrowded housing, poor nutrition, or, more in general, inadequate maternal life style during pregnancy and insufficient prenatal care, are more likely to be associated with a low socioeconomic level. A clear inverse correlation with economic level, as determined from father's occupation, has been described in British and North American studies.[7,21,60,61] Yet, it failed to be demonstrated in reports from low-risk areas,[18,39] suggesting a greater sensitivity to environmental variables where the defects are more common. However, in a recent survey from Nigeria,[43] a country with a low incidence of NTD, a higher than expected percentage of fathers with low occupational status and low educational level was observed.

Discordant results may be related to methods of classification. Also, the kind of society the mother grew up in has been proposed to be possibly more important than that which she married into.[62] Moreover, the impact of different racial susceptibilities complicated the understanding of socioeconomic influences. In India, Sikhs are by far the most affected ethnic group, despite their high economic standard. According to the well-known high incidence of NTD in Ireland, the proportion of Irish in the different social classes in England and Australia should be taken into account when interpreting the risk related with economic status.

Besides the role of economic standards, the possible influence of life style has been considered. Jorde et al.[41] described a significant negative correlation between NTD and the percentage of Mormons in each Utah county. As Mormons also showed a lower incidence of cancer and cardiovascular diseases, life style factors, i.e., exposure to teratogens, differences in urban–rural residence, and occupational risk factors, have been suggested, although the support of a case-control study is mandatory.

Maternal Circumstances: Age, Parity, and Reproductive History

Apart from the well-known close relationship between advanced maternal age and some genetic syndromes such as trisomies, maternal age and parity are considered among the conditions able to modify the prenatal environment. The birth order effect is not easy to separate from that of maternal age because the amount of data needed to apply correct statistical standardization procedures is not always available. Moreover, the significance of birth order may be affected by the number of fetal and neonatal deaths in different series.

A strict connection between maternal age, parity, and NTD occurrence has not been sufficiently demonstrated as data from the literature are often conflicting, ranging from no significant evidence to contradictory figures.[51,61] A U-shaped relationship, i.e., an excess of first and late born as well as an excess of the youngest (<20 years) and of the oldest (>35 years) mothers, has been described, at least for high-risk countries,[9,21,22] whereas in low-risk areas a linear, a monotonic trend, increasing with age and parity, seems to be the most common finding.[39] The widely reported excess of miscarriages in families with an affected child[21] has been tentatively interpreted by Knox[25] with the assumption that NTD in later pregnancies are due to an interaction between the fetus and some trophoblastic material remaining from the previous abortion. Even though this hypothesis is compatible with the higher percentage of miscarriages observed before birth of the index patient,[51] the most widely accepted explanation is that aborted fetuses are fatally affected by the neural tube malformation,[21,63] in light of a family aggregation of the defect. Creasy and Alberman,[17] comparing the estimated prevalence of NTD at the eighth week of gestation among spontaneously aborted conceptuses without chromosomal anomalies with the prevalence in total births, calculated that only 24% of these are born alive, whereas 54% abort spontaneously and 22% are stillborn. Furthermore, Roberts and Lloyd,[64] having found an inverse relationship between previous spontaneous abortion rate and the birth incidence of NTD in different areas within South Wales, speculated that differences in miscarriage rate may account for geographic variations, but this finding has not been confirmed elsewhere.[7] Support for the "male miscarriage hypothesis" proposed by James[63] to explain the excess of abortions in affected families is not available, as the deficit of male sibs to be accordingly expected has not been encountered.[4,51]

Maternal Circumstances: Dietary Intake

Since the late 1960s attention has been focused on the possibility that poor diet could be involved in determining NTD.[7,21] In 1972 Renwick[65] suggested that eating blighted potatoes could possibly result in contamination by the fungus *Phytophthora infestans*, a theoretic causative factor. Although experimental studies have proved cytochalasin, a fungine metabolite, and other alkaloids derived from potatoe sprouts,[26] to be effective as teratogens,[66] further clinical trials and geographic surveys failed to confirm Renwick's observation.[7,21]

A clear correlation between poor maternal diet and the recurrence rate of NTD has been recently demonstrated by Laurence.[67] An inadequate dietary intake has been proposed in considering the social class distribution of NTD or the "epidemic" occurrence during period of economic depression, whereas the seasonal variation might be linked to a relative unavailability of fresh food products. In effect, a diet not globally poor but lacking in some essential elements and vitamins, particularly folic acid, has been considered a risk factor. The teratogenic effect of folic acid antagonist drugs is well known,[68] and, the interference of folic acid deficiency on rat embryo development was demonstrated by Nelson as early as 1960.[69] Hibbard and Smithells[70] found a higher frequency of pathologic results of a formimminoglutamic acid excretion test in mothers of affected infants. It is noteworthy that pregnancy itself may interfere with folate metabolism.[71] Central nervous system malformations have been observed in women suffering from gravidic megaloblastic anemia.[72] Moreover, as a lower concentration of folate and other vitamins was found during the first trimester of pregnancy in women who subsequently gave birth to children with NTD, a trial with periconceptional vitamin supplementation has been carried out by Smithells et al.[73,74] on women at risk because of previous affected pregnancies. A sevenfold reduction in the recurrence rate was observed in fully supplemented women compared to noncompliant women.[74] However, the great impact that the proven efficacy as such an easy, and relatively inexpensive, prevention could have on the overall occurrence of the disease, and the concern about the opportunity for a mass-prevention program, suggest some caution in interpreting the results and the need for further "fine-grained" surveys. Actually, the Smithells study was criticized for want of both a placebo-administered group and a randomized double-blind case-control method, as mothers without supplementation were a self-selected group.

Therefore, although positive results were also obtained by Laurence et al.[75] with folate periconceptional supplementation, a newly designed multicenter program has been developed by the British Medical Research Council, according to which women are assigned in a random and double-blind fashion to four groups, each receiving one of the following supplementations: folate and other vitamins plus minerals (as in the study by Smithells et al.); folate and minerals; other vitamins and minerals; minerals only (the last group possibly representing a placebo-administered one, as a true placebo group was not included because of the ethical concern for a case-control study). A three-group trial (multivitamins and folate, folate only, or multivitamins only) has been started in Dublin.[76] It is worth noting that, once again, as discussed above for other variables, in the field of pericon-ceptional multivitamin supplementation, a greater susceptibility to environmental factors has been found in high-risk versus low-risk areas, as well as in female versus male fetuses. In fact, in a recent study carried out by Seller and Nevin,[77] a 5.4-fold reduction in the overall recurrence rate has been found in fully supplemented women living in Northern Ireland, whereas a 2.4-fold decrease has been observed in southeastern England, these regions being placed respectively at the highest and lowest extremes of NTD birth prevalence in that country. Once confirmed, these observations could be an issue to design country-tailored prevention programs. It is noteworthy that Seller and Nevin found, in spite of the supplementation protocol, seven cases of recurrence, of which six were males. This supports the theory according to which, in conditions of multifactorial etiology, when an unequal sex incidence is present, the less affected sex has a greater genetic component in the etiology, thus being less sensitive to environmental manipulations.

Maternal Circumstances: Metabolic Disorders

The well-known higher incidence of malformations in the offspring of diabetic mothers applies also to NTD, as reported in several studies.[78,79] The role of intolerance to carbohydrates, even in the absence of overt diabetes, has been described by Wilson and Vallance-Owen, who found a significantly higher frequency of albumin–insulin antagonism in mothers of children with spina bifida.[80] The teratogenic effect of the altered carbohydrate metabolism may be ascribed to hyperinsulinism or to a greater maternal concentration of glucose and/or ketones.[81,82] Interest has also been raised regarding the role of zinc in developing embryos, as zinc is an essential factor in DNA synthesis and assembly and in the maintenance of the cytoskeleton (i.e., the microtubules), the alteration of which has been related to NTD. In addition to what we have already discussed about the possible correlation between a zinc-deficient diet and the incidence of NTD, it is interesting to note that an increased rate of affected births was described in women suffering from acrodermatitis enteropathica, until dietary zinc supplementation was started.[40] On the other hand, it has been reported that mothers of children with spina bifida failed to show the progressive decrease in hair zinc content during pregnancy that control mothers did.[83] This finding has been associated with maternal zinc deficiency. Zimmerman,[84] in 1984, postulated that these findings could be related to a defective fetal utilization of zinc, accounting for the observed fetal hyperzinchemia and elevated maternal albumin-bound zinc. A zinc supplementation in well-nourished women was, thus, not warranted. The correlation between zinc and vitamin A has also been investigated,[85] since vitamin A deficiency depresses the synthesis of the α_2-macroglobulin, responsible for zinc transport in blood. Experimental animal studies as well as occasional human reports have pointed out the teratogenic efficacy of either deficiency or excess of vitamin A.[85] A significantly higher vitamin A concentration was observed in the amniotic fluid of affected versus unaffected pregnancies, despite a lack of serum concentration differences. This has been related to an impaired regulatory mechanism of vitamin A transfer to the fetus. For all these reasons caution has been advocated in the use of vitamin A for periconceptional supplementation, until the teratogenic effect of its hyper versus hypo level is definitely clarified.[85]

Infectious, Physical, and Chemical Agents

The hypothesis that viral infection may represent a clue in the genesis of NTD, either directly or through the concomitant hyperthermic episode, has failed to be demonstrated consistently, even though influenza or fever in early pregnancy have been recalled by mothers of affected children.[51,59] Also, although successfully tested on experimental models, the effectiveness of hyperthermia resulting from exposure to high environmental temperatures (working conditions or hot saunas) in causing neural tube malclosures has been investigated[86] but not definitively proved.

Investigations on chemical agents possibly responsible for NTD have been mostly addressed to drug consumption. Little information is available on the effect of potentially toxic substances encountered during day-to-day life or work activities, apart from the report of a significantly more frequent exposure to organic solvents in mothers of neonates with NTD.[87] A correlation with the use of herbicides was tested in Sweden[88] without finding any positive result. In contrast, the causative role of folic acid antagonists, such as aminopterin, has been definitively proved.[68] A teratogenic effect of clomifene on the central nervous system has been claimed. However, it is difficult to separate the effect of the drug from that of ovulation disorders and subfertility initiating its administration, not to mention the possibility of an apparent infertility due to precocious abortions of malformed embryos.[89]

No other evidence followed the first report on a causative effect of hormonal exposure and several studies demonstrated no significant association between use of oral contraceptives and central nervous system malformations.[90]

Common drugs, as antihistamines, antibiotics, benzodiazepines, and antinflammatory compounds do not seem to be related to NTD occurrence and no significant correlation between maternal drug history and central nervous system anomalies was found in a recent survey on 764 mothers of affected children.[90]

Although an increased rate for epileptic women treated with barbiturates and fenilhydantoin has been suggested,[91] more recently the possible teratogenic effect of valproic acid has received widespread attention and has aroused concern about the use of this drug during pregnancy. Sodium valproate is teratogenic in rodents[92] and, from data collected so far,[97] NTD seem to occur in about 1% of mothers taking valproic acid (i.e., close to the recurrence rate in affected families).[93] However, the number of NTD occurring after exposure to valproate is still low and, because of the restricted risk group, an attentive multicenter survey is needed to obtain definitive evidence.

Recent Decline in NTD Prevalence

In the last decades a pronounced and fairly constant decline in the prevalence of NTD has been reported from many areas (United Kingdom, United States, Australia) (Fig. 6.2).[7,54,55,57,93,94] The previously discussed fluctuation in secular trends urges some caution, as other apparent recessions in the past were just the descending phase of a previous peak, and a new increase might be encountered. In fact, it is not easy to establish a baseline level from which one may confidently identify a peak or a trough. However, the present decline has been widespread and a downward trend is persistent since as early as the late 40s in the United States (Fig. 6.2).[56] Moreover, some positive reasons can be claimed to account for this reduction.

The availability since the 1970s of antenatal NTD screening test (α-fetoprotein and ultrasonography) could explain, to a certain extent, the recent trend. However, the number of pregnancy terminations reported from Britain (Fig. 6.3) and Australia accounts only for a fraction of the decrease recorded in those countries.[55,93,95] Moreover, a decline is registered in the United States although screening tests are not uniformly spread and, in any case, the decline was present well before the beginning of the screening programs (Fig. 6.2). On the other hand, it must be underlined that the reduction is irrelevant in the Irish Republic where antenatal diagnosis and abortion are not accepted because of the strong religious concern.[95]

Since about 5% of all cases of NTD are represented by familial recurrence,[55] the availability of genetic counselling might play a role in the general decline of the disease. A fall in the recurrence rate parallel to the one in the overall incidence has been reported by Seller and Hancock.[96] In contrast, in the Owens[55] study from Liverpool and Bootle, the recurrence rate remains fairly constant, although one might have expected this group to drop dramatically, at least because of the dedicated antenatal screening. If avoidance of conceptions in high-risk families and pregnancy terminations after a positive prenatal screening test are able to explain only a fraction of the present reduction, other factors must be involved. Since the present recession is too rapid to be accounted for by any modification in the genetic load, environmental variables must be considered:

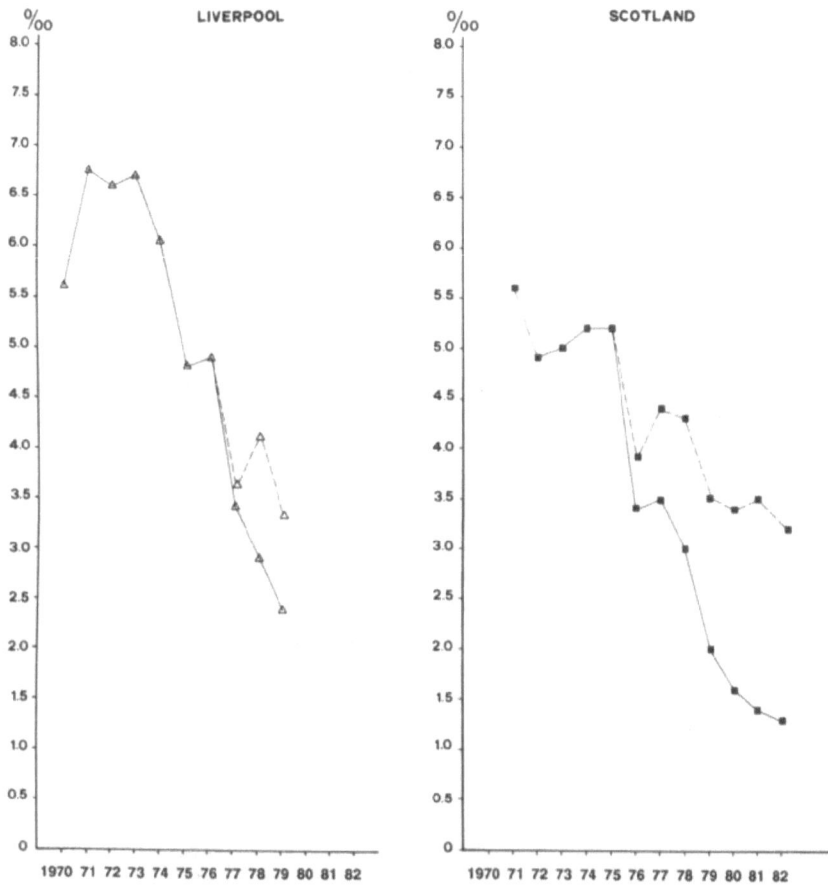

Figure 6.3. Time-trend of neural tube defects in Liverpool and Scotland.[54] The dotted lines indicate the total number of affected conceptuses, including pregnancy terminations.

1. Improved economic standards have led to better housing, increase in general welfare, and safer working conditions even in low social classes.
2. Increased public health intervention and parental awareness have led to a better prenatal care, closer medical control, and concern about life style during pregnancy.
3. The identification of risk factors involved in determining NTD have attracted attention to the exposure to possible teratogens, metabolic disorders, and poor or unbalanced dietary intake, and has promoted prevention programs of periconceptional supplementation.

If a change in environmental factors is determining the present decline, a most striking reduction might be observed in more susceptible groups and, more susceptible groups and, as proposed by Janerich and Piper,[33] an approach to the genetic baseline for a given population might be expected.

Conclusions

When coping with a not yet clarified etiology, unselected biases may at any moment represent a source of misinterpretation, not to mention the underlying risk of an apparent chance relationship. Ericson et al.[88] simulated an epidemiologic survey, letting a computer randomly assign malformation diagnoses across a single country and studying the obtained distribution among the different parishes. In one parish, located between two large industrial plants, abut 50% of the infants showed some kind of malformation. They state, "Had this random cluster occurred in real life, the local observation would have probably associated it with pollution from the two industries."[88]

Epidemiologic studies are precious in offering clues to the etiology, as investigating the sources of variation may lead to the identification of possible causative factors. This is not an end-point, as every relationship arising from epidemiologic surveys must always be verified through case-control and experimental studies. Again, the possible etiological agent, identified through experimental, epidemiologic, and clinical investigations, should be confirmed when subjected to epidemiologic controls under different circumstances. The effectiveness of appropriately designed programs of primary prevention may be decisive. (Fig. 6.4).

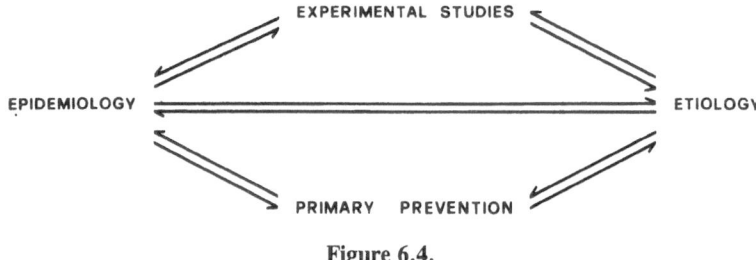

Figure 6.4.

Summary

An increasing number of studies conducted during the last decades have demonstrated that isolated NTD show common epidemiological patterns. They vary widely according to place and time of survey, as well as ethnic group, family, and maternal variables (socioeconomic status, age and parity, reproductive history, metabolic disorders, and diet during pregnancy). These variations appear to result from a combination of genetic and environmental factors adding up to a score that represents a threshold beyond which an embryo is prone to develop the disease. An evident decline in the occurrence of NTD has recently become apparent in many areas. Prenatal screening, genetic counselling, better prenatal care, and attention to exposure to possible risk factors during pregnancy, as well as an increased general welfare, have been proposed as reasons for this trend.

References

1. Record RG, McKeown T: Congenital malformations of the central nervous system. A survey of 930 cases. Br J Prev Soc Med 3:183–219, 1949.
2. Lesi F: The significance of congenital defects in developing countries. Med Today 3:26–40, 1969.
3. Neel JV: A study of major congenital defects in Japanese infants. Am J Hum Genet 10:398–445, 1958.
4. Field B: Neural tube defects in New South Wales, Australia. J Med Genet 15:329–338, 1978.
5. Naggan L, Mac Mahon B: Ethnic differences in the prevalence of anencephaly and spina bifida in Boston, Massachusetts. N Engl J Med 227:1119–1123, 1967.
6. Laurence KM, Carter CO, David PA: Major CNS malformations in South Wales. I: incidence, local variations and geographical factors. Br J Prev Soc Med 21:147–160, 1967.
7. Nevin NC: Prevention of neural tube defects in an area of high incidence. In: Dobbing J (ed): Prevention of Spina Bifida and Other Neural Tube Defects. Academic Press, London, 1983, pp. 127–144.
8. James WH: The sex ratio in spina bifida. J Med Genet 16:384–388, 1979.
9. Carter CO: Clues to aetiology of neural tube malformations. Dev Med Child Neurol 16 (Suppl. 32):3–15, 1974.
10. Smithells RW, D'Arcy EE, McAllister EF: The outcome of pregnancies before and after the birth of infants with nervous system malformations. Dev Med Child Neurol 1:6–10, 1968.
11. Williamson EM: Incidence of family aggregation of the major congenital malformations of the CNS. J Med Genet 2:161–172, 1965.
12. Roselli R, Velardi F: Embriologia. In: Di Rocco C, Caldarelli M (eds): Mielomeningocele. Casa del Libro Ed., Rome, 1983, pp. 3–26.
13. Holmes LB, Driscoll SG, Atkins L: Etiologic heterogeneity of neural-tube defects. N Eng J Med 294:365–369, 1976.
14. Khoury MJ, Erickson DJ, James LM: Etiologic heterogeneity of neural tube defects: clues from epidemiology. Am J Epidemiol 115:538–548, 1982.
15. Khoury MJ, Erickson DJ, James LM: Etiologic heterogeneity of neural tube defects. II. Clues from family studies. Am J Hum Genet 34:980–987, 1982.
16. Martin RA, Fineman RM, Jorde LB: Phenotypic heterogeneity in neural tube defects: a clue to causal heterogeneity. Am J Med Genet 16:519–525, 1983.
17. Creasy MR, Alberman ED: Congenital malformations of the central nervous system in spontaneous abortions. J Med Genet 13:9–16, 1976.
18. Czeizel A: Schisis association. Am J Med Genet 10:25–35, 1981.
19. Opitz JM, Gilbert EF: CNS anomalies and the midline as a "developmental field." Am J Med Genet 12:443–455, 1982.
20. Ilyina HG, Lurie IW: Neural tube defects in sibs of children with tracheo-oesophageal dysraphism. J Med Genet 21:73–74, 1984.
21. Elwood JM, Elwood JH: Epidemiology of anencephalus and spina bifida. Oxford University Press, New York, 1980, pp. 120–138.

22. Leck I: Epidemiological clues to the causation of neural tube defects. In: Dobbing J (ed): Prevention of Spina Bifida and Other Neural Tube Defects. Academic Press, London, 1983, pp. 155–182.

23. Windham GC, Bjerkedal T, Sever LE: The association of twinning and neural tube defects: studies in Los Angeles, California, and Norway. Acta Genet Med Gemellol 31:165–172, 1982.

24. Burn J, Gibbens D: May spina bifida result from an X-linked defect in a selective abortion mechanism? J Med Genet 16:210–214, 1979.

25. Knox EG: Fetus-fetus interaction. A model aetiology for anencephalus. Dev Med Child Neurol 12:167–177, 1970.

26. Renwick JH, Claringbold WDB, Earthy ME, Few JD, McLean ACS: Neural tube defects produced in syrian hamster by potato glycoalkaloids. Teratology 30:371–381, 1984.

27. Leck I: The geographical distribution of neural tube defects and oral clefts. Br Med Bull 40:390–395, 1984.

28. Baird PA: Neural tube defects in the Sikhs. Am J Med Genet 16:49–56, 1983.

29. Toriello HV, Warren ST, Lindstrom JA: Possible X-linked anencephaly and spina bifida: report of a kindred. Am J Med Genet 6:119–121, 1980.

30. Fineman RM, Jorde LB, Martin RA, Hasstedt SJ, Wing SD, Walker ML: Spinal dysraphia as an autosomal dominant defect in four families. Am J Med Genet 12: 457–464, 1982.

31. Baraister M, Burn J: Brief clinical report: neural tube defects as an X-linked condition. Am J Med Genet 17:383–385, 1984.

32. Stevenson AC, Johnson HA, Stewart MIP, Golding DR: Congenital malformations. A report of a study of series of consecutive births in 24 centres. Bull WHO 34:1–125, 1966.

33. Janerich DT, Piper J: Shifting genetic patterns in anencephaly and spina bifida. J Med Genet 15:101–105, 1978.

34. Windham GC, Sever LE: Neural tube defects among twin births. Am J Hum Genet 34:988–998, 1982.

35. Schinzel AAGL, Smith DW, Miller JR: Monozygotic twinning and structural defects. J Pediatr 95:921–930, 1979.

36. Myrianthopoulos NC: Congenital malformations: the contribution of twin studies. Birth Defects Orig Art Ser 14:151–165, 1978.

37. James WH: Twinning and anencephaly. Ann Hum Biol 3:401–409, 1976.

38. Edwards JH: Familial predisposition in man. Br Med Bull 25:58–64, 1969.

39. Strassburg MA, Greenland S, Portigal LD, Sever LE: A population-based case-control study of anencephalus and spina bifida in a low-risk area. Dev Med Child Neurol 25:632–641, 1983.

40. Hambridge KM, Neldner KH, Walravens PA: Zinc, acrodermatitis entropathica and congenital malformations. Lancet 1:577–578, 1975.

41. Jorde LB, Fineman RM, Martin RA: Epidemiology of neural tube defects in Utah, 1940–1979. Am J Epidemiol 119:487–495, 1984.

42. Segall A, Mac Mahon B, Hannigan M: Congenital malformations and background radiation in Northern New England. J Chron Dis 17:915–921, 1964.

43. Adeloye A, Oyewole A, Adeyokunnu AA: Epidemiological aspects of spina bifida cystica in Ibadan, Nigeria. Riv Neurosc Pediatr (J Pediatr Neurosci) 1:137–148, 1985.

44. Penrose LS: Genetics of anencephaly. J Ment Defic Res 1:4–15, 1957.

45. St. Leger AS, Elwood PC, Morton MS: Neural tube malformations and trace elements in water. J Epidemiol Commun Hlth 34:186–187, 1980.
46. Dorsch MM, Scragg RKR, McMichael AJ, Baghurst PA, Dyer KF: Congenital malformations and maternal drinking water supply in rural South Australia: a case-control study. Am J Epidemiol 119:473–486, 1984.
47. Knox EG: Anencephalus and dietary intakes. Br J Prev Soc Med 26:219–223, 1972.
48. Smithells RW, Chinn, ER: Spina bifida in Liverpool. Dev Med Child Neurol 7:258–268, 1965.
49. Leck I: Causation of neural tube defects: clues from epidemiology. Br Med Bull 30:158–163, 1974.
50. Dallaire L, Melancon SB, Potier M, Mathieu JP, Ducharme G: Date of conception and prevention of neural tube defects. Clin Genet 26:304–307, 1984.
51. Hunter, AGW: Neural tube defects in Eastern Ontario and Western Quebec: demography and family data. Am J Med Genet 19:45–63, 1984.
52. Pietrzyk JJ, Grochowski J, Kanska B: CNS malformations in the Krakow region. I. Birth prevalence and seasonal incidence during 1979–1981. Am J Med Genet 14:181–188, 1983.
53. Maclean MH, Mac Leod A: Seasonal variations in the frequency of anencephalus and spina bifida in the United Kingdom. J Epidemiol Commun Hlth 38:99–102, 1984.
54. Carstairs V, Cole S: Spina bifida and anencephaly in Scotland. Br Med J. 289:1182–1184, 1984.
55. Owens JR, Harris F, McAllister E, West L: 19-Year incidence of neural tube defects in area under constnt surveillance. Lancet ii:1032–1035, 1981.
56. MacMahon B, Yen S: Unrecognised epidemic of anencephaly and spina bifida. Lancet i:31–33, 1971.
57. Janerich DT: Epidemic waves in the prevalence of anencephaly and spina bifida in New York State. Teratology 8:253–256, 1973.
58. Koch M, Fuhrmann W: Epidemiology of neural tube defects in Germany. Hum Genet 68:97–103, 1984.
59. Laurence KM, Carter CO, David PA: Major CNS malformations in South Wales. II: Pregnancy factors, seasonal variations, and social class effects. Br J Prev Soc Med 22:212–222, 1968.
60. Carter CO, Evans K: Spina bifida and anencephalus in Greater London. J Med Genet 10:209–233, 1973.
61. Nesbit DE, Ziter FA: Epidemiology of myelomeningocele in Utah. Dev Med Child Neurol 21:754–757, 1979.
62. Sever LE, Emanuel I: Intergenerational factors in the etiology of anencephalus and spina bifida. Dev Med Child Neurol 232:151–154, 1981.
63. James WH: Birth ranks of spontaneous abortions in sibships of children affected by anencephaly or spina bifida. Br Med J 1:72–73, 1978.
64. Roberts CJ, Lloyd S: Area differences in spontaneous abortion rates in South Wales and their relation to neural tube defect incidence. Br Med J 4:20–22, 1973.
65. Renwick JH: Hypothesis: anencephaly and spina bifida are usually preventable by avoidance of a specific but unidentified substance present in certain potato tubers. Br J Prev Soc Med 26:67–88, 1972.
66. Linville G, Shepard T: Neural tube closure defects caused by cytocalasin B. Nature 236:246–252, 1972.

67. Laurence KM, James N, Miller M, Campbell H: Increased risk of recurrence of pregnancies complicated by fetal neural tube defects in mothers receiving poor diets and possible benefit of dietary counseling. Br Med J 281:1592–1594, 1980.

68. Thiersh JB: Therapeutic abortion with a folic acid antagonist, 4-amino pteroyl glutamic acid (4 amino PGA), administered by the oral route. Am J Obstet Gynecol 63:1298–1304, 1952.

69. Nelson MM: Teratogenic effects of pteroylglutamic acid deficiency in the rat. In: Wolstenholme WE, O'Connor M (eds): Ciba Foundation Symposium on Congenital Malformations. Churchill, London, 1960, pp. 134–152.

70. Hibbard ED, Smithells RW: Folic acid metabolism and human embryopathy. Lancet i:1254, 1965.

71. Rotham D: Folic acid in pregnancy. Am J Obstet Gynecol 108:149–152, 1970.

72. Fraser, JL, Watt HJ: Megaloblastic anemia in pregnancy and the puerperium. Am J Obstet Gynecol 89:532, 1964.

73. Smithells RW, Sheppard S, Schorah CJ, Seller MJ, Nevin NC, Harris R, Read AP, Fielding DW: Apparent prevention of neural tube defects by periconceptional vitamin supplementation. Arch Dis Child 56:911–918, 1981.

74. Smithells RW, Nevin NC, Seller MJ, Sheppard S, Harris R, Read AP, Fielding DW, Walker S, Schorah CJ, Wild J: Further experience of vitamin supplementation for prevention of neural tube defect recurrence. Lancet i:1027–1031, 1983.

75. Laurence KM, James N, Miller MH, Tennant JB, Campbell H: Double blind randomized controlled trial of folate treatment before conception to prevent recurrence of neural tube defects. Br Med J 282:1509–1511, 1981.

76. Elwood JM: Can vitamins prevent neural tube defects? Can Med Assoc J 129:1088–1092, 1983.

77. Seller MJ, Nevin NC: Periconceptional vitamin supplementation and the prevention of neural tube defects in south-east England and Northern Ireland. J Med Genet 21:325–330, 1984.

78. Mills JL: Malformations in infants of diabetic mothers. Teratology 225:385–394, 1982.

79. Milunsky A, Alpert E, Kitzmiller J, Younger M, Neff R: Prenatal diagnosis of neural tube defects. VIII. The importance of serum α-protein screening in diabetic pregnant women. Am J Obstet Gynecol 142:1030–1032, 1982.

80. Wilson JSP, Vallance-Owen J: Congenital deformities and insulin antagonism. Lancet ii:940–942, 1966.

81. Garnham EA, Beck F, Clarke CA, Stanisstreet M: Effects of glucose on rat embryos in culture. Diabetologia 25:291–295, 1983.

82. Horton WE Jr, Sadler TW: Effects of maternal diabetes on early embryogenesis. Alterations in morphogenesis produced by the ketone body, β-hydroxybutyrate. Diabetes 32:610–616, 1983.

83. Bergmann KM, Makosch G, Tews KH: Abnormalities of hair zinc concentrations in mothers of newborn infants with spina bifida. Am J Clin Nutr 33:2145–2150, 1980.

84. Zimmerman AW: Hyperzincemia in anencephaly and spina bifida: a clue to the pathogenesis of neural tube defects? Neurology 34:443–450, 1984.

85. Parkinson CE, Tan JCY: Vitamin A concentration in amniotic fluid and maternal serum related to neural-tube defects. Br J Obstet Gynecol 89:935–939, 1982.

86. Chance PF, Smith DW: Hyperthermia and meningomyelocele and anencephaly. Lancet i:769, 1978.

87. Holmberg PC: Central nervous system defects in children born to mothers exposed to organic solvents during pregnancy. Lancet ii:177, 1979.
88. Ericson A, Kallen B, Westerholm P: Clusters of malformations in Sweden: a study with central registers. Environ Res 30:466–479, 1983.
89. James WH: Clomifene, anencephaly and spina bifida. Lancet i:603, 1977.
90. Winship KA, Cahal DA, Weber JCP, Griffin JP: Maternal drug histories and central nervous system anomalies. Arch Dis Child 59:1052–1060, 1984.
91. Lowe CF: Congenital malformations among infants born to epileptic women. Lancet i:9–10, 1973.
92. Brown NA, Kao J, Fabro S: Teratogenic potential of valproic acid. Lancet i:660–661, 1980.
93. Danks DM, Halliday JL: Incidence of neural tube defects in Victoria, Australia. Lancet i:65, 1983.
94. Stein SC, Feldman JG, Friedlander M, Klein RF: Is myelomeningocele a disappearing disease? Pediatrics 69:511–514, 1982.
95. Kirke P: Epidemiological clues to the causation of neural tube defects: discussion. In: Dobbing J (ed): Prevention of Spina Bifida and Other Neural Tube Defects. Academic Press, London, 1983, pp. 191–192.
96. Seller MJ, Hancock PC: Is recurrence rate of neural tube defects declining? Lancet i:175, 1985.
97. Bjerkedal T, Czeizel A, Goujard J, Kallen B, Mastroiacovo P, Nevin N, Oakley G Jr, Robert E: Valproic acid and spina bifida. Lancet ii:1096, 1982.

CHAPTER 7

Neural Tube Defects: Prenatal Diagnosis and Genetic Counseling

Giovanni Neri

The practice of genetic counseling for neural tube defects (NTD) has changed substantially over the past 15 years with the advent of three major developments, i.e., second-trimester prenatal diagnosis, mass screening of pregnant women for elevated serum α-fetoprotein levels, and vitamin supplementation around the time of conception. On the other hand, the principles on which recurrence risk estimates are based have changed little, the multifactorial model of inheritance being the one that still fits best the epidemiologic data.

Each one of these aspects will be dealt with, with special emphasis on practical implications that are relevant to a modern and comprehensive approach to genetic counseling.

Occurrence and Recurrence Risks

Neural tube defects include three major entities — anencephaly, encefalocele, and spina bifida, the latter term denoting lesions of varying severity, from spina bifida occulta to meningomyelocele. These defects differ from each other for the respective location along the neural tube, but seem to share a common etiology and pathogenetic mechanism, as suggested by the occurrence of either form in different members of the same family. The idea that there is a genetic component in the etiology of NTD rests primarily on the observation that these malformations are not evenly distributed in the populations that have been investigated, but rather have a tendency to recur in certain families. The incidence among sibs of affected individuals is 10- to 30-fold higher than that in the general population, the difference being largest in those populations where the birth prevalence is lowest. There are, in fact, pronounced ethnic variations. Among caucasians birth prevalence varies from around 8/1,000 in Northern Ireland and Wales,[1,2] to 3/1,000 in London,[3] and fewer than 1/1,000 in Italy[4] and Finland.[5] A similarly low prevalence has been reported among orientals and blacks.[6,7]

On the other hand, the birth prevalence of NTD among first-degree relatives of affected index cases is approximately 5%, with minor variations depending on whether the family at risk is from a high- or from a low-prevalence population.[8]

The malformation in the affected relative can be either anencephaly or spina bifida, irrespective of that present in the index case.[9] Since NTD, especially anencephaly, seem to be more common in females, a distinction should be made between the two sexes in calculating recurrence risks. After birth of an affected male, the recurrence risk in sibs is 4.5% for males and 7.2% for females; after birth of an affected female, the corresponding figures are 3.9 and 6.4%, respectively.[10] A 3 to 5% prevalence of NTD was also found among children of individuals with spina bifida who survived to adulthood and reproduced.[11,12]

After a couple has had two affected children, the risk that a third child will be affected varies from 9% for males after two affected females, to 16% for females after two affected males.[10] In contrast, the risk decreases rapidly for more distant relatives: about 2% for nephews and nieces of index cases, and 1% for cousins.[8]

Ethnic variations, sex differences, and recurrence risks all fit best into a model of multifactorial etiology, comprised of heritable polygenic predisposition and environmental factors, whose effects are additive. NTD occur when the total score exceeds a critical threshold.[13,14]

Prenatal Diagnosis

α-Fetoprotein

In 1972 Brock and co-workers[15,16] demonstrated a markedly increased concentration of α-fetoprotein (AFP) in the amniotic fluid of mothers who gave birth to an infant affected by anencephaly or spina bifida cystica. The assay, originally applied to third-trimester pregnancies, was readily adapted to samples of amniotic fluid collected around the 16th week from the last menstrual period, and soon became the most widely used method of prenatal detection of NTD, as reviewed by Brock.[17]

AFP is initially produced by the yolk sac and then by the liver. It represents the main protein component of the fetal serum during the first trimester of gestation. Its concentration declines rapidly thereafter, from a peak of up to 3.0 mg/ml to 50 μg/ml or less in umbilical cord blood.[18] A small amount of AFP is normally excreted in the fetal urine and from there into the amniotic fluid, where it can be found at concentrations 100- to 200-fold lower than in the fetal blood.[19] The increased amount of AFP in the amniotic fluid when the fetus has an NTD is probably due to a direct leak from the fetal circulation through the open lesion. In fact, amniotic AFP concentration is normal in cases of spina bifida occulta, where the defect is covered by skin.[20] Measurements are usually done by immunoelectrophoresis.[16] Standard curves of AFP concentration in amniotic fluid and maternal serum used in our prenatal diagnosis unit are shown in Figure 7.1. An excellent review on the physiopathology of AFP has been published recently.[21]

Before the amniotic AFP assay could be safely applied as a routine test in prenatal diagnosis of NTD, two points had to be clarified: (1) the range of vari-

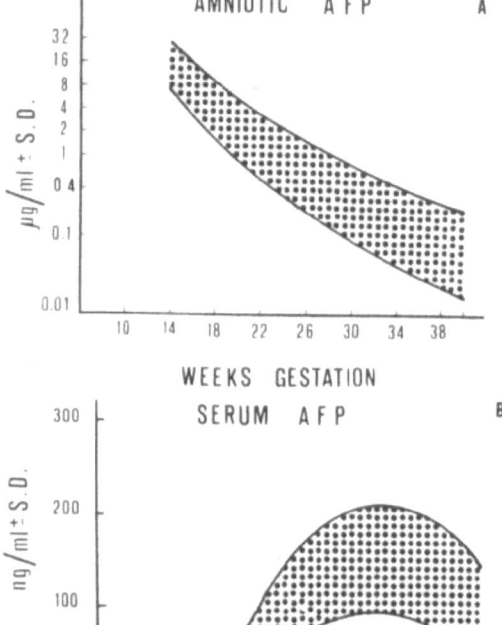

Figure 7.1. α-Fetoprotein concentrations during normal pregnancy in amniotic fluid (**A**) and maternal serum (**B**). Measurements were done by radioimmunoassay at the Prenatal Diagnosis Unit of the Catholic University School of Medicine, Rome. (Courtesy of Professor Umberto Bellati, Department of Obstetrics and Gynecology.)

ability of AFP concentration at various gestational periods in normal pregnancies and in pregnancies with NTD; and (2) the cut-off level between normal and abnormal range, compatible with a minimal proportion of false-positives and false-negatives. The Second Report of the UK collaborative study on AFP in relation to NTD,[22] based on 13,490 fluid samples collected by amniocentesis in the second trimester, provided reliable reference values for normal pregnancies and gave the following cut-off limits, expressed as multiples of the normal median (MoMs): 2.5 MoMs at 13 to 15 weeks, 3.0 MoMs at 16 to 18 weeks, 3.5 MoMs at 19 to 21 weeks, and 4.0 MoMs at 22 to 24 weeks. With this system, only 2% of all open lesions remained undetected (98% sensitivity) and 0.5% of all normal pregnancies turned out to be false-positives (99.5% specificity). These results and conclusions were confirmed by several other studies, such as that of Brock[23] on a series of 3,630 amniotic fluid samples.

Although relatively small, a 0.5% rate of false-positives is rather disturbing because of the large absolute number of pregnancies on which the AFP assay is performed, given the current practice to screen all amniotic fluids for AFP, regardless of the primary indication for prenatal diagnosis.

There are cases in which an elevated AFP is compatible with a normal fetus, such as when the amniotic fluid is contaminated by fetal blood, accidentally leaked during the operation of amniocentesis. In such cases it is advisable to repeat the procedure, after allowing enough time for the fluid to be cleared by contaminating blood. Another more subtle reason of abnormally elevated AFP levels is the undetected presence of an early aborted twin fetus (fetus papyraceous). It is well known[24] that fetal death and resorption causes an increased level of amniotic AFP which, in a case like this, would diffuse into the sac of the normal twin, from where the fluid is aspirated.[25]

However, false-positives are more often associated with an abnormal fetus. Since AFP normally reaches the amniotic fluid through the fetal kidney, impaired kidney function as in congenital nephrosis leads to a massive leak and therefore to elevated amniotic fluid concentrations.[26] Open lesions other than NTD, notably omphalocele, were also found to be in most cases associated with high amniotic levels of AFP.[27,28] Other less frequently reported cases of false-positives with an abnormal fetus are duodenal or esophageal atresia, gastroschisis, Meckel syndrome, Turner syndrome, etc.

All this considered, it has been calculated by Brock[17] that for low-risk populations (e.g., with 0.1% birth prevalence) the predictability of an NTD after a positive amniotic AFP test can be as low as 16% if the sensitivity of the test is adjusted to allow 2% of false-negatives and 0.5% of false-positives.

Other Methods

In view of these limitations, other methods for the prenatal detection of NTD have been proposed, two of which have gained wide acceptance. The one that proved to be by far the most reliable, possibly even more so than the AFP assay, is the acetylcholinesterase (AChE) test. AChE is an enzyme involved in the metabolism of neurotransmitters. It is bound to the membranes of neuronal cells, from which it passes into the cerebrospinal fluid, and into the amniotic fluid in case of an open neural lesion. Measurement is based on a colorimetric assay, after AChE has been separated from nonspecific cholinesterases by polyacrylamide gel electrophoresis.[29] Although this kind of assay is only qualitative, the presence of the AChE band is an all-or-none phenomenon and does not lend itself to ambiguous interpretation.[30]

A Collaborative Acetylcholinesterase Study[31] has demonstrated the high sensitivity, specificity, and valuable role of the AChE assay as an adjunct to the AFP assay for the prenatal detection of NTD, especially in situations with low a priori risk, where the meaning of a positive AFP assay always need to be validated by independent methods. This conclusion was substantially confirmed in a more recent series of 3,700 pregnancies.[32] The assay was shown to be equally useful in confirming the presence of an NTD in cases of borderline AFP levels,[33] and in recognizing those cases where AFP elevation is due to congenital nephrosis.[34]

The other method, also rather widely used, is based on the detection of rapidly adhering cells in the amniotic fluid.[35,36] These cells have been identified as macrophages derived from the fetal brain or spinal cord through an open lesion. Adhesion to the substratum occurs within 24 hours of plating of the cells, and four major morphological types can be recognized: long bipolar cells, cells with multiple processes, large vacuolated cells, and giant multinucleated cells.[37] However, not all laboratories have been equally successful in the implementation of this technique[33] and specificity for NTD does not seem to be very strict.[38]

Other proposed methods, based on the measurement of amniotic IgM,[39] α-2-macroglobulin,[40] fibrinogen degradation products,[41] S-100 protein,[42] and glial fibrillary acidic protein,[43] although they may be of value in the study of the development of the nervous system, did not prove of great practical value in prenatal diagnosis.

One final, obvious consideration is that prenatal diagnosis of NTD, whatever the assay used, should always be substantiated by ultrasound examination of the fetus, especially in a low-risk situation.[44] The accuracy and refinement reached by ultrasonography allowed in a recent series a 100% detection rate for anencephaly and 80% detection rate for open spina bifida.[45] This, in conjunction with similar progress in other areas of fetal medicine, makes ultrasonography a primary tool in prenatal diagnosis.

Population Screening

Prenatal diagnosis of NTD is usually offered only to high-risk mothers, i.e., those who had a previous child with anencephaly or spina bifida. However, affected fetuses of these mothers account for only 10% of all children born with NTD. Prenatal detection of the remaining 90% could be considered only if a noninvasive, low-cost assay were available.

In 1973 it was reported independently by two groups[46,47] that elevated levels of AFP in the amniotic fluid are paralleled by elevated levels in the maternal serum, although at a 1,000-fold lower concentration. The implication of this finding in connection with the prenatal diagnosis of NTD was quickly realized and led to a number of clinical trials, aimed at determining the effectiveness of this method for NTD prevention and its applicability to mass population screening. The issue received special consideration in Great Britain, where the birth prevalence of NTD is approximately 5/1,000. A UK collaborative study published in 1977[48] came to the conclusion that screening for maternal serum AFP (MSAFP) at 16 to 18 weeks of gestation could detect 88% of all cases of anencephaly and 79% of cases of open spina bifida. These encouraging results opened the way to a number of prospective studies, recently summarized by Ferguson-Smith,[49] through which several important points could be clearly established.

Since MSAFP concentration increases steeply from 13 weeks of gestation to peak at about 32 weeks, it is essential that the gestational age at the time when the assay is performed be precisely known. When a result is obtained that is clearly abnormal for that gestational age, one must first rule out two possibilities: (1) a twin pregnancy, usually accompanied by elevated MSAFP;[50] and (2) a missed or threatened abortion. Ultrasonography and clinical examination will usually clarify either situation and settle the issue. Overall, 30 to 40% of cases with elevated MSAFP are due either to miscalculation of the gestational age, or to twin pregnancy or to abortion. Of the remaining cases, approximately 90% are associated with the presence of a fetus with NTD, and 10% with another abnormality such as abdominal wall defects, chromosomal abnormalities, congenital nephrosis, etc.[49] Not all of these cases subsequently require amniocentesis. Some, like anencephaly, can be simply diagnosed by ultrasound. On average, no more than 1% of all cases screened for MSAFP will require amniocentesis. The proportion of apparently normal pregnancies terminated because of a false-positive AFP or AChE test in the amniotic fluid was in most series fewer than 1/20,000 screened pregnancies.[51]

It has been pointed out[52] that amniocentesis performed following an elevated MSAFP result carries a high risk (approximately 10%) of subsequent fetal loss by miscarriage. This may be due to the fact that an elevated MSAFP not associated with fetal abnormality is likely to be the indicator of an unrecognized threatened abortion and therefore of a preexisting risk to miscarry, independent of amniocentesis.[53]

Nearly 10 years of experience with MSAFP screening for the detection of NTD have been summarized at a consensus meeting,[51] with the conclusion that "MSAFP screening of pregnant women is advisable at least in populations with a birth prevalence of NTD of 1 in 1000 or higher". Screening programs are apparently effective in reducing substantially the birth prevalence of NTD,[49,54] and seem to be cost-effective, owing to the decreased number of surviving spina bifida patients who need lifelong support.[55,56] However, financial considerations are admittedly of limited value in an issue so heavily burdened by emotion and suffering. Human benefits and costs must also be considered,[57] as well as ethical implications, which make it especially important that each step of the screening program, and its consequences, be clearly understood and freely accepted by participating families.

Prevention

According to the multifactorial model of causation of NTD, a number of "risk genes" predisposes the embryo to the action of environmental factors, capable of interfering with the normal closure of the neural tube. The existence of such factors is largely conjectural, and their nature a very much debated matter. However, during the last 20 years some consistent evidence has been gathered, pointing to the possible role of adverse dietary factors. This was originally suspected on the basis of the observation that at least in the UK NTD are more prevalent among lower socioeconomic classes whose diet is poor, and display a seasonal variation, with a higher incidence among children conceived during winter and spring, when fresh food is more expensive and more difficult to obtain.

Laurence and co-workers were among the first to test this hypothesis, and showed in a retrospective study on a group of women who had had a previous child with NTD that there were no recurrences among those who switched to a good diet during the subsequent pregnancy, compared to a 10% recurrence among those who continued on a poor diet. These results were confirmed by a second study aimed at improving the diet of high-risk women in the course of a subsequent pregnancy. It was clearly shown that recurrences of NTD took place only among women who stayed on a poor diet.[59]

Circumstantial evidence that folic acid might be the crucial element missing or deficient in a poor diet led to a folic acid supplementation trial in which a group of high-risk mothers were treated periconceptionally (1 month before and 2 after) with 4 mg of folic acid per day, while a comparable group was given a placebo. Compliance to the supplementation regimen was checked by measuring folic acid concentration in serum. The overall quality of the diet was also taken into consideration, as done in the previous studies. An NTD recurrence rate of 6.4% was reported in the placebo group, versus 3.3% in the folate-supplemented group. However, all cases in the latter group occurred in women who were non-compliers, as judged by their serum folate levels. There were no recurrences among mothers on a good or a fair diet, irrespective of folic acid supplementation.[60]

Similar results were obtained by Smithells and co-workers,[61] who treated a group of high-risk women with a multivitamin complex, including folic acid, starting at least 28 days prior to conception and until the date of the second missed period. Although a control group treated with placebo was not included in the trial for direct comparison, recurrence of NTD among the offspring of the vitamin-supplemented women was significantly lower than expected for that population.

In spite of the fact that there still are a number of open questions concerning the role of vitamins, and which vitamins, in the prevention of NTD, and whether vitamin deprivation represents a risk factor also for populations outside the British Isles, there is no doubt that the results obtained so far are very encouraging and cannot be disregarded.

Genetic Counseling

The facts presented above represent the basis on which to formulate genetic counseling for the prevention of NTD. The risk of a first case for any couple is given by the birth prevalence of NTD in the population to which the couple belongs, and varies approximately from 5/1,000 in areas of high incidence to 1/1,000 or less in areas of low incidence. The risk of a second case, i.e., the recurrence risk for a couple who already had a previous affected child, is 10- to 30-fold higher than the occurrence risk, and varies usually from 3% in low-incidence areas to 5 to 8% in high-incidence areas. Similar risk figures apply to parents who are themselves affected by a mild form of spina bifida, compatible with procreation.

Besides the quantitative estimate, it is very important that the counselor clearly specifies the quality of the risk in a situation where the severity of the malformation varies from anencephaly to true meningocele. The former is lethal; the latter does not usually cause any serious disability. Therefore neither puts on the parents the lifelong burden of dealing with a severely disabled child. This leaves meningomyelocele and encephalocele as sole potential causes of serious handicap. However, a relatively large proportion of these infants are stillborn or will die in the first year of life. Taking all these circumstances into account, it has been calculated that for a couple who already had a child with NTD, the risk of having a second who will survive with a serious handicap is approximately 1.5%.[9]

If a couple has two previous children who are both affected by NTD, the risk for a third one to be similarly affected is about 10 to 15%, as to be expected for a multifactorial condition.

There is perhaps already enough evidence to reduce cautiously the above estimates of recurrence risk if it can be ensured that the woman will adhere to a good diet and/or vitamin supplementation, starting before conception and for at least 2 months thereafter. However, there is really no evidence that dietary improvement and vitamin supplementation have protective value outside those populations where trials were conducted.

Prenatal diagnosis has become an integral part of genetic counseling since it became an established clinical procedure more than 10 years ago. It is most commonly performed by measuring the concentration of AFP in the amniotic fluid at 16 to 20 weeks gestation. Determination of AChE is a useful adjunct. Ultrasound examination of the fetus should always be an essential part of the diagnostic procedure. Based on existing experience, it seems that the only consistent hazard associated with prenatal diagnosis is 1% risk of abortion consequent to amniocentesis.

Genetic counseling *must* be *nondirective*. This is particularly so in the case of prenatal diagnosis, which should be freely accepted or rejected by the informed couple, based on knowledge of the risks and benefits and on ethical considerations. There is not at the moment an effective prenatal treatment for a malformed fetus, and selective abortion has become common practice. The decision for or against it rests entirely on the parents and constitutes for them a grave moral dilemma. This is an important issue to raise in the course of the interview between the counselor and the couple, which should always precede the diagnosis.

Prenatal diagnosis is usually offered only to "high-risk" couples, namely those who had a previous child affected by NTD. However, only about 10% of NTD children are born to these couples, the other 90% being apparently sporadic. Low-risk couples can be counseled to an accurate fetal ultrasound and to measurement of maternal serum AFP at 16 weeks gestation.

Similarly, genetic counseling is in most cases sought by couples who already had an affected child and who, quite understandably, went through a period of great suffering. Therefore, the question of the recurrence risk, and of what can be done about it, must be approached tactfully, and yet in clear and comprehensible terms, allowing all the time needed for emotional readjustment and for a full understanding of the options available. Before prenatal diagnosis, fewer than 20% of high-risk couples receiving genetic counseling decided on another pregnancy within a year.[63] After prenatal diagnosis, this attitude seems to have changed drastically, with about 80% of couples opting for another pregnancy within a year.[8] It appears, therefore, that availability of prenatal diagnosis, although not affecting the decision on the number of subsequent children, made the decision easier to reach and the pregnancy more enjoyable.[64]

With much progress already made, it is now only to be hoped that additional clinical trials and more basic research on the causative role of environmental factors will allow a rapid progression from secondary to primary prevention of NTD.

Summary

Genetic counseling for the prevention of NTD is usually sought by, and offered to, those couples who already had a child with anencephaly, encephalocele, or spina bifida, and whose risk of having another one similarly affected is about 3 to 5%. This estimate could perhaps be reduced somewhat, if the woman adheres to a good diet or receives vitamin supplementation for 1 month before conception and 2 months thereafter. Prenatal diagnosis should be offered to all at-risk couples, by means of ultrasound visualization of the fetal head and spine and α-fetoprotein measurement in the amniotic fluid obtained by amniocentesis at 16 to 18 weeks' gestation. Ultrasound and maternal serum α-fetoprotein screening may be offered to all pregnant women, especially those from populations with high prevalence of neural tube defects.

References

1. Elwood JH, Nevin NC: Factors associated with anencephalus and spina bifida in Belfast. Br J Prev Soc Med 27:73–80, 1973.
2. Laurence KM, Carter CO, David PA: The central nervous system malformations in South Wales. I. Incidence, local variations and geographical factors. Br J Prev Soc Med 22:146–152, 1968.
3. Carter CO, Evans KA: Spina bifida and anencephalus in Greater London. J Med Genet 10:209–234, 1973.
4. Mastroiacovo P: Epidemiologia dei difetti del tubo neurale. Giorn Neurops Etá Evol 4:207–222, 1984.
5. Granroth G, Hakama M, Saxén L: Defects of the central nervous system in Finland: I. Variations in time and space, sex distribution, and parental age. Br J Prev Soc Med 31:164–170, 1977.
6. Emanuel I, Huang SW, Gutman LT, Yu FC, Lin CC: The incidence of congenital malformations in a Chinese population. Teratology 5:159–170, 1972.
7. Ogbalu MM, Leck I, Hillier VF: The prevalence of malformations at birth in Southern Nigeria. Paper presented at the Fifth International Conference on Birth Defects, Montreal, Canada, 1977.

8. Laurence KM: Prevention of neural tube malformations by genetic counselling and prenatal diagnostic surveillance. J Genet Hum 27:289–299, 1979.

9. Laurence KM: The recurrence risk in spina bifida cystica and anencephaly. Dev Med Child Neurol 11(Suppl 20):23–30, 1969.

10. Lalouel JM, Morton NE, Jackson J: Neural tube malformations: complex segregation analysis and calculation of recurrence risks. J Med Genet 16:8–13, 1979.

11. Carter CO, Evans K: Children of adult survivors with spina bifida cystica. Lancet ii:924–926, 1973.

12. Laurence KM, Beresford A: Fifty-one adults with spina bifida; continence, friends, marriage and children. Dev Med Child Neurol 17(Suppl 35):123–128, 1975.

13. WHO Scientific Group on Genetic Factors in Congenital Malformations: Genetic factors in congenital malformations. WHO Tech Rep Serv No 438, 1970.

14. Carter CO: Clues to the aetiology of neural tube malformations. Dev Med Child Neurol 16(Suppl 32):3–15.

15. Brock DJH, Scrimgeour JB: Early prenatal diagnosis of anencephaly. Lancet ii:1252–1253, 1972.

16. Brock DJH, Sutcliffe RG: Alpha fetoprotein in the antenatal diagnosis of anencephaly and spina bifida. Lancet ii:197–199, 1972.

17. Brock DJH: Amniotic fluid tests for fetal neural tube defects. Br Med Bull 39:373–377, 1983.

18. Gitlin D, Boesman M: Sites of serum alphafetoprotein synthesis in the human and in the rat. J Clin Invest 45:1826–1834, 1966.

19. Brock DJH: The molecular character of alphafetoprotein in C.N.S. malformations. Clin Chim Acta 87:315–320, 1974.

20. Laurence KM, Turnbull AC, Harris R, Jennison RF, Ruoslathi E, Seppala M: Antenatal diagnosis of spina bifida. Lancet ii:860, 1973.

21. Adinolfi M: Human alphafetoprotein 1956–1978. Adv Hum Genet 9:165–228, 1979.

22. Second Report of the UK Collaborative Study on Alpha-fetoprotein in Relation to Neural-tube Defects: amniotic-fluid alpha-fetoprotein measurement in antenatal diagnosis of anencephaly and open spina bifida in early pregnancy. Lancet ii:651–662, 1979.

23. Brock DJH: The use of amniotic fluid AFP action limits in diagnosing open neural tube defects. Prenat Diagn 1:11–16, 1981.

24. Kleijer WJ, De Bruijn HWA, Leschot NJ: Amniotic fluid alpha-fetoprotein levels and prenatal diagnosis of neural tube defects: a collaborative study of 2180 pregnancies in the Netherlands. Br J Obstet Gynecol 85:512–517, 1978.

25. Duncan SLB, Ginz B, Ward AM, Hingley SM: Amniotic fluid AFP in multiple pregnancy. Br Med J 1:1354, 1977.

26. Seppala M, Ranta T, Aula P, Ruoslathi E: Alpha-fetoprotein in normal and abnormal pregnancy. In Lehmann FG (ed): Carcino-Embryonic Proteins. Vol 1, Elsevier, Amsterdam, 1979, pp 191–197.

27. Brock DJH: Neural tube defects (AFP-analysis) in amniotic fluid and maternal serum. In Murken JD, Stengel-Rutkowski S, Schwinger E (eds): Proceedings of the Third European Conference on Prenatal Diagnosis of Genetic Disorders. Ferdinand Enke, Stuttgart, 1979, pp 87–93.

28. Wald NJ, Cuckle HS, Barlow RD, Smith AD, Stirrat GM, Turnbull AC, Bobrow M, Brock DJH, Stein SM: Early antenatal diagnosis of exomphalos. Lancet ii:1368–1369, 1980.

29. Smith AD, Wald NJ, Cuckle HS, Stirrat GM, Bobrow M, Lagercrantz H: Amniotic fluid acetylcholinesterase as a possible diagnostic test for neural tube defects in early pregnancy. Lancet ii:685–688, 1979.

30. Wyvill PC, Hullin DA, Elder GH, Laurence KM: A prospective study of amniotic fluid cholinesterases: comparison of quantitative and qualitative methods for detection of open spina bifida in early pregnancy. Prenat Diagn 4:319–327, 1984.

31. Report of the Collaborative Acetylcholinesterase Study: Amniotic fluid acetylcholinesterase electrophoresis as a secondary test in the diagnosis of anencephaly and open spina bifida in early pregnancy. Lancet ii:321–324, 1981.

32. Aitken DA, Morrison NM, Ferguson-Smith MA: Predictive value of amniotic acetylcholinesterase analysis in the diagnosis of fetal abnormality in 3700 pregnancies. Prenat Diagn 4:329–340, 1984.

33. Seller MJ, Cole KJ, Merritt BL: Alphafetoprotein, cholinesterases and rapidly adhering cells in the prenatal diagnosis of neural tube defects. Prenat Diagn 1:7–10, 1981.

34. Brock DJH, Hayward C, Seppala M: Distinguishing neural tube defects and congenital nephrosis by amniotic fluid assay. Lancet i:773, 1980.

35. Sutherland GR, Brock DJH, Scrimgeour JB: Amniotic fluid macrophages and anencephaly. Lancet ii:1098–1099, 1973.

36. Gosden CM, Brock DJH: Morphology of rapidly adhering amniotic fluid cells as an aid to the diagnosis of neural tube defects. Lancet i:919–922, 1977.

37. Gosden CM, Brock DJH, Eason PJ: The origin of the rapidly adhering cells found in amniotic fluids from foetuses with neural tube defects. Clin Genet 12:193–201, 1977.

38. Bobrow M, Evans CJ, Noble J, Patel C: Cellular content of amniotic fluid as predictor of central nervous system malformations. J Med Genet 15:97–100, 1978.

39. Cantuaria AA, Jones AL: Immunoglobulin M in human amniotic fluid and its possible association with neural tube malformations. Br J Obstet Gynecol 82:262–264, 1975.

40. Brock DJH: Amniotic fluid alpha-2-macroglobulin and the antenatal diagnosis of spina bifida and anencephaly. Clin Genet 8:297–301, 1975.

41. Purdie DW, Howie PW, Edgar W, Forbes CD, Prentice CRM: Raised amniotic fluid fibrinogen degradation products in fetal neural tube anomalies. Lancet i:1013–1014, 1975.

42. Sindic CJM, Freund M, Van Regemorter N, Verellen-Demoulin C, Masson PL: S-100 protein in amniotic fluid of anencephalic fetuses. Prenat Diagn 4:297–302, 1984.

43. Albrechtsen M, Bock E: Glial fibrillary acidic protein in amniotic fluids from pregnancies with neural tube defects. Prenat Diagn 4:405–410, 1984.

44. Persson PH, Kullander S, Gennser G, Grennert L, Laurell CS: Screening for fetal malformations using ultrasound and measurement of alpha-fetoprotein in maternal serum. Br Med J 286:747–749, 1983.

45. Roberts CJ, Evans KT, Hibbard BM, Laurence KM, Roberts EE, Robertson IB: Diagnostic effectiveness of ultrasound in detection of neural tube defects. Lancet ii:1068–1069, 1983.

46. Brock DJH, Bolton AE, Monaghan JM: Prenatal diagnosis of anencephaly through maternal serum alphafetoprotein measurement. Lancet ii:923–924, 1973.

47. Leek AE, Ruoss CF, Kitau MJ, Chard T: Raised alpha-fetoprotein in maternal serum with anencephalic pregnancy. Lancet ii:385, 1973.

48. Report of UK Collaborative Study on Alpha-fetoprotein in Relation to Neural-tube Defects: maternal serum-alpha-fetoprotein measurement in antenatal screening for anencephaly and spina bifida in early pregnancy. Lancet i:1323–1332, 1977.

49. Ferguson-Smith MA: The reduction of anencephalic and spina bifida births by maternal serum alpha-fetoprotein screening. Br Med Bull 39:365–372, 1983.

50. Ghosh A, Woo JSK, Rawlinson HA, Ferguson-Smith MA: Prognostic significance of raised serum alpha-fetoprotein levels in twin pregnancies. Br J Obstet Gynecol 89:817–820, 1982.

51. Special Report: Maternal serum alpha-fetoprotein screening for neural tube defects. Results of a consensus meeting. Prenat Diagn 5:77–83, 1985.

52. Bennet MJ: Fetal loss after second-trimester amniocentesis in women with raised serum-alpha-fetoprotein. Lancet ii:987, 1978.

53. Ferguson-Smith MA, Gibson AAM, Whitfield CR, Ratcliffe JG: Amniocentesis and the alpha-fetoprotein screening programme. Lancet i:39–40, 1979.

54. Roberts CJ, Hibbard BM, Elder GH, Evans KT, Laurence KM, Roberts A, Woodhead JS, Robertson IB, Hoole M: The efficacy of a serum screening service for neural tube defects: the South Wales experience. Lancet i:1315–1318, 1983.

55. Hagard S, Carter F, Milne RG: Screening for spina bifida cystica – a cost benefit analysis. Br J Soc Prev Med 30:40–53, 1976.

56. Sadovnick AD, Baird PA: A cost-benefit analysis of a population screening programme for neural tube defects. Prenat Diagn 3:117–126, 1983.

57. Chamberlain J: Human benefits and costs of a national screening programme for neural-tube defects. Lancet ii:1293–1296, 1978.

58. Laurence KM, James N, Miller M, Campbell H: Increased risk of recurrence of neural tube defects to mothers on poor diets and the possible benefit of dietary counselling. Br Med J 281:1542–1544, 1980.

59. James N, Laurence KM, Miller M: Diet as a factor in the aetiology of neural tube malformations. Zeit Kinderchir 31:302–307, 1980.

60. Laurence KM, James N, Miller M, Tennant GP, Campbell H: Double-blind randomised controlled trial of folate treatment before conception to prevent recurrences in neural tube defects. Br Med J 282:1509–1511, 1981.

61. Smithells RW, Sheppard S, Schorah CJ, Seller MJ, Nevin NC, Harris R, Read AP, Fielding DW: Apparent prevention of neural tube defects by periconceptional vitamin supplementation. Arch Dis Child 56:911–918, 1981.

62. Dobbing J: Prevention of Spina Bifida and Other Neural Tube Defects. Academic Press, London, 1983.

63. Morris J, Laurence KM: The effectiveness of genetic counselling for neural tube malformations. Dev Med Child Neurol 18(Suppl 37):157–163, 1976.

64. Laurence KM, Morris J: The effect of the introduction of prenatal diagnosis in the reproductive history of women at increased risk from neural tube defects. Prenat Diagn 1:51–60, 1981.

CHAPTER 8

Meningomyelocele: Surgical Treatment and Results

David C. McCullough

Meningomyelocele is both the most common and the most severe of the verte-brospinal dysraphic states. It is a complex central nervous system disorder with implications for the musculoskeletal and genitourinary systems. Management and outcome are strongly influenced by the extent of cerebral and spinal cord involvement in individual cases.

The cornerstone of management of meningomyelocele is thorough initial evaluation by a coordinated multidisciplinary team that will provide sophisti-cated counseling for parents and future continuity of care.[1] Experience and regu-lar communication between team members enable them to avoid therapeutic misadventures and to convey realistic appraisals and expectations to family members. For this reason, newborn infants with myelodysplasia should be referred to a specialized pediatric center for initial evaluation and management. Because prenatal ultrasonography has instigated the disclosure of gestational cases of spina bifida[2] such referral is also appropriate for counseling of mothers and families of potential patients diagnosed in utero.

Systematic efforts for repair of meningomyeloceles were first stimulated by the introduction in the 1950s of valve-regulated cerebrospinal fluid (CSF) shunts for hydrocephalus. Medical requirements of surviving children with relatively well-controlled hydrocephalus generated the multidisciplinary care programs of the 1960s. Pediatricians, neurosurgeons, urologists, and orthopedists began to col-laborate to provide coordinated, centralized treatment programs.

After extensive experience with centralized care of numerous myelodysplastic children, evaluation of results began to emerge in the 1970s. This afforded the first significant opportunity to analyze outcome in terms of the initial extent of the lesions, producing the concept of selective intervention.[3-7] This, in turn, generated a controversy that has endured well into the present era. Pronounce-ments of ethicists, clerics, jurists, administrators, and legislators have been added to those of clinicians in efforts to influence the medical management of infants born with spina bifida cystica.[6,8] Although certain aspects of therapy and progno-sis can be readily documented and comprehended at present, the lifelong impli-cations of the disorder remain under critical study. As the facts continue to reveal themselves, improved methods of initial evaluation and continuing therapy can be expected to emerge.

A Review of Therapy and Results

Selection: Results in Untreated Patients

The controversial issue of selection for therapy influences the evaluation of results and the therapeutic attitudes of clinicians. Prior to the development of satisfactory methods of treating hydrocephalus, the practice of selecting candidates for repair of meningomyeloceles appears to have been consistent.[9] With the potentially effective tools of implantable CSF shunts at hand neurosurgeons seriously began to attempt salvage of newborns with myelodysplasia. Lorber's review of a large number of unselected patients in 1971[6] inspired his recommendation that infants with certain "adverse criteria" be denied active care. This restrained the enthusiasm of many neurosurgeons, but in at least one positive aspect stimulated some of the first critical evaluations of the fate of both treated and untreated infants in other medical centers. Subsequent reports demonstrate that most untreated babies die within the first year[10,11] but some survive well beyond infancy.[9,12]

To this day reports of the outcome of selective therapy reveal an absence of strict adherence to the "adverse criteria" of Lorber. As many as 50%[11,13] or as few as 10%[14,15] go untreated. This obviously biases results in terms of complications, outcome for treated cases, and survival of the untreated. Without detailing the difficult subject of quality of life among the untreated, various reviews from 1966 through 1985 disclose 1-year mortality rates of 84 to 100%.[11,16-18] Cautious interpretation of such data is warranted, since many patients who are denied initial surgery may later come to repair.

Timing of Repair

Emergency operative intervention is seldom necessary in newborn infants with meningomyelocele, but delay beyond 48 hours definitely increases the possibility of central nervous system infection.[19,20] Late closure may also result in decreasing motor function in some patients. Charney et al. recently advocated the allotment of time for careful medical evaluation of newborn infants and counseling of parents.[16] Although the value of complete evaluation and appropriate instruction of responsible family members is unquestionable, most authorities agree that surgical repair within 24 to 48 hours is a reasonable practice.[19-21]

An early study of alternately treated and untreated infants disclosed consistent deterioration of motor function in patients in whom treatment was delayed and functional improvement in a remarkable number of patients who were treated early.[22] McLone et al.[23] found a 37% incidence of ventriculitis among infants with delayed repair compared to a 7% incidence in those treated early. In their selected series Charney et al.[16] claimed no significant consequences of delay on neurologic function, developmental disability, or ventriculitis. Those authors, however, attested to the importance of antibiotics in the prevention of ventriculitis in delayed cases.

Table 8.1. Myelomeningocele: operative and early[a] postoperative mortality

Author	Year	No. of cases	Mortality (%)
Unselective series			
Ingraham[25]	1943	279	12
Lorber[6b]	1971	524	15–19
Ames and Schut[24]	1972	171	4
Naglo and Hellstrom[26]	1976	59	0
McLone et al.[19]	1985	200	2
Selective series			
Althouse and Wald[3]	1980	93	6
Lorber and Salfield[11]	1981	42	10
Gross et al.[13]	1983	36	0
Charney et al.[16]	1985	96	4
McCullough[14]	1986	100	2

[a] 1–60 days.
[b] Two sequential series.

Operative Mortality

In series where selection of cases occurred the mortality rates from repair of meningomyeloceles ranged from 2 to 19%. In unselected series there was a similar mortality rate, ranging from 2 to 12%. Intraoperative death is currently exceedingly rare and early postoperative mortality (1 to 60 days) approaches 2% (Table 8.1).[3,6,11,13,14,19,24-26] Unusual anesthetic, hemorrhagic, and transfusion complications contribute slightly to intraoperative mortality, whereas postoperative deaths are usually caused either by infectious or respiratory complications.

Operative and Early Postoperative Morbidity

Infection

Early meningitis and ventriculitis are potentially extremely damaging. These either occur as primary complications or may be first disclosed after shunt therapy for hydrocephalus. Some surgeons advocate meningomyelocele repair and CSF shunting as initial combined procedures,[27] whereas others recommend primary shunting followed by meningomyelocele repair as necessary.[28] Although there is no evidence that either of these methods increases risks of infection, the standard practice remains first to repair the lesion and to insert the shunt during a later procedure.[21] Contemporary series establish the incidence of early infection as 3 to 10% when repair is performed within 48 hours of birth.[11,14,19] Including episodes of early ventriculitis after shunt insertion, the author has observed an incidence of 4% of cases (including one death).

The devastating effects of neonatal ventriculitis on intellect of survivors with myelodysplasia are well documented.[23,29] The mean intellectual quotient (IQ) in ventriculitis victims was at least 30 points lower than the IQ in noninfected patients. The younger infants with gram-negative infections suffer most.

Wound Complications

Local wound complications relate to the size of lesions, technique of repair, and the severity of uncontrolled hydrocephalus after repair. Aside from the subject of CSF leaks after repair (6 to 23% of cases[30,31]), the literature is sparse on the specific incidence of wound disruption or problems of healing. The plethora of innovative suggestions for the repair of large lesions would seem to indicate that a problem exists. Various publications have described Z-plasty,[32] relaxing incisions,[33] gradual mobilization of flaps with tension-producing foreign materials,[34] myocutaneous flaps,[35-37] free skin grafts,[21] excision of protruding pedicles, and primary kyphectomy.[9] In the hands of experienced neurosurgeons primary vertical or horizontal linear closure, aided by extensive undermining of adjacent skin, usually suffices to prevent wound disruption, CSF fistula, ulceration, or abscess formation.[14]

Neurologic Consequences of Repair

Preservation of vital remaining motor, sensory, or, if applicable, sphincter function represent crucial objectives of early repair of meningomyeloceles. The establishment of an accurate assessment of the preoperative neurologic status of each patient, as recommended by Stark,[38] provides a reasonable check on the delicacy of surgical technique. Supplemental electrodiagnostic testing may be helpful. Reigel et al.[39] use intraoperative evoked somatosensory potentials for monitoring repair. This methodology has not yet become standard. The author has used nerve stimulators to assist in the identification of viable neural elements, but has found the technique to be misleading and less useful than low-power optical magnification.

Few citations in the literature provide data on the subject of neural injury with meningomyelocele repair. Table 8.2 summarizes the subject with reference to improvement or deterioration of motor and sensory function associated with surgery. Recent data indicate that 4 to 7% of infants show increased deficit and 4 to

Table 8.2. Myelomeningocele: change in neurological deficit after repair

Author	Year	No. of cases	Improvement (%)	Deterioration (%)
Ingraham[25]	1943	132	7	11
Sharrard et al.[22]	1967	238	21	4
Guthkelch et al.[30]	1981	63	13	7
McLone et al.[19]	1985	200	37	—
McCullough[14]	1986	100	4	3

37% improve.[14,19,30] Although the record discloses significant gains, reports of improvement in extremely high percentages of patients may reflect overly pessimistic preoperative assessments.

Exacerbation of Hydrocephalus

Although approximately 90% of patients with meningomyelocele have ventriculomegaly at birth[40] only a minority have overt signs of hydrocephalus.[21] Clearly, the exacerbation of progressive hydrocephalus is a frequent consequence of repair of the spinal lesion.[25,41,42] Various mechanisms have been proposed, including infectious or chemical meningitis, packing of cerebellar–medullary tissue at the foramen magnum (producing IVth ventricle outlet or aqueductal obstruction), and removal of the sac that served as a CSF pulse pressure "sink" or an absorptive surface. Linder et al.[43] recently verified the augmentation of CSF pulse pressure in a patient after repair. Except for the theoretic absorptive role of the sac any of the proposed mechanisms may contribute to acceleration of hydrocephalus. This issue is somewhat academic in that repair is generally desirable and over 70% of patients will eventually require shunt therapy.[14]

Long-Term Results: Survival and Handicap

Longevity and Quality of Survival

The severity of hydrocephalus, levels of paralysis, and associated birth defects are important influences on the mortality and morbidity in spina bifida cystica. But experienced clinicians dispute the teaching that ultimate quality of life is consistently predictable from assessment of deficit in neonates.[42,44] Complications of hydrocephalus, brain stem, and cranial nerve deficits and central nervous system infection primarily determine early mortality while sequelae of the neurogenic bladder influence late mortality. Table 8.3 demonstrates that survival has increased in sequential series. Mortality in treated cases is curbed by policies of selective intervention. In unselected series current mortality figures after 1 to 12 years of follow-up range from 14 to 19%.[19,24,25] When selection is practiced, 1- to 15-year mortality is 3 to 14%.[3,11,13,21]

Morbidity among survivors relates to hydrocephalus and complications of its treatment, but also to the extent of paralysis and to orthopedic conditions such as spinal kyphosis and hip dysplasia. Published data reveal that the intellectual capacities of survivors have steadily improved in both the selective and unselective series.[11,13,14,16,20,27] Significant learning disabilities (IQ below 80) can be expected in 15 to 35% of patients.

With modern urologic management, emphasizing the early institution of intermittent clean catheterization and pharmacotherapy, urinary complications and incontinence have progressively declined. Now, various investigators report that 50 to 90% of children with spina bifida cystica are continent of urine.[19,45] Over 70% of children will become ambulatory with or without assistive devices and most remain so at least into the middle teenage years.[14,19]

Table 8.3. Myelomeningocele: combined early and late mortality in treated cases

Author	Year	No. of cases	Years follow-up	Mortality (%)
Unselective series				
Lorber[6]	1971	524	3–12	41–63[a]
Ames and Schut[24]	1972	171	4–9	19
Naglo and Hellstrom[26]	1976	59	5–12	18
McLone et al.[19]	1985	200	1–10	14
Selective series				
Althouse and Wald[3]	1980	93	5	23
O'Brien and McLanahan[21]	1980	63	1–9	8
Lorber and Salfield[11]	1981	42	5–10	14
Gross et al.[13]	1983	36	1–6	3
McCullough[14]	1986	100	1–15	4

[a] Two sequential series.

Respiratory Problems

Pharyngeal constrictor or laryngeal muscle paralysis secondary to the Chiari II malformation present potentially life-threatening complications of the disorder. McLone et al.[19] stated that 13% of their patients had severe stridor and respiratory disorders. Early swallowing problems may result in aspiration, and laryngeal palsies may be associated with periods of apnea and serious airway obstruction. The clinical management of these patients is controversial. Park et al.[46] performed posterior fossa-cervical decompressions in 17% of their large series of patients. Although their postoperative mortality rate was high, those authors argued that failures could be attributed to delayed intervention. I have witnessed stridor in 4% of my patients, with one neonate expiring of aspiration and one infant requiring tracheostomy. Using careful respiratory care and monitoring, all the other patients have survived with the stridor subsiding after the first year of life.[14]

Tethered Cord

There are insufficient long-term data to evaluate the importance of spinal cord tethering in the production of late progression of neurologic deficit in meningomyelocele patients. In his series of 102 patients with symptomatic tethering, Reigel[47] noted that 90 had previously repaired meningomyeloceles. The mean age at presentation was 10 years. Diverse associated pathology included lipomas, granulomas, dermoids, teratomas, diastometomyelia, and stitch granulomas (sutured neural placodes). Recently, some surgeons have advocated inversion of neural placodes as part of initial repair procedures to prevent late tethering.[31,48] Except for one equivocal analysis by Guthkelch et al.[30] there is no reliable body of evidence to establish the value of this technique.

Hydromyelia and Scoliosis

Subtle progressive neurologic deficit and spinal curvature may be consequences of hydromyelia that appear many years after primary repair of meningomyeloceles.[49,50] Some patients respond to efficient ventricular CSF shunting, but others may require cystoperitoneal diversion, direct drainage, or foramen magnum decompression.[27,50] The recently introduced magnetic resonance imaging (MRI) procedure should prove to be a powerful tool in screening for this complication.

Evaluation and Management

Transport and Early Protective Care

Infants delivered with signs of myelodysplasia deserve evaluation by a qualified spina bifida team. After initial determination of cardiorespiratory stability, they may be transported in a warming isolette with appropriate monitoring. The lesion itself, whether closed or open and leaking, should be covered with moist sterile saline-gauze dressings surrounded by a protective soft gauze doughnut and overlaid with a plastic sheet. If an intravenous line has been started prior to transport, prophylactic antibiotics should be started and continued throughout the period of evaluation and early treatment.

Evaluation by the Spina Bifida Team

After arrival at the treating facility the neonate should be examined in a comfortable, warm environment by the pediatrician and neurosurgeon. The general physical examination should be thorough in the search for associated birth defects such as congenital heart disease and gastrointestinal and genitourinary system anomalies. All of these are relatively infrequent, but influence the prognostic information that should be conveyed to parents. Radiographic and sonographic diagnostic studies are performed only if the initial physical examination suggests systemic anomalies.

The neurologic and musculoskeletal evaluation should be performed under normothermic conditions, with the infant as alert and content as possible. Head circumference, fontanel tone, and cranial defects (such as cranium bifidum) should be noted and recorded. Most newborns with spinal dysraphism do not have macrocephaly, although ventriculomegaly is the rule rather than the exception.[26,40] The size and location of the myelodysplastic lesion is next determined, followed by the character of spinal and lower extremity skeletal deformities (Fig. 8.1). Talipes equinovarus, tibial dysplasia, and hip dysplasia are common paralytic deformities that will require attention. Determination of the neurologic deficit largely results from observation. Stimulation of levels well above the site of the lesion usually produce active motion among the remaining innervated muscle groups. Movements elicited from stimulation of lower extremities may be of

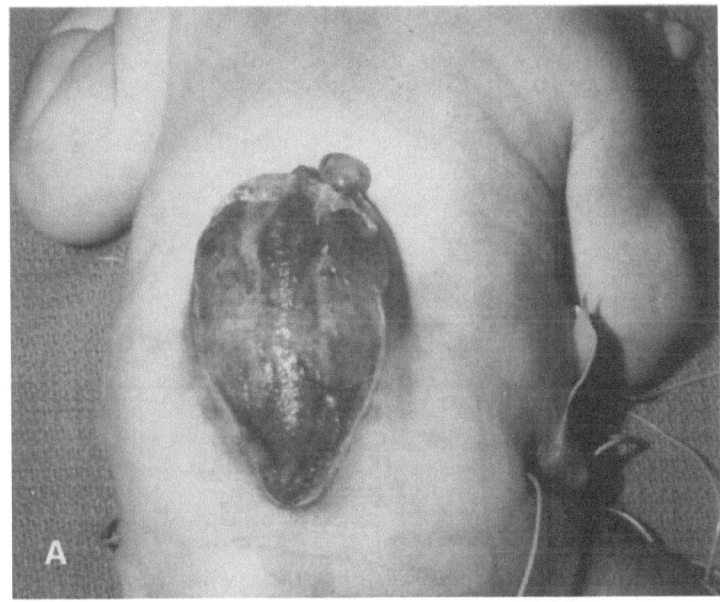

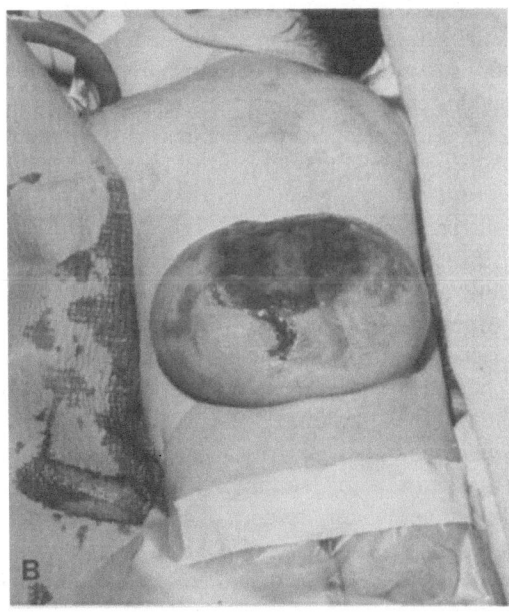

Figure 8.1. Examples of various configurations in meningomyeloceles in newborns. **A:** Large thoracolumbar lesion which is entirely membranous in its covering. Associated kyphosis. **B:** Cystic lumbosacral defect with central placode and generous skin cover.

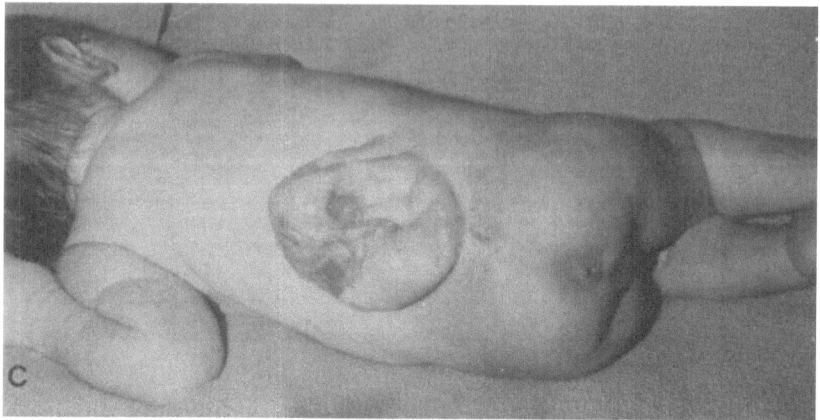

Figure 8.1C. Collapsed and leaking lumbar lesion with redundant skin.

a reflex nature and are misleading for the interpretation of future volitional motor abilities. Sensory stimulation with pinprick should include close observation for startle or grimace, indicative of conscious appreciation of pain. Although some patients have asymmetric deficits, motor and sensory levels are usually consistent or similar. Electromyography is not mandatory, but may provide a reliable check on surgical technique or future deterioration.

Most meningomyelocele patients have poorly developed gluteal creases and at least somewhat patulous anuses. In spite of this, the anal wink response is often present in the early hours after delivery. This, again, probably represents isolated reflex activity.

If convenient, or if there are serious prognostic questions before repair, spinal films and cranial sonography or computed tomography (CT) should be performed to establish better the level and extent of spinal involvement and the severity of the hydrocephalus. If the level of paralysis is severe or the macrocephaly profound, parents may have serious questions concerning the viability of the child. In that case, it is appropriate to take the time to complete the team evaluation by assessing renal function and accomplishing a preoperative orthopedic consultation, so that maximum data are available for counseling. Unless there is nearly total absence of cerebral tissue on CT, I recommend early repair. If parents feel they may be unable to cope, temporary alternative or foster parenting is offered, ordinarily with no permanent obligation of parents to give up the child for adoption.

After the initial assessment is completed, the neurosurgic consultant discusses the recommendations, operative risks, and long-term outlook with the father or available family member. Arrangements are made for the pediatrician and spina bifida coordinator to visit both the mother and the father in the referring maternity unit, to initiate counseling relative to the condition, its implications, and management. This is accomplished within 24 to 48 hours after referral. The information conveyed at this initial meeting is repeated frequently over the ensuing weeks. The concept of the supporting multidisciplinary care system is emphasized along with the philosophy of support of the highest quality independent existence for patient and family.

Infants referred late without repair or after a "trial of life" are frequently infected. In such cases the wounds and CSF should be cultured and appropriate antibiotic therapy started during the period of evaluation. Surgical repair should not be undertaken in the face of frank infection. Shunts should not be inserted until the ventricular fluid is proven sterile.

Operative Repair

Under general endotracheal anesthesia with appropriate overhead warming lights the patient is positioned prone on chest bolsters. Intravenous lines should be adequate to accommodate blood transfusion. The wound area is widely prepared and draped. The central neural placode and membrane are cleansed with sterile saline irrigations and the surrounding skin is cleaned and then painted with iodinated solutions. The surgeon uses optical magnification with loupes. For electrocoagulation a bipolar system should be available.

The membranous portion of the sac is separated circumferentially from the surrounding viable skin with sharp iris scissors (Fig. 8.2A). Hemostats are applied to the subcutaneous tissue for retraction, and subcutaneous bleeders are obliterated with bipolar coagulation. The central membrane of the sac with the midline placode and neural elements are then gently dissected inferiorly into the spinal canal (Fig. 8.2B). Here the surgeon inspects for tethering connections and diastametomyelia (spurs) and removes them if they are present.

Next the membranous sac and adjacent central granulation tissue are carefully trimmed from the placode (Fig. 8.2C). Fine bipolar coagulation obliterates bleeding points. The placode is temporarily wrapped in oxycellulose sheets. The dura mater is identified and disconnected from elements of the sac that are usually adherent to underlying tissues from surface skin down through the epidural space. Leaves of dura are developed from each side to be used in a comfortable (but not redundant) closure. Fine clamps are placed on the dural edges. Returning to the placode, the hemostatic sheets are removed and the placode is inverted with fine 7-0 sutures applied at the edges of the glistening, smooth pia–arachnoid tissue, approximated over the midline and tied (Fig. 8.2D). If there is no identifiable linear placode, the existing neural elements are simply left within the confines of the spinal canal. Dura is closed with a continuous 4-0 suture (Fig. 8.2E). The lumbosacral fascia is then mobilized from each side of the midline. Not infrequently the displaced pedicles are extremely prominent. If so, they are dissected and removed to prevent a fulcrum effect on overlying tissues. If the fascia is prone to fraying, the rather hearty remaining elements of sac that

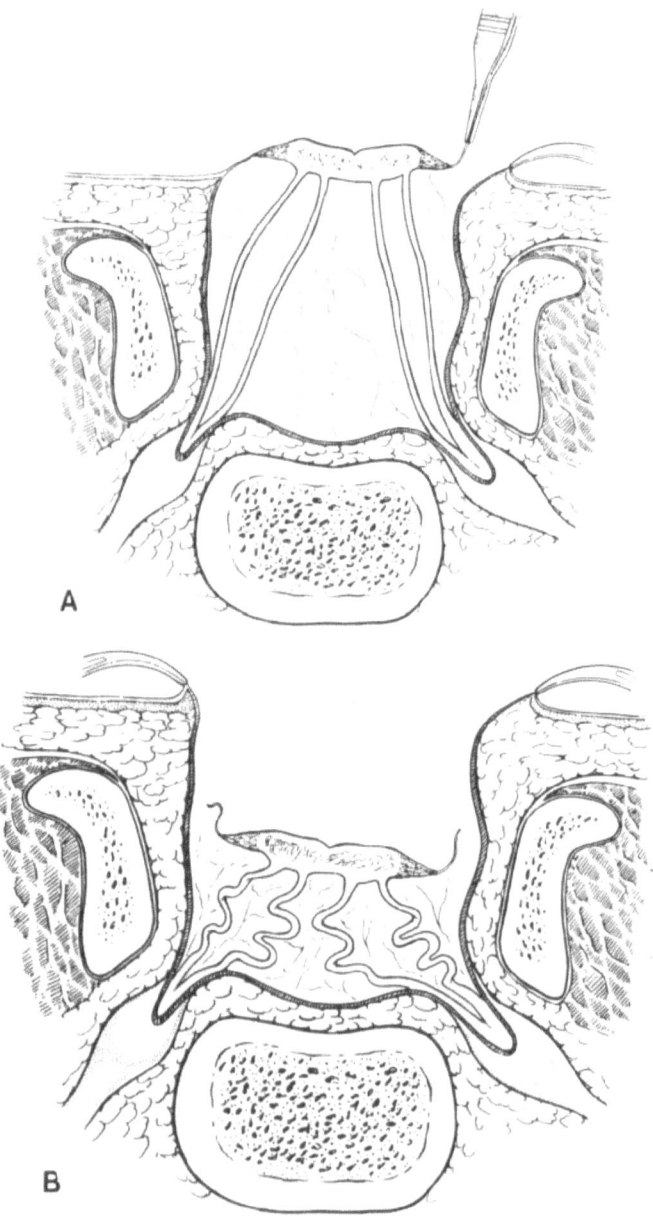

Figure 8.2. Cross-sectional diagram of operative repair of meningomyelocele: **A**: Initial detachment of central membrane from surrounding viable skin. **B**: Central membrane and neural elements have been detached and separated down into the spinal canal.

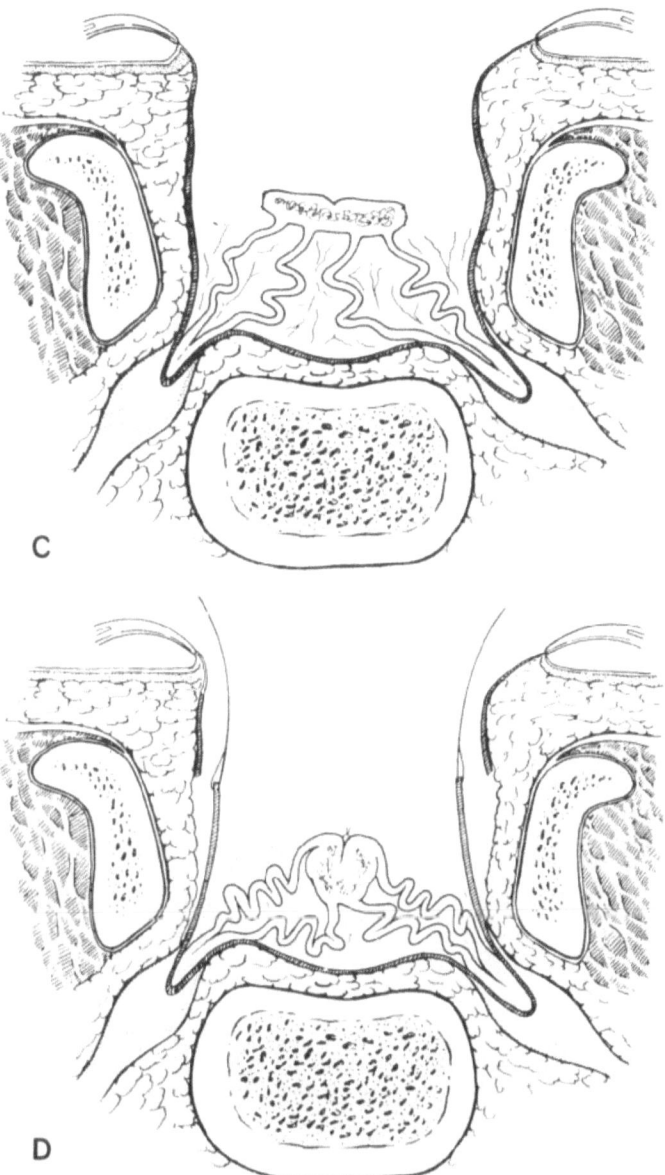

Figure 8.1C. Membranous surface portion of sac and central granulation tissue separated from central placode which remains attached to neural elements. **D**: Placode inverted and dura mobilized and temporarily retracted.

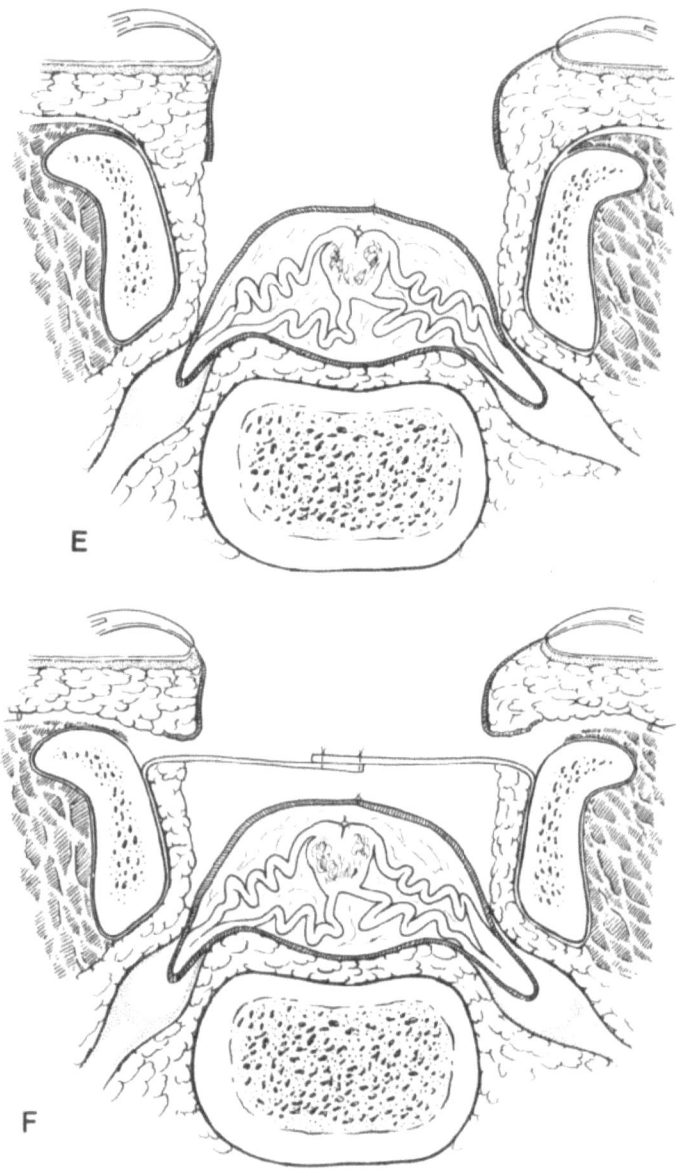

Figure 8.1E. Dura has been closed with a continuous suture. **F**: Fascia mobilized and turned medially for overlapping closure.

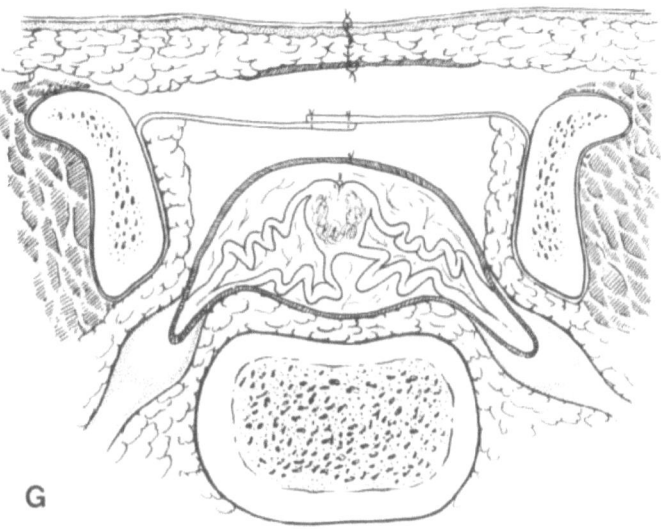

Figure 8.1G. Completed repair including skin and subcutaneous closure.

were left on the subcutaneous tissues can be used as the third level of closure. The fascia or the remaining sac elements are raised as flaps overlapping at the midline and approximated with 4-0 absorbable sutures (Fig. 8.2F).

Finally, the subcutaneous tissue is widely undermined until the skin edges can be comfortably approximated at the midline for vertical closure or brought together for horizontal closure. This usually necessitates the removal of excess tissue at either end of the wound to eliminate "dog ears." After this final trimming, the subcutaneous layer is sutured with interrupted 4-0 absorbable stitches and the skin with interrupted 5-0 synthetic sutures (Fig. 8.2G). Skin approximation is seldom difficult if undermining has been adequate. Only occasionally are Z-plasty procedures required. A waterproof sterile dressing is applied, using pressure to prevent accumulation of blood and serum in the dead space.

Postoperative Care and Evaluation

In the early postoperative period, infants may be nursed in any comfortable position. If there is any tendency toward CSF leak or subcutaneous fluid collection they are kept horizontal. Feedings should be initiated after careful determination of competence in swallowing without aspiration. Prophylactic antibiotics are continued for 48 hours.

Orthopedic evaluation is usually accomplished during the next few days. If serial cast applications are required, these may then be initiated. Further urologic assessment involves repeated palpation for bladder size, renal sonography, and voiding cystourethrogram. Early postoperative urinary retention may necessitate intermittent catheterization. If hydronephrosis with reflux is detected a temporary suprapubic cystostomy is performed.

Continuing evaluation of hydrocephalus requires frequent inspection of repair sites, head measurements, assessment of anterior fontanel tone, and serial cranial ultrasonography, as necessary. If there is obvious progressive hydrocephalus a ventriculoperitoneal shunt is inserted during the first week. The appropriate time for shunting remains a matter of surgical judgment. In my experience 70% of meningomyelocele patients require shunting; and, in over 50%, this becomes apparent within 10 days of repair.

Most patients may be discharged from hospital care in 10 to 14 days, after further parent orientation. Frequent visits to the spina bifida clinic are useful during the first 6 months to further counsel the parents, evaluate the status of hydrocephalus, and attend to early orthopedic requirements. Developmental testing and infant stimulation programs are utilized. The spina bifida coordinator keeps close counsel with community programs to ensure that appropriate services are rendered in the home area.

Projected Neurosurgery Care

Long-term neurosurgery follow-up should be within the setting of the spina bifida clinic. Obviously, the management of hydrocephalus remains a primary consideration. Parents are educated to be alert for signs of symptomatic hydrocephalus or shunt dysfunction. In my experience, an average of two shunt revisions are required within the first decade of life. Each examination should include examination of the optic fundi, extraocular movements, head size and growth rate, and questioning for symptoms suggestive of increased intracranial pressure or subtle ventriculomegaly. Periodic CT scanning appropriately monitors the anatomic changes and may provide a baseline for future scanning during symptomatic periods.

The urologist initiates intermittent clean catheterization, and continually monitors for urinary tract infections and hydronephrosis; the orthopedist seeks to prevent, and correct, deformities; the neurosurgeon remains alert for signs of the tethered cord, hydromyelia, and acquired brain stem compression. Stridor and serious swallowing difficulties may appear during the first few weeks of life and may require judicious airway management. Foramen magnum decompression carries a high mortality rate in infants with myelodysplasia. Apnea monitoring, airway toilet, or even tracheotomy may be more efficacious. After careful management during the first year of life the condition is usually self-correcting.

The potential incidence of cord tethering after meningomyelocele repair is still uncertain. Progressive development of orthopedic deformities or frank increase in neurologic deficit dictates myelography and re-exploration if the anatomic evidence is secure. Progressive scoliosis or upper extremity involvement suggests hydromyelia. Again, myelography or MRI aids in confirmation. None of these problems will be expeditiously detected unless the patient receives careful serial neurologic examinations at each clinic visit.

Perhaps the most severe of the unsolved problems of myelodysplastic patients is that of kyphosis (gibbus), which is usually present at birth, but progresses. Reigel has advocated primary kyphectomy, presumably to facilitate closure of large thoracolumbar lesions.[9] In spite of early kyphectomy the deformity usually recurs. Often, the cutaneous repair site erodes in later life. Most orthopedists prefer to defer kyphectomy procedures as long as possible to permit enough growth for reasonable prospects of optimum trunk length. However, in spite of the time of repair and because of the severe paralysis and prefixed deformity, sustained correction seldom results.

As patients mature, the neurosurgeon and his colleagues should begin to educate them in the elements of care for which they will be responsible during their adult lives. This requires cooperation with local schools and community agencies involved in education and services for the handicapped. Those having learning disabilities continue to provide serious challenges. Meaningful employment and adequate medical services are at present rather evasive possibilities for the increasing population of handicapped older patients.

Summary

As the most common of the dysraphic disorders, meningomyelocele represents a challenge that can be most satisfactorily addressed by an experienced multidisciplinary team, providing early comprehensive evaluation, appropriate family counseling, expert neurosurgical intervention, and aggressive long-term follow-up care. After initial evaluation and parent education, expeditious closure of the lesion should be accomplished in multiple layers with efforts to prevent future spinal cord tethering. Hydrocephalus, which occurs as a manifestation of the Chiari II malformation in 90% of patients, should be assessed and treated at an early stage with ventriculoperitoneal shunting. Patients with mild hydrocephalus should be followed indefinitely as potential candidates for exacerbation of the progressive disorder. Respiratory disorders associated with the hindbrain anomaly remain a controversial subject. While some clinicians advocate early brain stem decompression, such procedures carry a high mortality rate which recommends conservative approaches. The incidence of late neurologic deterioration referable to the spinal cord, including hydromyelia and tethering, is uncertain. However, the possibility of these complications dictates vigilance, careful serial examinations, and intervention when confirmed by neuroradiologic studies.

Through the auspices of a coordinated spina bifida program the medical, educational, and social needs of these multiply handicapped patients should be met to ensure the highest possible levels of independence and eventual self-care. Currently it can be expected that over 90% of patients will survive into adulthood. Most will have shunts for hydrocephalus. About 70% of survivors will have at least normal intellect. But many with normal IQ will require specific educational assistance. The majority can be kept continent of urine with intermittent catheterization and pharmacotherapy. At least into the late teenage years most patients will ambulate with assistive devices. Congenital thoracolumbar kyphosis, which is usually progressive, represents a major complication refractory to therapeutic measures. Independent employment and satisfactory medical services remain problematic for the growing numbers of adult survivors.

References

1. Freeman JM: Practical Management of Meningomyelocele. University Park Press, Baltimore, 1974.
2. Chervenak FA, Duncan C, Ment L, Tortora M, McClure M, Hobbins JC: Perinatal management of meningomyelocele. Obstet Gynecol 63:376–380, 1984.
3. Althouse R, Wald N: Survival and handicap of infants with spina bifida. Arch Dis Child 55:845–850, 1980.
4. Black PMcL: Selective treatment of infants with meningomyelocele. Neurosurg 5:334–338, 1979.
5. DeLange SA: Selection for treatment of patients with spina bifida aperta. Dev Med Child Neurol 16:27–30, 1974.
6. Lorber J: Results of treatment of meningomyelocele: an analysis of 524 unselected cases with special reference to possible selection for treatment. Dev Med Child Neurol 13:279–303, 1971.
7. Stein SC, Schut L, Ames MD: Selection for early treatment in meningomyelocele: a retrospective analysis of various selection procedures. Pediatrics 54:553–557, 1974.
8. Freeman JM: To treat or not to treat: ethical dilemmas of treating the infant with meningomyelocele. Clin Neurosurg 20:134–146, 1973.
9. Reigel D: Spina bifida. In: McLauren RH (ed): Pediatric Neurosurgery: Grune & Stratton, New York, 1982, p 23.
10. Lorber J: Early results of selective treatment of spina bifida cystica. Br Med J 4:201–204, 1973.
11. Lorber J, Salfield SAW: Results of selective treatment of spina bifida cystica. Arch Dis Child 56:822–830, 1981.
12. Fetham SL, Tweed H, Perrin S: Practical problems in selection of spina bifida infants for treatment in the USA. Z Kinderchir 28:301–306, 1979.
13. Gross RH, Cox A, Tatyrek R, Pollay M, Barnes WA: Early management and decision making for the treatment of meningomyelocele. Pediatrics 72:450–458, 1983.
14. McCullough DC: Spinal dysraphism. meningomyelocele. In: Horwitz N, Rizzoli H: Postoperative Complications in Neurological Surgery, Vol. 3: Williams & Williams, Baltimore, 1987, pp 138–144.
15. Shurtleff DB, Hayden W, Loeser JD, Kronmal RA: Myelodysplasia: decision for death or disability. N Engl J Med 291:1005–1011, 1974.
16. Charney E, Weller S, Sutton L, Bruce DA, Schut LB: Management of the newborn with meningomyelocele: time for a decision making process. Pediatrics 75:58–64, 1985.
17. Hide DW, Williams HP, Ellis HL: The outlook for the child with a meningomyelocele for whom early surgery was considered inadvisable. Dev Med Child Neurol 14:304–307, 1972.
18. Laurence KM: The survival of untreated spina bifida cystica. Dev Med Child Neurol 11:10–19, 1966.
19. McLone DG, Dias L, Kaplan WE, Sommers MW: Concepts in the management of

spina bifida. In: Humphreys RP (ed): Concepts in Pediatric Neurosurgery, Vol. 5: Karger, Basel, 1985, p 97.

20. McLone DG: Results of treatment of children born with a meningomyelocele. Clin Neurosurg 30:407–412, 1983.

21. O'Brien MS, McLanahan CS: Review of the neurosurgical management of meningomyelocele at a regional pediatric medical center. In: Epstein F (ed): Concepts in Pediatric Neurosurgery, Vol. 1, 19: Karger, Basel, p 202.

22. Sharrard WJM, Zachary RB, Lorber J, Bruce AM: A controlled trial of intermediate and delayed closure of spina bifida cystica. Arch Dis Child 38:18–22, 1963.

23. McLone DG, Czyzewski D, Raimondi AJ, Sommers RC: Central nervous system infections as a limiting factor in the intelligence of children with meningomyelocele. Pediatrics 70:338–342, 1982.

24. Ames MD, Schut L: Results of treatment of 171 consecutive meningomyeloceles – 1963 to 1968. Pediatrics 50:466–471, 1972.

25. Ingraham FD: Spina Bifida and Cranium Bifidum: Harvard, Cambridge, 1943.

26. Naglo AS, Hellstrom B: Results of treatment in meningomyelocele. Acta Pediatr Scand 65:565–569, 1976.

27. Epstein F: Meningomyelocele: "pitfalls" in early and late management. Clin Neurosurg 30:366–384, 1983.

28. Shurtleff DB, Foltz EL: A comparative study of meningomyelocele repair or cerebrospinal fluid shunt as primary treatment in 90 children. Dev Med Child Neurol 13:57–64, 1967.

29. Hunt GM, Holmes AE: Factors relating to intelligence in treated cases of spina bifida cystica. Am J Dis Child 130:823–827, 1976.

30. Guthkelch AN, Pang D, Vries JK: Influence of closure technique on results in meningomyelocele. Childs Brain 8:350–355, 1981.

31. McLone DG: Technique for closure of meningomyelocele. Childs Brain 6:65–73, 1980.

32. Cruz NI, Ariyan S, Duncan CC, Cuono CB: Repair of lumbosacral meningomyeloceles with double Z-rhomboid flaps. J Neurosurg 59:714–717, 1983.

33. Habal MB, Vries JK: Tension free closure of large meningomyelocele defects. Surg Neurol 8:177–180, 1977.

34. Winston KR, Schuster SR, Mickle P: Management of large skin defects in newborn children with myelodysplasia: a new method. J Pediatr Surg 13:303–306, 1978.

35. Clark DH, Walsh JW, Luce EA: Closure of myelorachischisis defects with reverse latissimus dorsi myocutaneous flaps. Neurosurgery 11:423–425, 1982.

36. McDevitt NB, Gillespie RP, Woosley RE, Whitt JJ, Bevin AG: Closure of thoracic and lymbar dysraphic defects using bilateral latissimus dorsi myocutaneous flap transfer with extended gluteal fasciocutaneous flaps. Childs Brain 9:394–399, 1982.

37. Munro IR, Neu BR, Humphreys RP, Lauritzen CG: Limberg-latissimus dorsi myocutaneous flap for closure of meningomyelocele. Childs Brain 10:381–386, 1983.

38. Stark GD: Neonatal assessment of the child with meningomyelocele. Arch Dis Child 46:539–548, 1971.

39. Reigel DH, Dallmann DE, Scarff TB, Woodford J: Intra-operative evoked potential studies of newborn infants with meningomyelocele. Dev Med Child Neurol 18:42–49, 1976.

40. Lorber J: Systematic ventriculographic studies in infants born with meningomyelocele and encephalocele. The incidence and development of hydrocephalus. Arch Dis Child 37:381–389, 1961.

41. Doran PA, Guthkelch AN: Studies in spina bifida cystica—I General survey and reassessment of the problem. J Neurol Neurosurg Psychiatry 24:331–345, 1961.
42. Laurence KM, Evans RC, Weeks RD, et al: The reliability of prediction of outcome in spina bifida. Dev Med Child Neurol 37:150–156, 1976.
43. Linder M, Nichols J, Sklar FH: Effect of meningomyelocele closure on the intracranial pulse pressure. Childs Brain 11:176–182, 1984.
44. Hunt G, Lewin W, Gleave J, Gairdner D: Predictive factors in open meningomyelocele with special reference to sensory level. Br Med J 4:197–201, 1973.
45. Mulcahy JJ, James HE: Management of urinary incontinence in infancy and childhood. In: Epstein F (ed): Concepts in Pediatric Neurosurgery, Vol. 1. Karger, Basel, 1981, p 216.
46. Park TS, Hoffman HJ, Hendrick EB, Humphreys RP: Experience with surgical decompression of the Arnold–Chiari malformation in young infants with myelomeningocele. Neurosurgery 13:147–152, 1983.
47. Reigel DH: Tethered spinal cord. In: Humphreys RP (ed): Concepts in Pediatric Neurosurgery, Vol. 4: Karger, Basel, 1983, p 142.
48. Venes JL, Stevens EA: Surgical pathology in tethered cord secondary to myelomeningocele repair. In: Humphreys RP (ed): Concepts in Pediatric Neurosurgery Vol. 4: Karger, Basel, 1983, p 165.
49. Hall P, Lindseth R, Campbell R, Kalsbeck JE, Desousa A: Scoliosis and hydrocephalus in myelocele patients. J Neurosurg 50:174–178, 1979.
50. Park TS, Carl W, Maggiolo M, Mitchell DC: Progressive spasticity and scoliosis in children with myelomeningocele. J Neurosurg 62:367–375, 1985.

CHAPTER 9

Hamartomas and the Dysraphic State

Anthony J. Raimondi

Vertebrospinal congenital anomalies, the opposite of vertebrospinal injuries, are common, becoming clinically obvious either at birth, in the toddler (when the child begins to walk), and during the enormous growth spurt that occurs during the transition from juvenile into adolescent years. In broad terms, these anomalies may be subdivided into two groups: (1) those associated with the dysraphic state, and (2) those characterized by congenital tumors or anomalies without defects in the posterior vertebral arch. This chapter discusses only the former.

Hamartomas and the Dysraphic State

Surgical anomalies of the dysraphic state include myelocele, meningomyelocele, meningocele; lipomeningocele, lipomeningomyelocele; some hamartomas (lipoma, dural fibrolipoma, leptomyelolipoma, anterior spina bifida, enterogenous cysts) extending from the intramedullary area into the subcutaneous space; and diastematomyelia. With the rarest of exceptions, these do not exist as pure, anatomic anomalies. Rather, one almost invariably blends imperceptibly into another and, in many instances such as lipomeningomyelocele and hamartomas, several may coexist.

Before undertaking an operative procedure, one asks himself what specifically he expects to attain: closure of a defect to protect against infection, anatomic reconstruction to restore function, resection of mass to relieve compression, or sectioning of a tethering structure to eliminate stretching.

Despite some rather startling claims made many years ago (and subsequently corrected) by Sharrard, it is a well accepted fact that closure of a myelocele, meningocele, or meningomyelocele in a newborn does not result either in improved neurologic function or in increasing the possibilities of subsequent rehabilitation. Similarly, the particular closure technique used does not affect subsequent neurologic function. The closure simply provides the central nervous system (CNS) protection from infecting organisms. Therefore, the procedure and the timing of its performance are to be interpreted only on the basis of protecting the CNS from bacterial and physical damage.

When the lipomatous portion of a lipomeningomyelocele, or a medullary lipoma, compresses the medulla spinalis, removing it affords similar—but not identical—beneficent results as removing a neurinoma or meningioma. The results are similar, not identical, because it is not possible at present to remove the intramedullary portion of the lipoma. Consequently, the decompression is never complete and the potential for lipoma regrowth and expansion is always present. Removal of a diastematomyelic spur, when it is pathogenetic of spinal cord deficit, may be considered palliative, as may severing of the filum terminale when it is pathogenetic of a conus medullaris syndrome. "Prophylactic" surgery for removal of subcutaneous lipoma, supported by some neurosurgeons but opposed by most, must be evaluated critically as must "prophylactic" resection of asymptomatic diastematomyelia. In light, then, of the previous comments, techniques for the surgical treatment of the individual developmental anomalies associated with the dysraphic state are described, with the realization that one anomaly may blend imperceptibly into others. Nowhere in the field of pediatric neurosurgery do "feelings" so disrupt objective analysis of indications, treatment, and results as in the dysraphic state. What a pity!

Any decision to perform surgery on a patient suffering from one or more anomalies of the dysraphic state is predicated on a detailed understanding of the developmental anatomy and pathology of the clinical entity: Precise terminology assists one neurosurgeon to communicate his observations and concepts to another. The reader is referred to the works of Duckworth et al.,[2] Lebedeff,[3] von Recklinghausen,[4] Morgagni,[5] Patten,[6] James and Lassman,[7] Ingraham and Matson,[8] Talwalker and Dastur,[9] Emery and Lendon,[10] and Rokos.[11]

Amyelia

The clinical entity known as *amyelia* is significant to the neurosurgeon only from one point of view: providing evidence that muscle masses may develop and dorsal roots may be found within the spinal canal of severely deformed fetuses and newborns *who have no spinal cord at all*. This allows one to understand that neural elements may be present within the dysraphic area independent of a medulla spinalis, that the presence of somatosensory evoked potentials between the lower extremities and the spinal area *is not* indicative of a functional spinal cord.

Defects in Closure of the Spinal Cord and Posterior Vertebral Arch

In this chapter I present briefly and for orienting purposes a classification of the dysraphic state and brief comments on its treatment. This is done to offer a conceptual distinction and grasp of pathoanatomic similarities between spina bifida aperta, the closed forms of dysraphism, and the hamartomatous lesions. It is

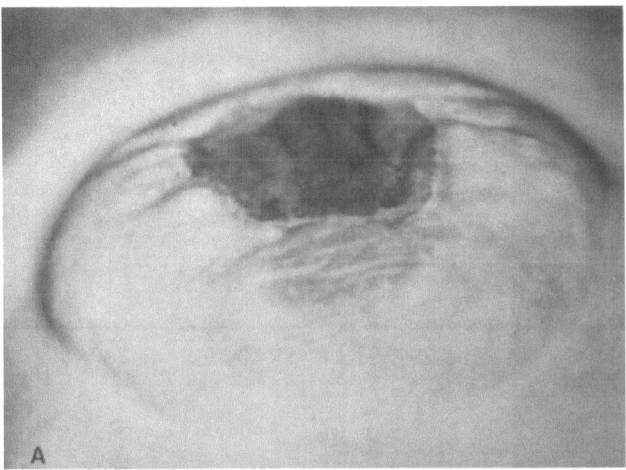

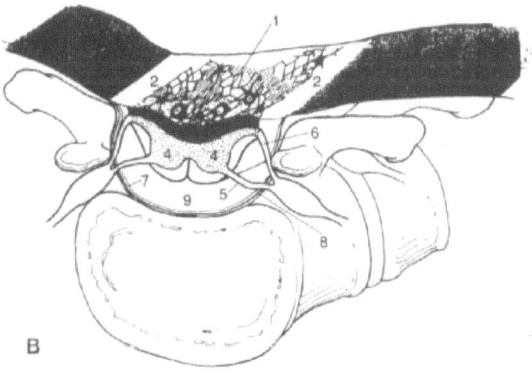

Figure 9.1.A. Myelocele. The myelocele may exist as either a simple myelocele (no cyst present), a scarred myelocele (easily confused with the placode of a meningomyelocele), or a cystic myelocele (in which there is a subarachnoid cyst between the ventral surface of the unclosed cord and that portion of the arachnoid and dura abutting upon the posterior longitudinal ligament. This figure illustrates a cystic myelocele with some scarring. **B**: Simple myeloschisis (myelocele) is herein represented diagramatically. The surface of this lesion (1) is a composite of glial scar, ectopic neurons, patches of ependyma, and degenerative changes. This is the "medullovasculosa," which is bordered by a zone of tissue devoid of neural or epithelial tissue (2) which, in turn, is surrounded by the "zona epitheliosa" (3). Note the enclosed spinal cord (4) with ventral (5) and dorsal (6) roots. The arachnoid (7) and dura (8) rest along the ventral surface of the spinal canal (9).

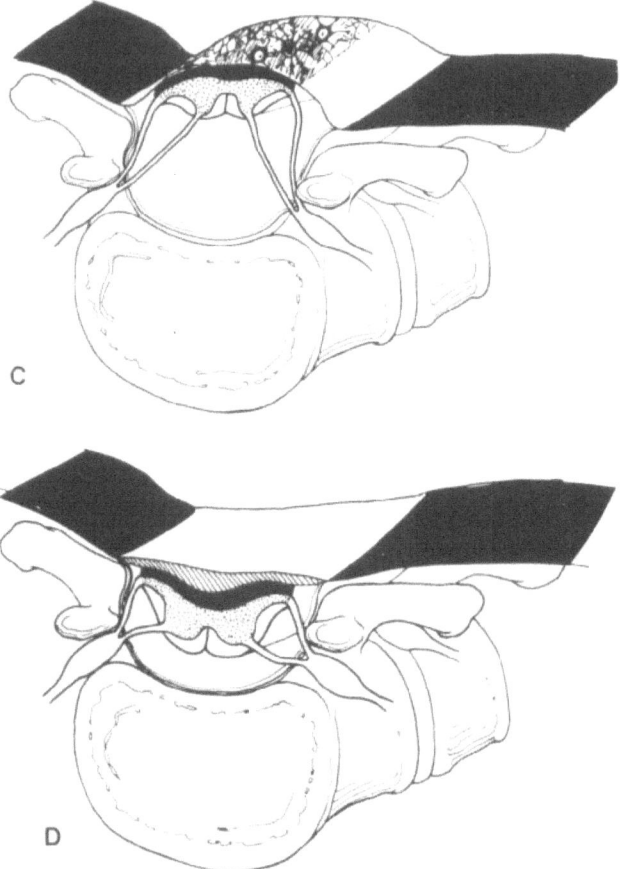

Figure 9.1C. Cystic myeloschisis, on the other hand, has a large cystic cavity, subarachnoid, located between the ventral surface of the unclosed cord and the arachnoid and dura mater abutting upon the posterior longitudinal ligament. **D**: The scarred myelocele, which may be confused with the placode of the meningomyelocele, consists of a myeloschisis, simple or cystic, covered by granulation tissue, which is organized and epithelialized.

unfortunate that we generally speak indiscriminately of "M-M" as though all children born with a sac on their back had the same congenital anomaly. This confuses treatment and prognosis. With this in mind, the following classification, taken from the 1976 edition of Greenfield's *Neuropathology*,[12] is recommended:

Myelocele

Myelocele (Fig. 9.1) is failure of closure of the neural tube (myeloschisis), resulting in a flattening of the spinal cord. The defect is covered by granulation tissue that is highly vascularized and surrounded by a translucent membrane that establishes continuity between it and the peripheral skin. If the flattened cord lies normally within the ventral aspect of the spinal canal, it is referred to as *simple myeloschisis*. If it is floating on an arachnoidal cyst that separates it from the ventral aspect of the spinal canal it is *cystic myelocele*. If the vascularized granulation tissue covering the myeloschisis organizes and epithelializes, simple myeloschisis or cystic myelocele may be *confused* with meningomyelocele when, in fact, it is a *scarred myelocele*. This confusion of two distinctly different dysraphic states has led some authors to suggest that it is possible to reconstruct the unclosed spinal cord in meningomyelocele. The placode of meningomyelocele is quite different, *nonfunctional*, pathologic tissue!

The developmental pathologic anatomy of the myelocele results in flattening of the spinal cord, which has not closed into a tubular structure, with medial location of the ventral horns and roots and lateral location of the dorsal horns and roots. Consequently, all roots exit from the ventral surface of the malformed cord. On the dorsal surface there may be glial scars, dysgenetic ependyma, ectopic islands of neural tissue, and extensive areas of degenerative changes. This is important to remember since closure of a myelocele necessitates separating this nonfunctional, pathologic tissue, the scarred portion similar to the placode, from the underlying opened cord and nerve roots (dorsal and ventral), prior to dural and fascial imbrication. This is accomplished by brushing the dysgenetic tissue away with wet cotton "fluffies" or, if adherent, by microdissection using $3\times$, or, at most, $6\times$ magnification. One must not close exposed, contaminated granulation or epithelial tissue (scar tissue, placode surface) into the spinal canal; infection or a dermoid tumor may result.

Meningocele

In *meningocele* (Fig. 9.2) the hernia sac consists only of meninges, covered by skin or epithelialized tissue, and the posterior spinal arch defect is limited to one vertebra. The spinal cord is located normally within the spinal canal, resting upon its ventral surface. Nerve roots may float into the hernia sac or be tethered to its neck. When the posterior arch defect involves two or more vertebrae, the spinal cord itself may be attached (tethered) to the neck of the hernia, closely resembling the meningomyelocele.

Surgical Technique

If the meningocele is covered with skin at the time of birth, one may profitably wait until the child is several months old to repair it. If, on the other hand, it consists of a thin layer of epidermis, it is best to repair it immediately lest it rupture and serve as a portal of entry for bacteria.

An elliptical incision is extended along the midline from superior to inferior, to the base of the meningocele, where it should skirt either side of the pedicle, taking care to leave enough skin for the closure. At the inferior portion of the pedicle, the skirting incisions from either side of the pedicle are brought into the

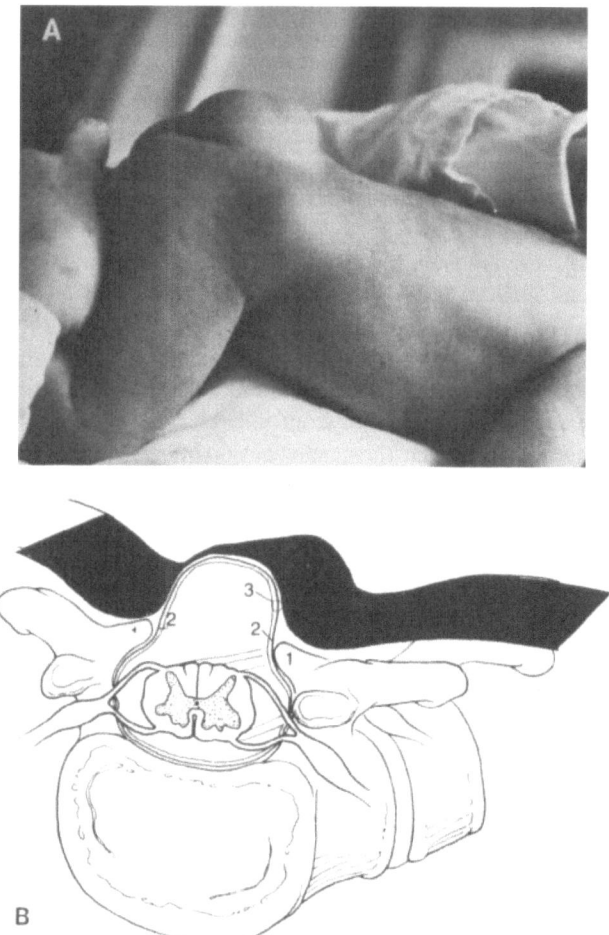

Figure 9.2.A. This child has a lumbosacral meningocele completely covered with skin. **B**: The simple meningocele results from a small defect in a single arch (1). The neck of the hernia (2) is the narrowest point through which the dura and arachnoid (3) herniate. The sac is a simple meningocele, extending through the neck, dorsal to normal cord and roots.

midline from whence a single incision is extended inferiorly for a distance of about 2 cm. Only the epidermal and dermal layers of the skin should be cut, with an attempt to avoid incising the underlying pachy- and leptomeninges. The skin bleeding is stopped as one progresses to extend the incision superior and inferior to the meningocele. This permits the surgeon to expose the fascia, and facilitates exposure of the underlying dura and *the inspection of its contents for neural elements*. If the meningocele is covered completely by skin, one may make the incision around the pedicle in a line of his choosing, allowing adequate skin flap for a cosmetically desirable closure. If, however, it is covered by a thin layer of

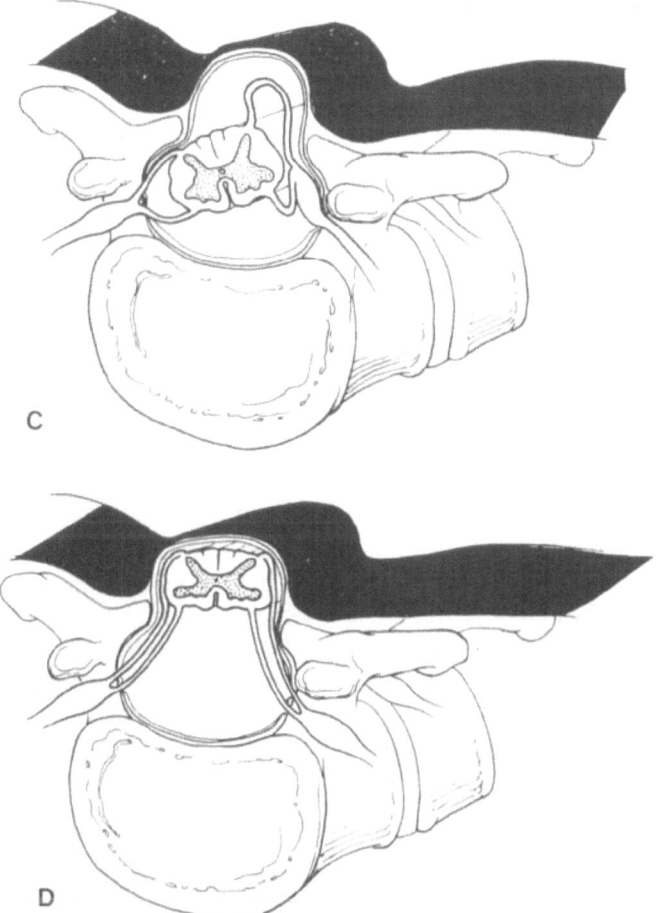

Figure 9.2C. When there is a wide defect in a single arch, the meningocele may entrap one or more nerve roots, tethering the cord indirectly. **D**: The meningocele which herniates through a wide defect in two or more arches has meninges and cord within the center of the sac. The cord attaches to the meninges, tethering itself at the most caudal level of the dysraphism.

epidermis, one should make the incision along the line of transition between full-thickness skin and epidermis, postponing the planning of the skin closure until after the meningeal component of the meningocele has been repaired. In those instances in which the meningocele is covered only by a thin layer of epidermal tissue, the dura will be opened unavoidably when one cuts along the transition of full-thickness skin into epidermis.

In both instances, once the skin incision has been completed and the loose subcutaneous connective tissue separated from the underlying fascia, the exposed dura, whether intact (as in the case of meningoceles covered with skin) or dysgenetic (as in the case of meningoceles covered with epidermis) is opened. An Adson–Brown forceps is used to grasp the dura and put it under slight traction prior to cutting it with a tenotomy scissors. Magnification is essential to ascertain that no neural elements are damaged. The egress of cerebrospinal fluid (CSF) occurs immediately if the meningocele is covered only by an epidermal layer, but not until the arachnoid is opened if the covering is full-thickness skin. In the former event, the surgically isolated portion of skin is separated from the underlying dura and discarded. The dura is then cut in the midsagittal plane, from the inferior to the superior extremities of the dysplastic posterior vertebral arch, and then incised perpendicular to the sagittal cut on both sides, superiorly and inferiorly. This fashions two trapdoors. The arachnoid should be intentionally opened only to free and reduce the tethered roots (small hernia neck) or spinal cord (large hernia neck) in the event they are present. Whether it is intentionally or inadvertently opened, it should be closed before reconstructing the dura.

One of the two fashioned dural trapdoor openings is then laid snugly over the arachnoid and sewn to the inner surface of the dura on the opposite side, maintaining the normal dural circumference, using 4-0 or 5-0 sutures. If it is necessary to imbricate the dura at the superior and inferior durotomies to eliminate the pouch, this should be done with interrupted sutures. The dural trapdoor from the other side is then brought over the now closed and imbricated dura, sewing it down so as to provide additional support to the area of prolapse. Fascia from the paraspinal muscle masses is then fashioned into a flap on either side, and, in turn, imbricated one over the dura first and then the other over the fascial flap, giving a four-layer closure. The skin is closed with interrupted mattress sutures.

Meningomyelocele

In meningomyelocele, the spinal cord is herniated into a sac of intact meninges that is located in the subcutaneous space. It may either be flattened out over a ventral arachnoidal cyst (*cystic meningomyelocele*), or it may be located normally within the spinal canal but have at its center an enormous hydromyelic cavity (*meningomyelohydrocele*) which distends and deforms its dorsal surface, pushing it into the hernia sac. Thus, the meningomyelohydrocele has three layers within the hernial sac: dura, arachnoid, and deformed dorsal surface of closed spinal cord.

In the cystic meningomyelocele, dysgenetic neural tissue (consisting of any combination of portions of spinal cord, conus medullaris, and nerve roots) is pathoanatomically continuous with the epidermal membrane externally and spinal cord elements centrally. There is no functional continuity, the placode is not a functionally or anatomically intact structure, nor does it hold anatomically intact neural elements. It is as much dysgenetic neural tissue as are the epithelial sac and dysraphic vertebral arch, respectively, dysgenetic skin and somites.

One should speak of surgical closure, not surgical repair of a meningomyelocele. It is impossible to repair (that is to say, to restore anatomic and functional integrity). The procedure, therefore, closes the opening between the spinal canal and the environment, bringing neural and connective tissue elements, respectively, *into* the spinal canal and *onto* one another. This seals CSF within the spinal canal, and bacteria and foreign substances from it.

The operative procedure consists of making an incision along the point of transition between skin and epithelial membrane, stopping individual bleeders as one proceeds by applying small-toothed hemostats to the underlying connective tissue, or by using very low-voltage bipolar coagulation. Once the skin has been incised, full thickness, around the entire circumference of this transitional area, it is separated from the underlying loose subcutaneous connective tissue until the paravertebral muscle fascia is identified. One then dissects immediately beneath the approximately 1 mm lip of dermoepithelial membrane transition tissue, until the subarachnoid space is entered, at which time CSF wells out of the field. This occurs when the flattened cord is floating on a ventral arachnoid cyst (cystic meningomyelocele), or it has a grossly dilated central canal with the thinned posterior cord adherent to the meninges (meningomyelohydrocele).

Cystic Meningomyelocele

The *cystic meningomyelocele* (Fig. 9.3) is a dysraphic state with ventral arachnoid cyst and a closed, deformed, cord, the placode. If one identifies a placode along the dorsal surface of the sac, and is certain that this is not a *scarred myelocele*, he should proceed to open dura and arachnoid, dissect the epithelialized placode from the underlying roots (maintaining these latter intact if possible), discard the epithelialized placode, and then reduce nerve roots and intact spinal cord into the spinal canal, if possible, before proceeding with the meningeal, fascial, and skin closure. No effort should be made to force the herniated spinal cord and/or cauda equina into a narrow spinal canal.

Tenotomy or iris scissors are used to cut the arachnoid around the circumference and the now centrally placed, totally isolated, epithelial membrane surrounding placode, separating this from the full-thickness skin. When the epithelial membrane and centrally placed placode are elevated, one will see dysgenetic nerve roots adherent to the undersurface of the placode. The epithelialized tissue and dysgenetic placode are then cut from the underlying posterior roots that may be adherent to it. The nerve roots are allowed to fall back into the intact inferior half of the neural arch, and the now-freed placode and epithelial membrane discarded.

If it is possible to identify arachnoid on either side, the two edges should be sewn to one another at this time. One should not attempt to force nerve roots or other dysgenetic neural tissue into the spinal canal since this may result either in compression of these elements or adhesions between the neural and mesenchymal components of dysraphic tissue. Subsequently, the dura should be freed from the paraspinal muscle fascia on either side, as described above for meningocele, fashioning as generous trapdoor dural flaps as possible. These latter are brought first one over the arachnoid and underlying nerve roots, and then the other over it. The dural flaps are sewn to dura with interrupted 5-0 sutures,

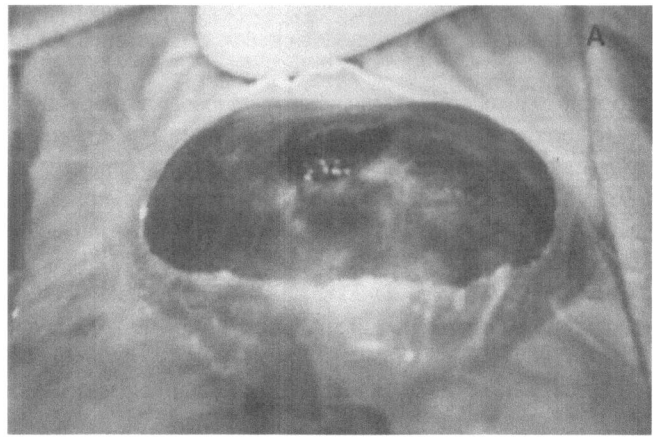

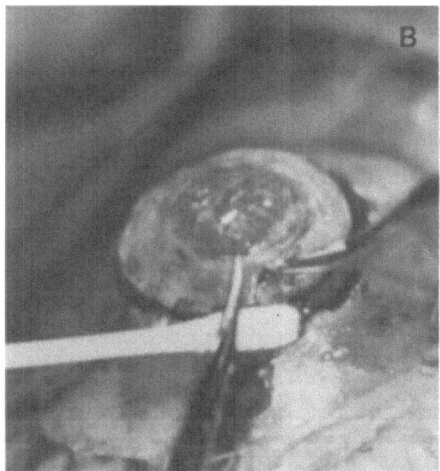

Figure 9.3.A. This photograph illustrates a cystic meningomyelocele, with epithelialization of the sac, which has been prepped. The skin over the thoracolumbosacral areas and the buttocks has been covered with adherent plastic material. **B**: The surgical procedure has begun: the separation of the epithelialized meningocele sac from the surrounding skin as the first stages of dissection of the placode.

making every effort to attain a seal. The first trapdoor dural flap is brought across the congenital defect and sewn to dura on the opposite side, superiorly and inferiorly, taking care to avoid producing a constriction. The second dural flap is laid over the former, and sewn down similarly. Then, as described under *meningocele*, fascial flaps are fashioned and sewn one over the other, giving four imbricated layers of closure.

Meningomyelohydrocele

If the central canal is blown out into the hernia sac, its disrupted and dysgenetic ependymal layer and the membranized dorsal portion of the spinal cord fuse with the arachnoid and dura to form the sac (Fig. 9.4). This latter may be more or less

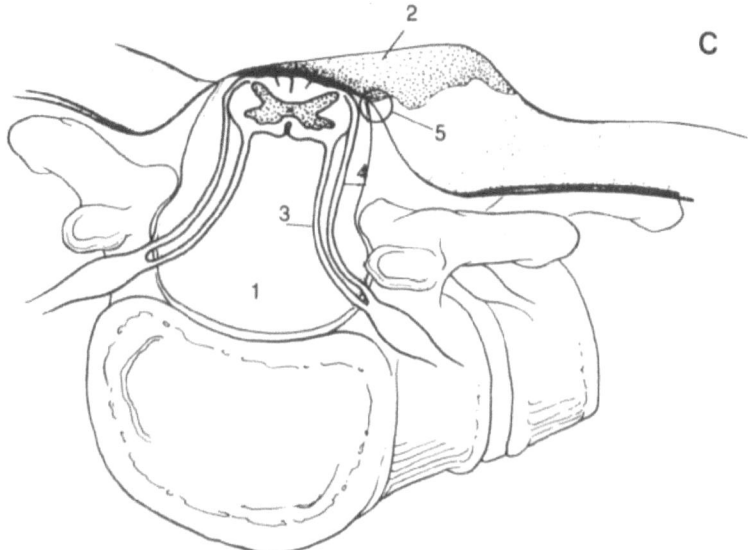

Figure 9.3C. This is a diagramatic representation of the meningomyelocele, which has a ventral arachnoid cyst (1) and a closed, deformed cord-placode (2). The ventral (3) and dorsal (4) roots follow an almost vertical course because of the cyst. Arachnoid, dura, and epithelium fuse at the lateral border of the placode (5).

epithelialized, though it is never covered completely by skin. At times, cloacal extrophy exists as an associated anomaly.

Repair of meningomyelohydrocele consists of identification of as many individual anatomic elements of the sac as possible (though one seldom is able to identify more than a single fibroepithelial appearing membrane), and then closure over the ventrally displaced and flattened spinal cord. If one extends the dissection into the area immediately medial to the paraspinal muscle masses, he may be able to identify arachnoid, which has a glistening surface. If so, this should be closed and then the dura, in turn, identified, freed from the adjacent paraspinal muscle fascia, and closed with imbricating sutures. The fascial and skin closures are the same as for a meningomyelocele and meningocele.

Concerning skin closure of all forms of the dysraphic state, depending on the size of the defect and the degree of posterior vertebral arch dysplasia, one may find it necessary to perform a Z-plasty to effect closure. Spurs of bone should be rongeured to avoid compression necrosis of the skin. The skin is best closed with interrupted 4-0 mattress sutures, placing them alternatively at the superior and inferior edges, working one's way from peripheral to central, whether or not a Z-plasty is necessary. Thus, one may continuously correct for uneven segments of skin by lengthening or shortening the interval between sutures on one side or the other.

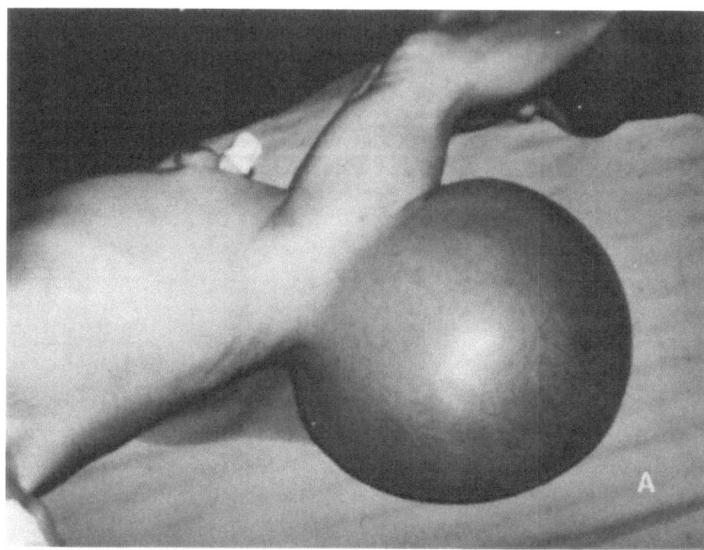

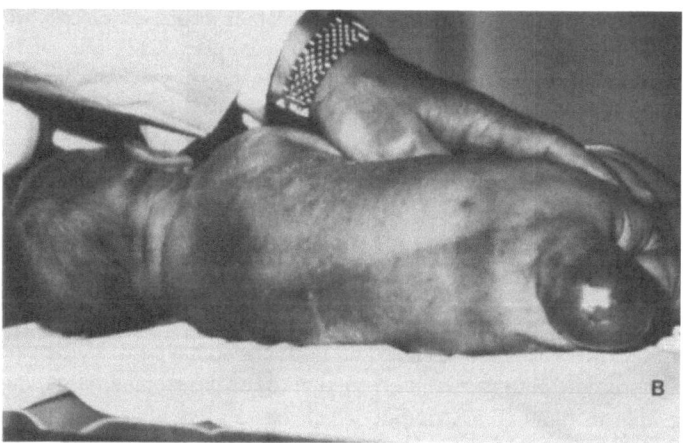

Figure 9.4A. Meningomyelohydrocele. One notes that the meningomyelohydrocele in this child has broad pedicles extending from the lumbosacral junction to the mid-thigh, all of which is covered by skin. **B**: This is a child with meningomyelohydrocele and with anatomical and functional integrity of the sphincters and pelvic diaphragm.

Distematomyelia

Diplomyelia is invariably present, to a greater or lesser degree, when there is either a diastematomyelic spur or a fibrous band. In essence, the spinal cord is cleft over a variable distance, with each independent medullary segment being covered by its own lepto- and pachy meanings, by a spur that generally has bone at its base, cartilage at its tip, and a connecting fibrous band extending from the

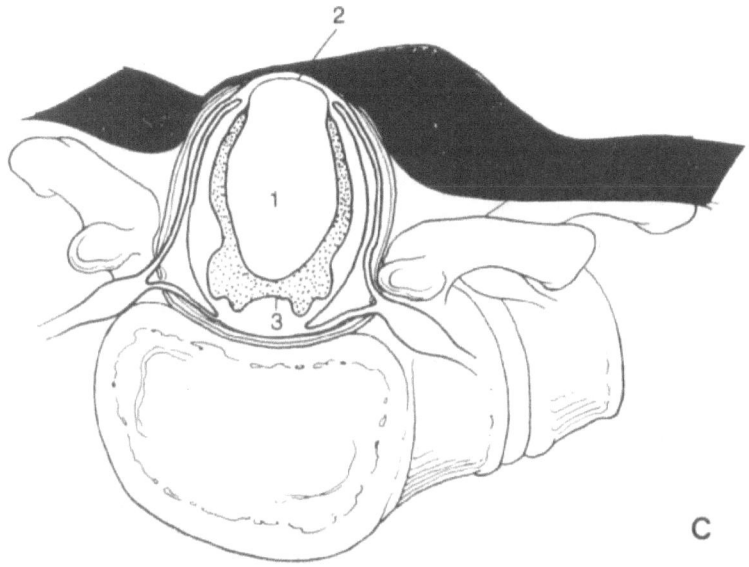

Figure 9.4C. This diagrammatic representation of meningomyelohydrocele reveals that the spinal cord has been blown out around the enormously dilated central canal (1), so that the dorsal cord (2) is converted into a membrane and the ventral cord (3) is flattened.

cartilagenous tip to the dorsal segment of the vertebral arch. Occasionally, a lipoma may be present in this pathologic tissue. This septum, or septum and lipoma, in its simplest terms, is the point of division between the two spinal cord segments, and is pathogenetic only in that the spinal cord may press against it as the child grows, or flexes and extends the vertebral spine. Consequently, one may have intermittent episodes of neurologic deficit, or, more commonly, slowly progressive neurologic deficit, referable to the spinal cord. The deficit is not radicular in nature, as one sees in the lipoma: it is medullary, upper motor. At times, the bony spur is not present but, rather, the cleft between the double spinal cords contains a more or less dense fibrous band that stretches from the ventral to the dorsal surfaces of the spinal canal. The net result, when clinically obvious, is the same since the fibrous band is strong enough to compress the spinal cord.

A lipoma may be within the spur or attached to it. Hence, *one could be justified in considering diastematomyelia as an intermediate congenital anomaly between the dysraphic state and hamartomous lesions.*

Irrespective of any other consideration, it is recommended that the diastematomyelic spur, osteocartilagenous or fibrous, with lipoma if present, be resected immediately when the diagnosis is made, even if the diagnosis is one of serendipity. The risks of surgery are so minimal, the opportunity to resect completely the spur so good, and the possible damage to the thoracic spinal cord, the level at which the diastematomyelic spur most often occurs, is so great that this course of action is considered fully justified.

The operative procedure consists of performing a three-level *laminotomy* centered over the diastematomyelic spur. Care must be taken in removing the laminar flap, since one should avoid attempting to roll the flap away from the underlying diplomyelic deformity until he is certain that either there is a no fibrous band connecting the diastematomyelic spur to the posterior surface of the spinal canal or, if one is present, that it be cut away before the laminar flap is lifted from the field. Once this is done, the surgeon has a view of the spinal cord, a single spinal cord above and below the diastematomyelic spur, with a segment of diplomyelia, each covered by intact dura mater, on either side of the spur. With few exceptions, one may state that the spur is extradural, so that its removal does not necessitate opening the dura mater. In fact, this is to be avoided. When lipoma is present, however, it is generally intradural. In these cases, one must open the dura and remove it!

If the "spur" consists of no more than a fibrous band, the operation will have terminated when the lamintomy flap is lifted from the field, since the surgeon already will have transected the bridging, anchoring, fibrous band running from the ventral to the dorsal surfaces of the spinal canal. He might choose to inspect the cleft between the diplomyelic segment of the spinal cord, to assure himself that there is not a cartilagenous or bony segment protruding from the ventral surface of the spinal canal, one that could potentially be pathogenetic.

When the diplomyelic spur is an osteocartilagenous spur, the surgeon should remove it with the finest tipped rongeur available, biting away one- or two-millimeter fragments at a time. The disadvantage of using a high-speed drill, even one with a diamond burr, to do this rests in the necessity to retract the diplomyelic segments of the spinal cord laterally, thus running the risk of compressing the spinal cord. It is preferable, therefore, to use the fine-tipped rongeur, inserting it so that the jaws open in the longitudinal (sagittal) plane, avoiding the risk of damaging the spinal cord in its narrowest, most vulnerable, horizontal plane. There is generally little or no bleeding associated with the removal of the spur, so one need not be concerned. After the diastematomyelic spur has been removed, the operative procedure is considered completed.

Dysraphic Hamartomas

What are commonly referred to as lipoma or dermoid tumors in neurosurgical parlance are, in fact, heterogeneous groupings of congenital and developmental anomalies which belong in the neuropathologic category of *hamartomas* in dysraphic children. The dysraphic hamartomas may be **lipomatous**, **dermoid**, or **endodermal**.

The simplification of grouping all lipomatous hamartomas into "lipoma" and "lipomeningocele" has resulted in recommending surgery for every child with a subcutaneous fatty tumor, and in very confusing interpretations of surgical results. It is suggested, therefore, that one speak of *lipomatous hamartomas*, and that they then be subclassified as: (1) *lipoma*, (2) *lipomyelolipoma*, (3) *dural fibrolipoma*, and (4) *lipomeningocele*.

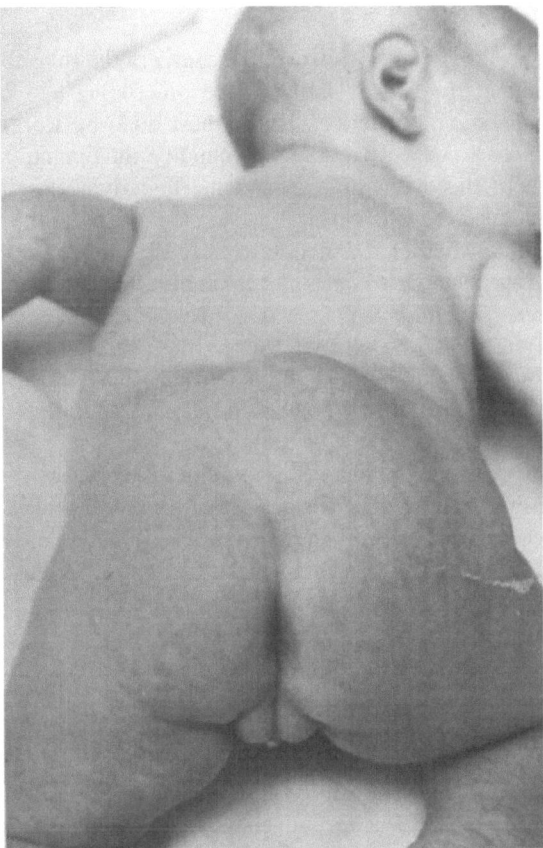

Figure 9.5. This child has a subcutaneous lipoma located at the lumbosacral junction and extending widely into the right buttock and both flanks. Masses presenting clinically such as this may either be (1) limited entirely to the subcutaneous tissue, in which case they are simply subcutaneous lipomas; (2) extend between, or through, the posterior vertebral arches, attaching themselves to the dura mater (in which case they are dural fibrolipomas); or (3) penetrate the dura to enter medulla spinalis (myelolipoma) and, occasionally, the nerve roots (leptomyelolipoma).

Lipomatous Hamartomas

Lipomatous hamartomas, the so-called *lipomas*, are almost never cervical, very rarely thoracic, most commonly lumbar and sacral, present as subcutaneous masses, variable in size, which may remain in the midline or expand over one or both gluteal areas (Fig. 9.5). They almost invariably present either as subcutaneous masses, without neurologic deficit, or with varying degrees of radiculopathy. Myelopathy and upper motor neuron deficits are very unusual.

Surgical Technique

It is best to make a midline incision over the center of the subcutaneous lipoma, and then to retract the skin laterally before proceeding to resect the entire mass of subcutaneous fatty tissue. This is best done by working within the loose, subcutaneous, connective tissue surrounding the lipoma, freeing it completely from both the overlying skin and the underlying fascia of the paravertebral muscle masses. This enables the surgeon to elevate the entire lipoma, so as to determine whether it penetrates the (dysraphic) vertebral arches and intervertebral ligaments. If so, it is not a simple subcutaneous lipoma, but a *dural fibrolipoma, myelolipoma,* or a *leptomyelolipoma.* If such an extension exists, the lipoma should be severed, cutting the subcutaneous component of the lipoma from the hourglass extension into the spinal canal. One may cut this with impunity, since nerve roots are never located within this portion of the lipoma.

With the subcutaneous lipomatous mass removed, one has excellent visualization of the dysraphic and normal posterior vertebral arches, so that they may be cleared of paravertebral muscle masses by subperiosteal dissection, using periosteal elevators. It is recommended that one strip muscular and periosteal tissue from at least two spinous arches beneath the hourglass extension of the lipoma, and three above it. *The performance of laminectomy, to expose the spinal canal is discouraged*, especially because these children already suffer the destabilizing effects of the dysraphic state, greatly predisposing them to scoliosis. Consequently, one is advised to perform a *laminotomy*, a procedure that not only contributes significantly to diminishing postoperative scoliosis, but also one that allows the surgeon to expose as extensive an area of the spinal canal as he chooses. It is recommended that the laminotomy be extended from two vertebrae below the hourglass extension of the lipoma to the superior surface of the arch of the third vertebra above this transvertebral extension of lipoma.

Once the laminotomy has been performed and the epidural bleeders stopped, one may inspect the underlying dura above and below the transdural extension of tumor. Some surgeons recommend opening the dura from above downward, reasoning that they prefer to expose normal spinal cord first and then to work toward the lipoma. Others prefer just the opposite, for just the opposite reasons. It is a matter of surgical judgment and familiarity: what works well for one surgeon is not necessarily correct for another.

In either event, whether beginning to work from the spinal cord downward, or from below the lipoma upward, individual nerve roots must be identified, so that one is obliged to work with magnification and to proceed slowly in dissecting the lipoma from within the spinal canal. In essence, the entire indication for the procedure rests with successful decompression of the spinal cord and the roots coursing through or being splain over the lipoma. One does not, and cannot, resect completely all lipomas: some (the *myelolipomas* and *leptomyelolipomas*) grow within the center of the spinal cord, which telescopes the finger-like extension of lipoma from its center. Others, the *lipomeningocele dural fibrolipomas*, may occasionally be separated from the cord and roots. These facts, in essence, are the crux of disagreement between those neurosurgeons recommending elective removal of lipoma and those who prefer to observe the child, reserving recommendation for surgery until neurologic deficits appear. It is not possible to know preoperatively whether one can remove a lipomatous hamartoma completely since it may extend into the spinal cord, engulf the spinal cord and nerve roots, or simply compress neural (cord and/or root) elements.

The use of the laser eliminates traction on the lipoma, and, consequently, traction of the spinal cord and nerve roots. Intraoperative SSEPs are helpful.

Once one has removed all of the lipoma or dural fibrolipoma he is *comfortable* with removing (this, and only this, should represent the end-point of his operative procedure), the dura is closed. Inspection of the cul-de-sac allows one to ascertain that a tongue of fatty tumor is not left attached to neural elements at one end and dura at the other, lest the cord subsequently become tethered. It is often impossible to close the dura without bringing a fascial graft into place. The laminotomy flap should be brought back into position, anchored down, and the paraspinal muscles, in turn, sewn to the interspinous ligaments. Redundant skin is resected and the remainder of the closure is effected with inverted mattress sutures. The very negative aspect of this procedure is the possibility of postoperative adhesions between dura and cord—tethering the cord.

By far the single most common **dysraphic hamartoma**, the *lipoma*, is generally located within the region of the filum terminale and cauda equina. These masses either remain confined within the subarachnoid and subdural spaces, or perforate the meninges at one discrete point to expand through the defect in the posterior vertebral arch and within the subcutaneous spaces.

The indications for surgery are either aesthetic or neurologic. If the child is perfectly normal neurologically, the indication for surgery is aesthetic. If a neurologic deficit becomes apparent, however, surgery is to be recommended. Some neurosurgeons, especially at the present time, are recommending elective resection of the lipoma even in children without neurologic deficit. There is no evidence that the children they operate electively do not subsequently develop a neurologic deficit. *In fact, quite the opposite is true.* For the present, consequently, it appears that the recommendation for elective surgery or for observing the child is one of judgment of the individual neurosurgeon, that one cannot assure a family either that the child will not subsequently suffer progressive neurologic deterioration or, if he does, that it will not be as severe as if he were not operated "prophylactically." The author prefers to observe asymptomatic children, and to operate only those who develop signs.

The dural fibrolipoma is extremely difficult to distinguish immediately from the *myelolipoma* and the *leptomyelolipoma* (Fig. 9.6), which may expand from within the conus medullaris out into the *cul-de-sac*, engulfing completely the

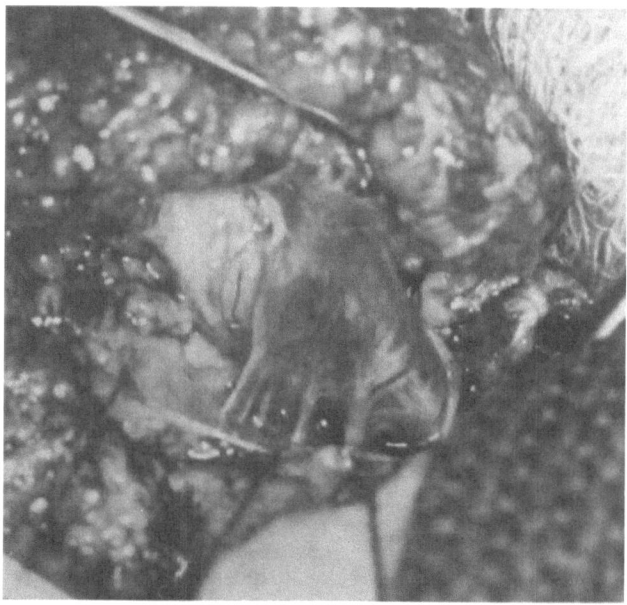

Figure 9.6. This is a leptomyelolipoma. One notes the Penfield dissector holding the subcutaneous fatty mass away from the tongue-like extension of fatty tissue, lipoma, into the conus medullaris and nerve roots. What does one do? Amputate the fatty tissue at the entrance into the conus? Pursue the lipoma into the conus and nerve roots? If the fatty tumor has not been removed from the medulla spinalis and nerve roots, what positive function has the surgery served?

filum terminale and varying numbers of dorsal and ventral nerve root components of the *cauda equina*. These latter tumors are difficult, if not impossible, to deal with surgically since they are composed of fatty tissue, nerve fibers, meningeal strands, and fibrous bands. One simply is not able to distinguish a fibrous band from a meningeal strand from a nerve fiber, or from an entrapped nerve root.

Dural fibrolipomas, on the other hand, are quite easy to identify and resect completely since they expand as well-delimited tumor masses, dumb-bell fashion, within the intra- and extradural compartments, on either side of the dysraphic posterior vertebral arch. These are similar in histology and point of origin to the lipomas which may be found within mesenchymal tissue, and dura, separating the two halves of a diastematomyelia.

The *lipomeningocele* (Fig. 9.7) is, in essence, a dural fibrolipoma that has expanded into both the extra- and intradural compartments *and* that has a cystic component at either end of the dumb-bell. Lemire et al.[12] consider this entity as one in which the fatty mass expands on either side of dura, which it penetrates as a fibrous stalk, but state little more. The author has chosen to use the surgi-

Figure 9.7.A. Lipomeningocele. This child had a lipomeningocele with lipomatous mass on either side of the dysraphic spinal column and both intraspinal and subcutaneous meningocele (digit-like structure). **B**: Lipomeningocele. This myelographic study shows the spinal cord as a less dense structure extending to the posterior surface of the spinal canal, to which it is adherent. Both intraspinal and extraspinal cysts are present, and one notes the space-filling defect from the lipomatous tissue.

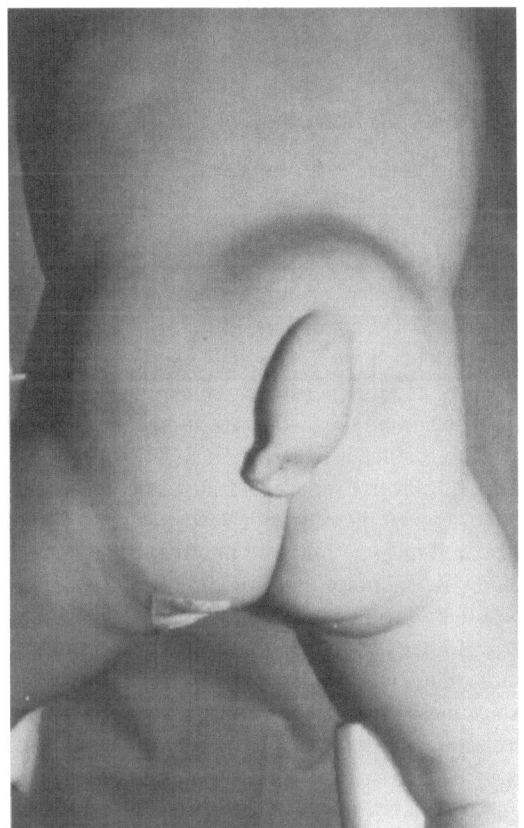

A

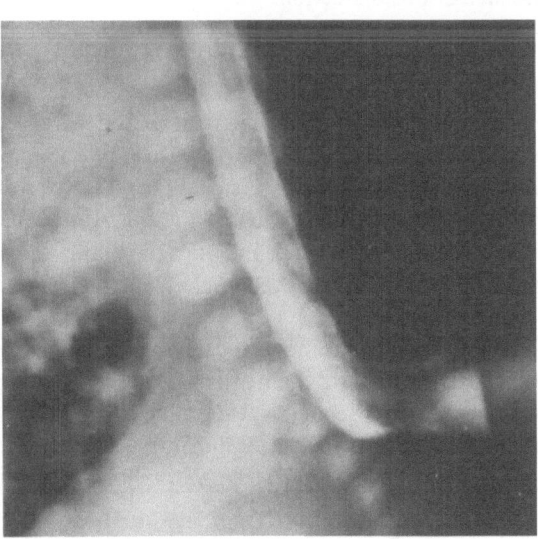

B

cally more valuable classification which has evolved from the works of James and Lassman, and Karch and Urich.[13]

Dermoid Hamartomas

These hamartomas are announced clinically by a tuft or a patch of hair, abnormal pigmentation of the skin, a dimple or pit, or sinus tract that is connected to an intraspinal dermoid tumor. There may be digit-like growths along the midsagittal plane of the body.

The surgical technique for removing them consists of isolating the dermal sinus, if present, and performing an elliptical incision around it, taking care not to open it or empty its contents into the surgical field. Once the ellipse of skin has been cut and the incision extended into the subcutaneous area, it is best to tie a ligature around the sinus tract and cut away the portion in contact with the skin so as to remove it from the field. The dissection then extends around the sinus tract, or fibrous band, separating this latter from the surrounding tissue, and continues toward the posterior vertebral arch. If the tract extends through the vertebrae, it must be followed into the spinal canal and, subsequently, through the dura if it penetrates this structure. If one is obliged to enter the spinal canal, it is best to perform a laminotomy, and to plan to reconstruct the posterior vertebral arches after the dermal tumor has been removed. Opening the dura allows the surgeon to evaluate the extent of intradural tumor and to remove it, if possible. Since these tumors almost invariably consist of dermal elements, hair, epithelial rests, etc., it is impossible to predict what one will find. When the dermoid tumor is associated with a lipoma, the mass may invade the cord making resection impossible. Removing dermoid elements from the surface of the roots and spinal cord, avoiding attempts to dissect tumor from within either of these neural elements is the essence of this dissection.

Endodermal Hamartomas

The endodermal hamartomas are associated with ventral meningocele, a result of failure of the two sides of the vertebral body to fuse to one another. A hernia sac extends into the retroperitoneal lumbar or sacral (very rarely retropleural) areas. At times, there is a fistulous connection to the gut. Consequently, one may encounter rudiments of intestinal tissue in either the hernia sac or spinal canal. Also, mucus-producing columnar epithelium may line the ventral surface of the spinal canal.

Surgical closure of the anterior meningocele entails identifying and opening the meningeal lining of the neck of the hernia sac, inserting a plug of bone graft into the defect in the vertebral body(*ies*), and then using either a periosteal or *fascia lata* graft to close the dural defect. If the intra-abdominal (retroperitoneal) mass is of significant size, the general surgeon should remove it through a laparatomy.[14]

References

1. Sharrard WJW, Zachary RB, Lorber J, Bruce AM: A controlled trial of immediate and delayed closure of spina bifida cystica. Arch Dis Child 39:18–22, 1963.

2. Duckworth T, Sharrard WJ, Lister J, Seymour N: Hemimyelocele. Dev Med Child Neurol Suppl 16:69–75, 1968.

3. Lebedeff A: Über die Entstehung der Anencephalie mit Spina Bifida bei Vögeln und Menschen. Virchows Arch Pathol Anat Physiol 86:263–298, 1881.

4. von Recklinghausen F: Untersuchungen über die Spina bifida. Teil 2: Über die Art und die Entstehung der Spina bifida ihere Beziehung zur Rückenmarks- und Darmspalte. Virchows Arch Pathol Anat Physiol 105:296–332, 1886.

5. Morgagni GB: De Sedibus et Causis Morborum, (transl. Alexander B), Miller and Cadell, London, 1769.

6. Patten BM: Embryological stages in the establishing of myeloschisis with spina bifida. Am J Anat 93:365–395, 1953.

7. James CCM, Lassman LP: Spinal dysraphism. The diagnosis and treatment of progressive lesions in spina bifida occulta. J Bone Joint Surg 44:828–840, 1962.

8. Ingraham FD, Matson DD: Neurosurgery in Infancy and Childhood. Charles C Thomas, Springfield, IL, 1954.

9. Talwalker VC, Datsur DK: Meningoceles and meningomyeloceles (ectopic spinal cord). Clinicopathological basis of a new classification. J Neurol Neurosurg Psychiatry 33:251–262, 1970.

10. Emery JL, Lendon RG: The local cord lesion in neurospinal dysraphism (meningomyelocele). J Pathol 110:83–96, 1973.

11. Rokos J: Pathogenesis of congenital malformations of the central nervous system with special reference to spina bifida and Arnold–Chiari malformation. MD Thesis. University of Birmingham, England, 1973.

12. Lemire RJ, Loeser JD, Leech RW, Ellsworth CA Jr: Normal and Abnormal development of the Human Nervous System. Harper & Row, Hagerstown, MD, 1975.

13. Karch SB, Urich H: Occipital encephalocele: a morphological study. J Neurol Sci 15:89–112, 1972.

14. Raimondi AJ: Pediatric Neurosurgery: Theory and Art of Surgical Techniques. Springer-Verlag, New York, 1987.

CHAPTER 10

Nursing Care of Children with Spinal Dysraphism

Theresa Cunningham Meyer

Spinal dysraphism is a term used to describe those congenital anomalies that occur in the early weeks of gestation, during and after the closure of the neural tube.[1,2] Children with any form of spinal dysraphism most often require complex medical and nursing care.

Pediatric neurosurgical nursing is in itself a subspecialty, requiring astute observational and nursing skills. When one considers the multisystem involvement in the patient with spinal dysraphism, the nursing implications are challenging. Nurses must have knowledge of the types of spinal dysraphism, their clinical presentation, and the preoperative and postoperative management of these patients. The purpose of this chapter is to discuss the nursing implications of caring for the child with meningomyelocele, lipomeningocele, and the tethered cord syndrome. Emphasis is on the patient with meningomyelocele, as nursing care of the meningomyelocele patient broadly applies to all dysraphic states. However, there are additional patient needs with each entity which must be incorporated into an individualized plan of care. These are considered separately. The focus is on nursing management during the initial hospitalization, with discussion of preoperative and postoperative care.

Meningomyelocele

Meningomyelocele results from abnormal closure of the posterior neural tube.[3] It is characterized by a saclike protrusion which consists of an open neural placode. The external surface of this neural tissue is bathed by cerebrospinal fluid. It is important to note that the presence of this cerebrospinal fluid does not indicate rupture of the meningomyelocele.[4] The site of the sac may occur at any point along the spinal cord (Fig. 10.1).[5,6]

Initial Assessment and Preoperative Care

When the neonate with a diagnosis of meningomyelocele arrives on the unit, a thorough nursing assessment is required due to multisystem abnormalities that

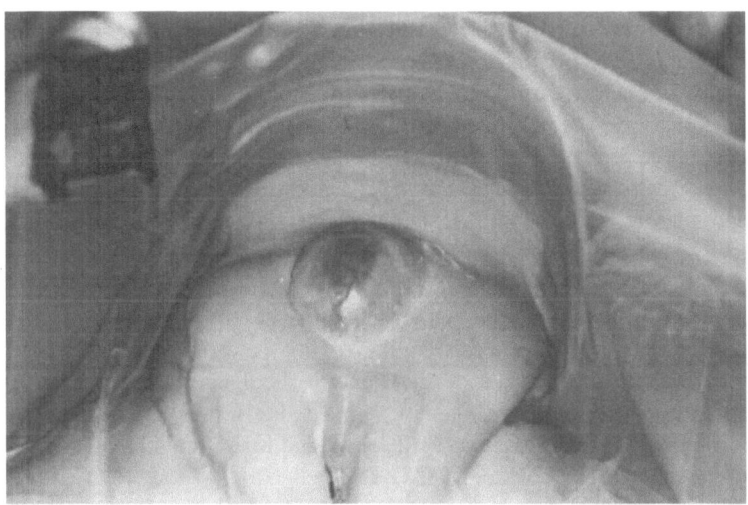

Figure 10.1. An open meningomyelocele at the lumbosacral region.

may present. During this initial period, the neonate is also being examined by the multidisciplinary team, including the orthopedic surgeon, neurosurgeon, urologist, neonatologist, and physical therapist. This can be a chaotic phase, so it is imperative that the nurse have a systematic means of assessment and recording of the infant's status at regular intervals.

The infant is placed prone in a warmed environment, such as an isolette or radiant warmer. Although assessment of the meningomyelocele site is a priority, initial assessment and stabilization of the infant's respiratory status should not be neglected. With the meningomyelocele site covered with sterile saline dressings, the respiratory status is assessed and an initial set of "vitals" taken. After stabilization of the infant, the meningomyelocele site is assessed. The size of the lesion and its appearance, including type and amount of drainage, should be noted.[5-7] The site is then covered with sterile nonadherent dressings soaked in normal saline.[6,8,9] Some authors recommend soaking the site with chemical or antimicrobial solutions.[5,7] Others recommend that these solutions not be applied to exposed neural tissue.[4] These saline dressings should be changed frequently enough that the site is kept moist. Sterile technique is used when changing the dressings. Approximately 90% of children born with meningomyelocele have an enlarged ventricular system, but only 80 to 90% require shunting for hydrocephalus.[10] The neonate should be assessed for signs of increased intracranial pressure and hydrocephalus. A head circumference is taken and the fontanel and sutures assessed. Are the sutures split or overriding? Are the fontanels flat and soft or bulging and tense?[6] The pupils are checked for equality and reaction to light, and extraocular movements (EOMs) are noted. The nurse should observe for sunsetting eyes, which may be an indication of increased intracranial pressure.[5]

In the neonate with meningomyelocele there is usually complete or partial paralysis of the skeletal muscles associated with the level of the lesion and a corresponding loss of sensory function.[11] Congenital hip flexion and knee-extension contractures, hip dislocation, and varieties of club foot are associated with meningomyelocele. They are due to intrauterine muscle imbalance.[12,13] Mobility of the neonate should be noted along with any associated abnormalities. Are spontaneous movements of the lower extremities noted?[7] Does the patient respond to tactile or painful stimuli? All of these observations should be recorded. Physical Therapy is notified and a preoperative muscle test performed.

Over 90% of children with meningomyelocele have a neurogenic bladder and bowel incontinence. Anal relaxation and prolapse are associated with lower motor neuron lesions.[3] The preoperative voiding pattern is assessed. Does the patient dribble urine or void a steady stream?[6] The bladder is palpated to check for distention. The patient should be on accurate intake and output, with a specific gravity done at least every 4 hours. Anal tone should be assessed, with pattern and consistency of stools also noted.

Lastly, but of equal importance, is the family assessment. If the neonate has been transferred to a pediatric center and the father has accompanied the infant to the hospital, he must be informed of the child's status and plan of care. When he meets with the neurosurgeon, the nurse should be in attendance to clarify any questions that might later arise. Communication with the mother at the referring hospital should be established and continued at regular intervals. During this time the team social worker also becomes involved with the family. It is important to remember that this can be an overwhelming and often devastating time for the parents. Therefore, much of what is said to the parents will not be retained and will have to be repeated.

Postoperative Care

The open meningomyelocele is closed within the first 24 hours.[14,15] The infection rate will increase if the closure is delayed beyond 48 hours.[16] Postoperatively, the goal is to prevent infection and minimize tension on the suture line. The patient is placed prone, but the extremities are not restrained. The patient can be positioned from side to side once the risk of cerebrospinal fluid leakage or wound breakdown has decreased. This positioning of the patient must be evaluated on an individual basis. Although use of the Bradford frame or "gingerbread board" is still advocated,[7,16] in this author's experience these are not used. They interfere with the child's mobility of extremities and restrict stimulation, which are vital during this newborn period. The integrity of the incision can be maintained with careful positioning and without restraining the infant. It should be noted that these same precautions should be used when feeding, weighing, or allowing the parents to hold the infant.

During the postoperative period and with each subsequent hospitalization, nursing actions are directed toward six problem areas: (1) skin integrity; (2) neurologic status; (3) mobility; (4) bladder and bowel function; (5) nutrition;

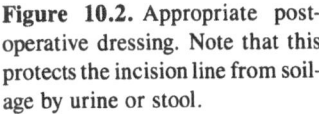

Figure 10.2. Appropriate post-operative dressing. Note that this protects the incision line from soilage by urine or stool.

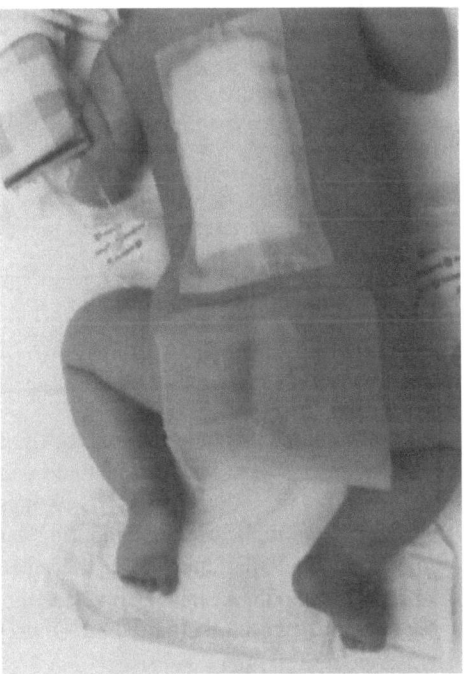

(6) family interactions. Each area is discussed separately, and discharge-teaching incorporated into these areas.

Skin Integrity

At the time of dressing changes, the wound should be inspected for any drainage, cerebrospinal fluid leakage, or areas of aseptic necrosis.[16] If the back wound is edematous and within a short time becomes flat, leakage of cerebrospinal fluid from the wound should be suspected. At this time, frequent observations of the wound should be made for leakage. A plastic drape should be placed below the meningomyelocele-site dressing. This drape should lie over the buttocks to protect the wound from soilage with urine and stool (Fig. 10.2).[9]

If the patient is discharged with the sutures still present, the family should be taught to change the dressing daily and as needed. Emphasis should be placed on correct positioning of the patient until the sutures are removed. Parents should also be aware of sensory deficits in the lower extremities and be taught to avoid extreme temperatures and to inspect the infant's skin daily.[12]

Neurologic Status

As stated previously, the infant must be monitored for signs of increased intra-cranial pressure. If hydrocephalus is present and a shunt is inserted, it is impera-

Table 10.1. Signs and symptoms of shunt malfunction

Infants	Toddlers	School-age children	Adults
Bulging or tense fontanel	Vomiting	Headaches	Headaches
Vomiting	Lethargy	Vomiting	Vomiting
Irritability	Irritability	Lethargy	Lethargy
Change in appetite	Seizures	Seizures	Seizures
Lethargy	Headaches	Irritability	Swelling or redness along shunt tract
Sunsetting eyes	Swelling or redness along shunt tract	Swelling or redness along shunt tract	
Seizures		Decreased school performance	
Swelling or redness along shunt tract			

tive that the nurse be able to recognize the signs and symptoms of a shunt malfunction (Table 10.1). The nurse should palpate the shunt tract and observe for edema, erythema, or tenderness. Dressings and suture lines are observed for drainage. The complications of shunting can be an important cause of death in meningomyelocele patients[17] and, therefore, discharge teaching in this area is vital. Parents should be taught to assess the fontanel, head circumference, and shunt tract daily with the infant's bath. By school-age the child himself should be taught to assess the tract daily.

With teaching it should be stressed that every child is different and some may display subtle signs of malfunction, such as personality or behavioral changes, or a decline in school performance.[18] Any abnormality should be reported to the pediatrician or neurosurgeon involved in the child's care.

The Chiari II malformation is a primary cause of mortality in the patient with meningomyelocele.[14] It is characterized by downward displacement of the vermis into the cervical spinal canal, causing compression of the underlying brain stem. This displacement may, or may not, be associated with displacement of the cerebellar tonsils. Almost all patients have occasional problems secondary to this malformation. Problems associated with the Chiari II malformation are respiratory stridor, inability to suck, difficulty with swallowing or drooling, and regurgitation of fluids through the nose.[10] Reflux with aspiration may be present.[19] Other signs of the Chiari II malformation are brief apneic episodes with cyanosis, which may become prolonged.[10] Nurses must observe the infant closely for any of the problems associated with this malformation. Emergency equipment, such as oxygen, suction, and an oral airway should be kept at the bedside.

Mobility

It is important that passive range-of-motion exercises be instituted within the first few weeks of life to prevent contractures.[12] The infant is repositioned frequently to prevent skin breakdown.[5,16] The infant should receive tactile, auditory, and verbal stimulation to ensure optimal development. Parents should be taught range-of-motion exercises by the physical therapist before discharge. They are also instructed in appropriate methods of stimulation and are encouraged to hold the infant in such a way as not to put any pressure on the suture line.

Bladder and Bowel Function

Postoperatively, the patient remains on accurate intake and output. By doing this, the nurse is alerted to urinary retention. In our institution we do not Credé the bladder as it can contribute to urethral reflux.[20] If the patient is retaining urine, intermittent clean catheterization is instituted. The introduction of intermittent clean catheterization[21] has provided a viable alternative to urinary diversion.[19,22] It ensures emptying of the bladder and may be used in cases of urinary retention, reflux or overflow incontinence.[22] The combination of intermittent catheterization and pharmacologic agents can eliminate retention and enhance social continence as the child grows older.[12] Intermittent clean catheterization should be performed every 4 hours, except during the night. The exception to this is if the patient is on intravenous fluids, or continuous-drip nasogastric feeding, with potential for bladder distention, at which time it should be performed around the clock. After 1 week of age the patient should undergo an intravenous pyelogram and a voiding cystourethrogram.

If the child is discharged home on intermittent catheterization, both parents should be taught this technique and the rationale for it. The nurse should stress the importance of doing it regularly to prevent overdistention of the bladder which causes decreased blood flow to the bladder tissue and, thus, decreased resistance to bacteria.[21]

In the neonatal period the most common bowel problem is constant stooling. The infant should be kept clean to prevent skin breakdown.[15] During infancy constipation may begin to be a problem. Increasing distention and atonia of the intestinal wall may interfere with later bowel management. During this initial postoperative phase, teaching should be done regarding prevention of constipation and dietary methods to regulate the bowel.[12] An actual bowel program will be instituted at a later time.

Nutrition

Obesity in the child with meningomyelocele is a major problem which can interfere with ambulation and contribute to skin breakdown.[15,18] During the postoperative period the dietician determines the neonate's caloric needs and meets with the family before discharge. Teaching should be done regarding the possibility of reflux and other feeding problems related to the Chiari II malformation. Parents should be taught to feed the infant with the head elevated. Slow feedings are encouraged.

Family Interactions

Throughout this chapter, discharge teaching has been incorporated into the nursing care. Discharge teaching can be difficult when dealing with the patient with meningomyelocele. It is necessary to give adequate information about possible complications, and yet it is important to encourage the parents to feel comfortable with their newborn child. To foster confidence in their caretaking abilities, we require a 24-hour stay for the parents before discharge. During this time the parents are responsible for complete care of the child. This allows them the security of having medical and nursing staff available for questions during the child's daily care. It also provides the nursing staff with an opportunity to evaluate the parents' care.

Lipomeningocele

Spinal lipomeningoceles are a common form of spinal dysraphism and can occur in any age group.[23,24] In the first year of life, most infants with lipomeningoceles are asymptomatic and present because of the skin covered mass on the back which is viewed as a cosmetic deformity.[4] Some clinicians think that if left untreated, the mass may lead to progressive and insidious neurologic denervation of one or both extremities. Lipomeningoceles can lead to changes in bladder and bowel function, including incontinence, recurrent urinary tract infections, urine retention, hydronephrosis, and severe pyelonephritis.[25,26] Care of the patient with lipomeningocele is based on the same rationale as the patient with meningomyelocele. This dysraphic state requires the expertise of all subspecialties involved in the care of the patient with meningomyelocele.[27] A major difference between these two entities is that patients with lipomeningoceles have not been shown to have hydrocephalus or the Chiari II malformation.[4,23,26]

Preoperative Care

Preoperative evaluation of the patient with lipomeningocele includes studies listed in Table 10.2.[25,27] If the infant is under 1 year of age there is incomplete ossification of the spine and plain radiographs are difficult. In these cases ultrasonography is used.[25,28]

It is important that the patient and family be aware of the preoperative evaluation and what each test involves. They should realize that with many of these examinations the patient will be NPO and require intravenous fluids.

Post myelogram, the patient is observed very closely with frequent monitoring of vital signs. Headache, nausea, and vomiting are the most frequent complaints encountered after a metrizamide myelogram.[29] Movement of all four extremities is assessed, along with bladder and bowel function. If metrizamide is the contrast material used, the patient should be on bedrest with the head elevated 30 to 45 degrees. This prevents movement of the dye into the intracranial regions, and thus decreases the risk of seizures.[29] Phenothiazine drugs should not be administered for 48 hours after the injection of the metrizamide as these drugs can increase the risk of seizures.

Table 10.2. Preoperative work-up of lipomeningocele and tethered cord syndrome

1.	Radiography
2.	Myelography
3.	CT
4.	Intravenous pyelogram
5.	Voiding cystourethrogram
6.	Urodynamic studies
7.	Muscle testing

From refs. 24, 27.

Postoperative Care

Treatment consists of a laminectomy to remove the mass, involving a midline skin incision.[4,26] Again, postoperatively the goal is to maintain the integrity of the skin. Schut[26] advocates maintaining the patient in the prone position with the head lower than the buttocks for 72 hours. In the author's experience, the patients are best kept flat for 72 hours and log-rolled from side to side. Postoperative complications to observe for are wound dehiscence, wound infection, or cerebrospinal fluid leakage.[1] Parents should be informed that the wound might appear swollen due to a temporary leakage of cerebrospinal fluid into the subcutaneous tissue.[23] The degree and rapidity of elevation to the sitting position after the initial 72 hours varies with each individual case and the appearance of the wound. Movement of the extremities is assessed with vital signs and any deterioration in function should be reported immediately.

Postoperatively, the patient will have an indwelling catheter for a varying period of time. After removal of the catheter, a urine culture should be obtained. The patient is also observed for urinary retention. Intermittent catheterization might be required for a period of time, but this is usually a temporary phenomenon with the patient regaining his preoperative voiding pattern.

Tethered Cord Syndrome

The tethered cord syndrome is fixation of the distal spinal cord in an abnormal position, which can produce stretch, distortion, and ischemia of the spinal cord.[30] Presenting symptoms include scoliosis, leg or back pains especially with exercise, bladder and bowel incontinence, and progressive motor or sensory deficits in the lower extremities.[31] Tethering can be produced by various lesions including lipoma, diastematomyelia, and can occur after repair of meningomyeloceles.[4,30]

The preoperative evaluation and postoperative care are similar to those for the patient with lipomeningocele. In addition, postoperatively, the patient may have a low-grade fever and irritability for 24 to 48 hours. This is in reaction to blood in the spinal fluid and will resolve.[30] Parents should be informed that this might occur.

Summary

The nursing care of the patient with meningomyelocele, lipomeningocele, and tethered cord syndrome is similar, but each clinical entity has unique features. With each syndrome, maintenance of skin integrity of the wound and prevention of infection is a priority. All require assessment and maintenance of optimal mobility and of bladder and bowel function. The child with meningomyelocele requires additional knowledge. Nurses must recognize the symptomatology of increased intracranial pressure and of the Chiari II malformation. Nurses with such knowledge are essential to the care required by these challenging patients.

References

1. James H, Williams J, Brock W, Kaplan G, Sang UH: Radical removal of lipomas of the conus and cauda equina with laser microneurosurgery. Neurosurgery 15:340–343, 1984.
2. Till K: Spinal dysraphism. A study of congenital malformations of the lower back. J Bone Joint Surg 51:415–422, 1969.
3. Reigel D: Spina bifida. In: McLaurin R (ed): Pediatric Neurosurgery Grune & Stratton, New York, 1982.
4. McLone D, Naidich T: Myelodysplasia and tethered spinal cord. In: Tachdjian M (ed): Pediatric Orthopedics. W.B. Saunders, Philadelphia, 1988.
5. Hausman K: Neurological crisis. In: Vestal K, Miller McKenzie C (eds): High Risk Perinatal Nursing, W.B. Saunders, Philadelphia, 1983, pp 399–411.
6. Pressman S: Myelomeningocele: a multidisciplinary problem. J Neurosurg Nursing 13:333–336, 1981.
7. Matthews UF: Manual of Pediatric Nursing Care Plans. Little, Brown, Boston, 1979.
8. Pillitteri A: Neonatal Newborn Nursing, 3rd edit. Little, Brown, Boston, 1985.
9. Sporing E, Walton M, Cady C: Pediatric Nursing Policies, Procedures, and Personnel. Medical Economic Books, Oradell, NJ, 1984.
10. Epstein F: Myelomeningocele: "pitfalls" in early and late management. Clin Neurosurg 30:366–384, 1983.
11. Moore K: The nervous system. In: Moore K (ed): The Developing Human W.B. Saunders, Philadelphia, 1982, pp 375–412.
12. Badell-Ribera A: Myelodysplasia. In: Molnar G (ed): Pediatric Rehabilitation (pp 176–206). Wilkins & Wilkins, Baltimore, pp. 1985, 176–206.
13. Brocklehurst G: Spina Bifida for the Clinician. J.B. Lippincott, Philadelphia, 1976.
14. McLone D, Dias L, Kaplan W, Sommers M: Concepts in the management of spina bifida. Concepts Pediatr Neurosurg 5:97–106, 1985.
15. Passo S: Malformations of the neural tube. Nursing Clin North Am 15:5–21, 1980.
16. Mori K: Anomalies of the Central Nervous System. Thieme-Stratton, New York, 1985.

17. Myers G: Myelomeningocele: the medical aspects. Pediatr Clin North Am 31:165–175, 1984.
18. Colgan M: The child with spina bifida. Am J Dis Child 135:854–858, 1981.
19. McLone D: Results of treatment of children born with a myelomeningocele. Clin Neurosurg 30:407–412, 1983.
20. Mulcahy M, James H: Management of urinary incontinence in infancy and childhood. Concepts Pediatr Neurosurg 1:216–229, 1981.
21. Lapides J, Diokno A, Silber S, Lowe B: Clean, intermittent self-catheterization in the treatment of urinary tract disease. J Urol 107:458–461, 1972.
22. Schoenberg H, Meador M: Analysis of 48 children with myelodysplasia. J Urol 127:749–750, 1982.
23. Hoffman H, Taecholarn C, Hendrick E, Humphreys R: Management of lipomyelomeningoceles. J Neurosurg 62:1–8, 1985.
24. James H, Walsh J: Spinal dysraphism. Curr Prob Pediatr 11:1–25, 1981.
25. James H, Schieble W, Kerber C, Hilton S: Comparison of high resolution real time ultrasonography and high resolution computed tomography in an infant with spinal dysraphism. Neurosurgery 13:301–305, 1983.
26. Schut L, Bruce D, Sutton L: The management of the child with a lipomyelomeningocele. Clin Neurosurg 30:464–476, 1983.
27. McLone D, Mutluer S, Naidich T: Lipomeningoceles of the conus medullaris. Concepts Pediatr Neurosurg 3:170–177, 1983.
28. Fernback S, Naidich T, McLone D, Shkolnik A: Sonography of congenital anomalies of the caudal spine. Perinatol Neonatol 8:50–59, 1984.
29. Nebe D: Diagnostic studies. In: Snyder M (ed): A Guide to Neurological and Neurosurgical Nursing. New York: John Wiley & Sons, New York, 1983, pp 41–71.
30. Reigel D: Tethered spinal cord. Concepts Pediatr Neurosurg 4:162–164, 1983.
31. Fedun P: Tethered cord syndrome. J Neurosurg Nursing 14:144–149, 1982.
32. McLone D, Reigel D, Sommers M, Frisbie C: An Introduction to Hydrocephalus. Chicago: American Heyer-Schulte Corp., 1982.

CHAPTER 11

The Orthopedic Aspects of Spinal Dysraphism

Luciano S. Dias

In this chapter we discuss the orthopedic problems and management of the two most common types of spinal dysraphism: spina bifida and lumbosacral lipomas.

Spina Bifida

The overall management of the spina bifida child has evolved significantly in the past 17 years. With new techniques in neurosurgical treatment, the mortality rate has declined to a very low level.[1] Urologic care has also changed; the use of intermittent catheterization and drugs has kept a significant number of children away from serious urinary tract infections and severe renal function impairment.

Orthopedic management has also changed. With better knowledge of orthopedic pathology, new and better surgical techniques, and new types of orthoses, the ambulation ability of the spina bifida child has increased.[2]

It is needless to emphasize that the orthopedic management is part of a team approach. In addition to a highly skilled pediatric orthopedic surgeon, there is a need for a well-trained group of paramedical personnel consisting of a pediatric orthopedic nurse, a physical therapist, and an orthotist. Close, accurate communication between the orthopedic surgeon and neurosurgeon is imperative for a good outcome in orthopedic care.

We have recently reviewed 198 spina bifida children who have been treated at our institution from the first day of life by the same orthopedic and neurosurgical team. Throughout this chapter, we will be referring to some of our experiences with this selected group of children.

Factors Producing Limb Deformity and Abnormal Posture During Gait

Orthopedic deformities can be subdivided into two types: congenital and acquired. Of 198 spina bifida children, 42% had no orthopedic deformities at birth. These deformities are more common in the high level child. At birth, at the high lumbar and thoracic levels, only 16.7% were free of deformities, but at the

Figure 11.1. Severe calcaneus foot secondary to spastic dorsiflexors.

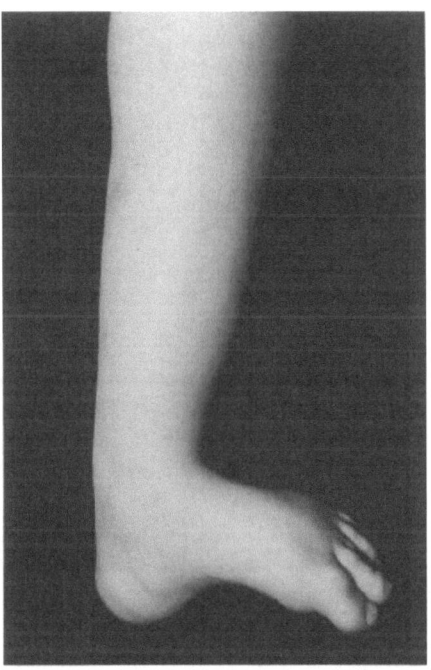

sacral level 52.4% had no deformities. The most common deformities are in the foot (54%). Congenital spinal anomalies, such as kyphosis and kyphoscoliosis, were present at birth in 7.5%. A typical example of a congenital deformity is a clubfoot or a teratologic hip dislocation.

Acquired deformities are usually secondary to muscle imbalance due either to lower or upper motor neuron lesions.[3,4] The persistent muscle imbalance leads to a gradual establishment of structural bony deformities. A typical example is the paralytic hip dislocation, seen in the low lumbar level, secondary to an imbalance between the hip flexors and abductors and the hip extensors and abductors. Another example is the calcaneal deformity secondary to an imbalance between the ankle dorsiflexors and plantar flexors (Fig. 11.1). A muscle imbalance can also be caused by spasticity which, to our knowledge, should not be present at birth. The spastic muscle leads to very early deformities, especially of the foot and knee. The two main causes of spasticity are either tethered cord or upper neuron lesion.

Acquired deformity can also occur secondary to an habitual posture assumed after birth. It usually occurs in the older child with flaccid paralysis of the lower extremities. For example, with the child lying in the supine position, the gravity force rotates the hip outward, in abduction and flexion, leading to a gradual development of a hip flexion–abduction–external rotation contracture (Fig. 11.2). It is the role of the orthopedic surgeon and physical therapist to prevent

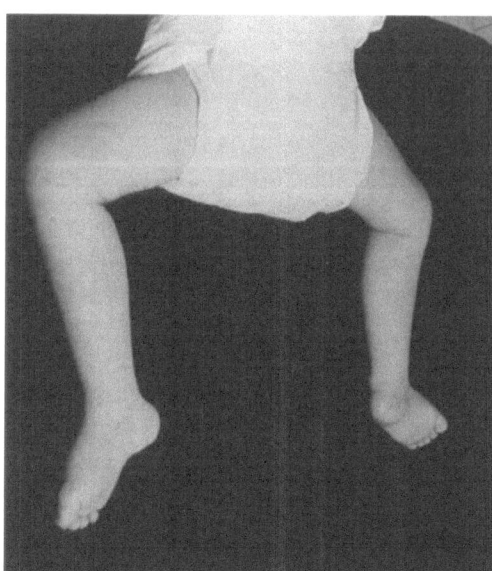

Figure 11.2. The hip position in abduction, flexion, and external rotation is characteristic of a high lumbar and lower thoracic level lesion.

these postural deformities as well as to correct muscle imbalances to prevent the development of severe structural deformities that can then interfere with mobility and gait.

Factors Related to Ambulation

Motor Level

The level of the lesion in the spinal cord and its effect on motor function have a direct effect on the walking ability of the spina bifida child. Perhaps a more rational and practical approach to the motor level is to consider spina bifida children in three main groups: (1) the high lumbar and thoracic level, in which quadriceps function is absent; (2) the low lumbar level, in which quadriceps function is present but gluteus medius and maximus functions are absent; and (3) the sacral level in which quadriceps and gluteus medius functions are present. It has been well documented[3] that quadriceps function is paramount in determining the level of community ambulation in a spina bifida child. The absence of quadriceps requires the use of a high brace, usually with a pelvic band. These children rarely attain the community ambulation level in adult life. Sixteen percent of children between the ages of 3 and 12 with a high lumbar and excellent upper extremity function and trunk balance were community ambulators. On the other hand, the low lumbar level, in spite of the absence of gluteus (in the presence of normal upper extremity function and trunk balance) coexisted with community ambulation in 94% of the children. The sacral level spina bifida child with gluteus medius and maximus should be able to ambulate without any external support.

Community ambulation was achieved in 100% of these children. In our selected population of 198 children, one-third were in the high lumbar-thoracic level group, one-third in the low lumbar level group, and one-third in the sacral level group. It is important to know that the level of the lesion should remain the same throughout the entire life of the child with spina bifida. Any change in motor level is a result of a pathology occurring at the spinal cord level, quite frequently, tethered cord. For this reason, it is imperative that the spina bifida child have a muscle test at birth and then once a year to document the stability of the motor level and motor function. It is also important to document, initially, the absence of any spasticity involving the lower extremities.

Trunk Balance

Besides the level of the lesion and degree of paralysis involving the lower extremities, trunk balance and upper extremity function are to be considered a main factor in ambulation ability. At least 30% of spina bifida children have some impairment of the sitting balance.

A functional and effective classification of sitting balance could be described as the ability to sit with or without hand support. A child has normal sitting balance when no hand support is needed, mild impairment when at least one-hand support is necessary, moderate impairment when two-hand support is needed, and severe impairment when no sitting ability is present. About 7% of spina bifida children have severe impairment of trunk balance: in this group no community ambulation is possible. All are either exercise ambulators in a special parapodium or nonambulators. About 15% have a moderate degree of impairment of the sitting balance and, again, none of these patients have the ability to walk independently. Fourteen percent had a mild impairment of the sitting balance and of these patients some will be able to walk as community ambulators.

There is an apparent coincidence of the number of shunt revisions and sitting balance. In children with normal sitting balance, the number of shunt revisions was 3.2; in children with severe involvement of the sitting balance, the average number of shunt revisions was 8.4. The instability of the central nervous system (CNS), reflected by the increased number of shunt revisions, is an indicator of the CNS function in relationship to trunk balance. A recent review of 36 children with no shunt revealed that 34 of the 36, regardless of their motor levels, were community ambulators. Looking at a group of 19 children who had more than 10 shunt revisions, 53% had normal trunk balance and 47% had either a moderate or severe impairment of sitting balance. In a group of children who had only one shunt revision, 85% were community ambulators. However, it must be remembered that sacral levels have a lower incidence of hydrocephalus, and that thoracolumbar levels have a higher incidence both of hydrocephalus and hydromyelia. Therefore, one cannot correlate directly hydrocephalus, shunt revision, and ambulation without factoring in meningomyelocele level and primary CNS damage.

Spasticity

Spasticity of the upper and/or lower extremities plays a major role in the ambulation potential of the spina bifida child. A recent study by Mazur and Menelaus[5] has shown quite clearly this correlation. Of 14 patients in whom spastic upper and lower extremities were present, only one was a community ambulator. Of patients in whom the upper extremity function was normal and there was flaccid lower extremity paralysis, 86% were community ambulators.

Body Weight

Another known factor affecting ambulation is body weight. This is particularly true for the upper lumbar and thoracic level child. It has been well documented in the literature, as well as in our own experience, that it is between the ages of 10 and 14 years that a number of high-level spina bifida children who are ambulating well with high braces will choose to be in a wheelchair because of the effects of obesity. Obesity is a common problem due to lack of physical activity. To maintain active walking ability throughout adult life, the spina bifida patient should not be overweight. An early approach to this problem is important. A dietician should be a very active member of the spina bifida clinic. Wheelchair exercises and participation in sports should be instituted.

Orthopedic Deformities

For a child to ambulate, the spine should be balanced over the pelvis, the pelvis balanced over the knees, and the feet need to be plantigrade.

Orthopedic deformities, beyond a certain limit, are important factors affecting ambulation ability. Among these deformities[6] are scoliosis and hip flexion contracture. A severe scoliosis affects trunk balance and this affects ambulation. A severe hip flexion contracture, especially in a high-level child, shifts the center of gravity forward to such a degree that a major force must be placed at the upper extremity to maintain trunk alignment and walking.

In summary, several factors can affect the walking ability of the spina bifida child. The most important is the level of the lesion. In reviewing 38 adults, all with good quadriceps function, we have found that there was a 95% correlation between quadriceps strength and the level of community ambulation. Only two were not community ambulators. One had bilateral foot amputation and the second was markedly obese.

Tethered Cord Syndrome

Radiologically, every spina bifida child may have a tethered cord. From the clinical standpoint a tethered cord demonstrates itself as a loss of motor function, or more frequently, as spasticity involving the lower extremity musculature. The most common site where spasticity is seen is at the knee flexors, medial hamstrings, and ankle dorsiflexors and evertors. Another clinical sign of tethered cord is scoliosis. In reviewing 51 patients with tethered cord at our clinic, 27 had an associated scoliosis; another three had an associated hydromyelia and tethering. It is interesting to note that the great majority of these patients presented with scoliosis in the first 4 years of life. The incidence of tethered cord syndrome is higher in the high lumbar and thoracic level child.

As our clinical experience increases, the incidence of tethered cord syndrome in spina bifida is rising. Nine percent of 198 spina bifida children studied by us had tethered cord syndrome; another 5% of our patients had a significant loss of motor function in the first 4 years of life. We feel at this point that these were patients in whom the tethered cord syndrome was not recognized initially. One may estimate that the incidence of clinical tethered cord syndrome in the first 10 years of life is around 20%.

Hydromyelia

It is well known that in spina bifida, hydromyelia can cause a spine curvature. It has been well documented that the surgical treatment of hydromyelia can lead to a gradual decrease of the scoliosis. In our review of 198 cases, 5% presented with hydromyelia within the first 10 years of life.

Orthotic Management

At least 90% of spina bifida children require some form of orthosis. Only the very low sacral level (S3), with good gastro-soleus strength, will not require an orthosis. A careful assessment of the child and his needs is important. A special orthotic team, consisting of an orthopedic surgeon, an orthotist, and a physical therapist, is indicated. The orthosis should be lightweight: the use of thermal setting plastic, such as polypropylene, has been an important advance in the orthotic management of the spina bifida child.

The type of brace is directly related to the degree of paralysis. The high lumbar and thoracic level child requires either a reciprocating gait orthosis (Fig. 11.3) if his trunk balance and upper extremity function is good,[7,8] or a parapodium such as the Orlau (Fig. 11.4), Toronto, or Rochester if not. The low lumbar level spina bifida child with good quadriceps function requires a below-knee brace (AFO) to provide ankle and foot support. On occasion, a knee-ankle-foot brace (KAFO) may be needed to provide some knee stability, or a twister cable may be attached to the AFO to control any rotational malalignment. The sacral level spina bifida child may need a below-knee brace if the gastro-soleus is weak.

Wheelchairs are, for the high lumbar-thoracic level, an important adjunct to the child's mobility. Lightweight wheelchairs, adjustable for growth, have been a major advance in recent years. Special sitting is required for children with severe spine curvatures or with severe impairment of trunk balance.

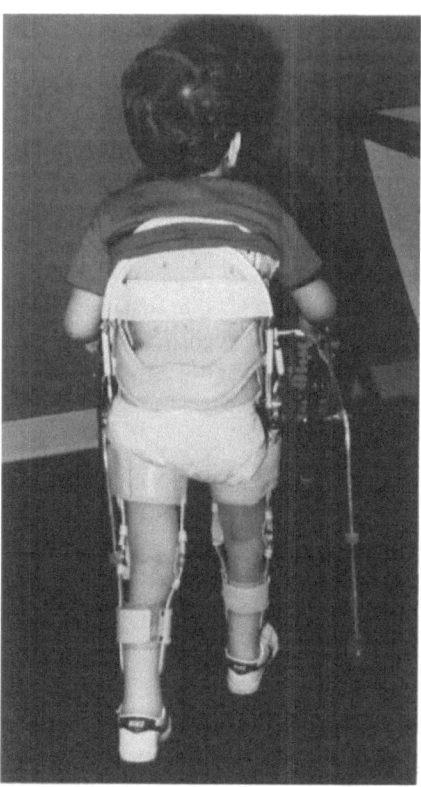

Figure 11.3. High-level spina bifida child with reciprocating gait orthosis.

General Principles of Surgical Management

Quite frequently a spina bifida child, during the growing years, needs surgical treatment of the deformities. The average number of operations is higher in the low lumbar level child because of major muscle imbalance at the hip and foot. In the first 10 years of life, a low lumbar level child may require five orthopedic procedures, a high lumbar-thoracic level child 3.5, and a sacral level child in whom muscle imbalance is less frequent, 2.5 surgeries.

Surgery has one main objective: to correct a deformity that is interfering with function. So, before undertaking major orthopedic surgery, one must analyze the child's ability to walk and his mobility for future walking ability in adult life. To minimize the number of hospitalizations, it is important to correct several deformities at the same time.[3] For instance, a thoracic level child with a hip flexion-abduction contracture and a knee flexion contracture should have correction of these deformities under the same anesthesia. It is important to have short periods of immobilization, since osteoporosis, a frequent complication of prolonged casting, may lead to pathologic fractures at cast removal. A spina bifida child, when

Figure 11.4. High-level spina bifida child with an Orlau parapodium. Note the swivel device on the parapodium base.

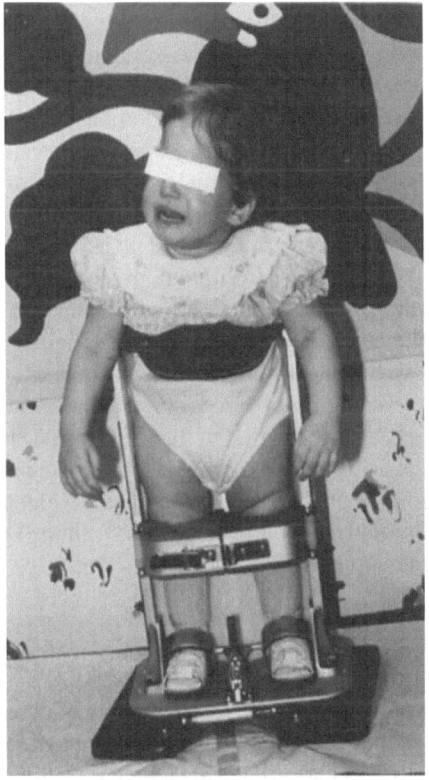

immobilized in a hip spica cast, should be allowed to stand for several hours a day to decrease osteopenia.

Early surgical intervention, correcting muscle imbalance and contractures, prevents the development of structural deformities in the bone. Usually, in children under the age of 6, most of the operations are soft tissue procedures. In the older child with structural deformities, besides correction of any muscle imbalance bony procedures are required.

A typical example of function dictating the type of surgery to be performed is the paralytic hip dislocation. In a high lumbar-thoracic level child, who will require an extensive orthosis for ambulation, a hip dislocation does not require surgical reduction. In these patients only soft tissue contractures at the hip level should be corrected (to prevent pelvic obliquity and scoliosis). On the other hand, a low lumbar level child with hip dislocation can have a functional effect on walking ability; so, in these patients, surgical reduction of the hip in association with tendon transfers and tendon releases is indicated.

It is important after any surgical intervention to prevent recurrence of the deformity, to use night splinting and have a close orthopedic follow-up.

The Spina Bifida Adult

Very few studies are available in the orthopedic literature about the spina bifida adult.[8,9] We recently reviewed, in the Chicago area, 71 spina bifida adults. Sixty percent were community ambulators and 25% were wheelchair-bound. The walking ability in this group was directly related with the motor level. Ninety-five percent of the community ambulators had quadriceps function. On the other hand, physical independence was not related to motor level. A number of the adult spina bifida, wheelchair-bound patients were independent physically. Whereas 85% had either high school or college education, only 35% of those over the age of 21 had a full-time job and 16% a part-time job. Seventy-five percent of the adults were still living with their parents. These numbers clearly show the psychological and economical dependence of the spina bifida adult, the low correlation between degree of education and productive employment.

If the overall goal of the spina bifida child is to promote mobility and independence, it is imperative that from early in life we educate the parents and children toward physical and psychological independence. It is also imperative that we provide these patients with job training and education to enable them to be active members in our society.

Lumbosacral Lipomas

Lumbosacral lipomas are a group of dysraphic conditions of the spine characterized by the incorporation of subcutaneous fat into the filum terminale, or the cauda equina, the lower portion of the spinal cord itself. They are often associated with defects in the posterior elements and are usually skin covered. Unlike meningomyelocele, the neuropathways are, for the most part, intact. The lipomas cause orthopedic and urologic manifestations by tethering the spinal cord to the surrounding structures. The resulting abnormalities are usually not present at birth, and develop later. They are often subtle in nature and of a less predictable pattern than those musculoskeletal anomalies caused by spina bifida. In the past 10 years, at the Children's Memorial Hospital Spina Bifida Clinic, we have seen and followed 127 patients who were treated for lumbosacral lipomas. We reviewed the first 57 patients. Two-thirds of these patients had orthopedic problems associated with the lumbosacral lipoma. A variety of orthopedic pathology can be seen associated with the tethering of the spinal cord secondary to the lumbosacral lipomas.

The most frequent deformities were seen in the foot (40%). An equinovarus deformity, a cavus foot with clawing of the toes, is quite common. In about 20% of our patients, the primary orthopedic problem was muscle weakness. Some have disturbance of gait, others present initially with scoliosis.

The orthopedic involvement is always asymmetric. All patients have good quadriceps function and are community ambulators. For this reason, it is imperative that the orthopedic treatment be directed toward correction of the deformities to maintain mobility and ambulation. Our experience has shown that even after the resection of the lipoma and release of the tethered cord, only 50% of the patients enjoy a partial recovery of muscle function. For this reason, any kind of tendon transfer or tendon lengthening procedure should be delayed until after 6 months, to allow recovery to occur. Of course, for structural deformities that interfere with function, the orthopedic treatment may be done at any time after the tethered cord release. In over 50% of our patients, orthopedic surgery was required to correct a major deformity that was interfering with function. Most of the problems requiring surgery were at the foot, necessitating either tendon release or transfers, and, on occasion, for structural deformities, bony procedures.

Retethering of the spinal cord in the surgical scar occurred in 16% of our patients. It was quite clear in our review that the retethering had a relationship with the neurosurgeon's previous experience. Of the lumbosacral lipomas that underwent surgical resection at our institution, the incidence of retethering was 5%. With the possibility of retethering in mind, it is clear that once surgery is performed, a continuous follow-up throughout life is necessary.

We strongly favor excision of the lipomas as soon as it is diagnosed. Of 13 patients seen by us for the first time over the age of 6 years, 12 already had an orthopedic problem related to tethering of the spinal cord. In other words, the older the patient the greater the chance for tethering of the spinal cord. Our present approach to the lumbosacral lipomas, when diagnosed at birth, is surgical excision within the first 6 weeks of life. Before surgical treatment an accurate muscle test should be done as well as a complete orthopedic examination. The child should have a muscle test, thereafter, on a yearly basis. Any change in function, any detection of a new deformity, should be considered as a clear sign of retethering of the spinal cord and a prompt neurosurgical evaluation is indicated.

References

1. McLone DG, Dias LS, Kaplan WE: Concepts in management of spina bifida. In: Concepts of Pediatric Neurosurgery, Vol. 5: S. Karger, Basel, 1984.
2. Schafer MF, Dias LS: Myelomeningocele: Orthopaedic Treatment. Williams & Wilkins, Baltimore, London 1983.
3. Menelaus MB: The Orthopaedic Management of Spina Bifida Cystica. E.S. Livingstone, 1980.
4. Sharrard WJW: The mechanism of paralytic deformity in spina bifida. Dev Med Child Neurol 4:310, 1962.
5. Mazur J, Menelaus MB: The significance of spasticity in the upper and lower limbs in myelomeningocele. J Bone Joint Surg 68B:213, 1986.
6. Lee EH, Carroll NC: Hip stability and ambulatory status in myelomeningocele. J Pediatr Orthop 5:522, 1985.
7. Lough: Ambulation of children with myelomeningocele: parapodium vs. parapodium with Orlau swivel modification. Dev Med Child Neurol 28:489, 1986.
8. Schmidt J: Clinical experience with the reciprocating gait orthosis in myelodysplasia. J Pediatr Orthop 6:157, 1986.
9. McLaurin RL: Spina Bifida: A Multidisciplinary Approach. Praeger, New York, 1986.

CHAPTER 12

Social, Psychologic, and Educational Problems

Sonya Oppenheimer

The goals of treatment for a child born with spina bifida include attainment of the highest possible level of functioning, maximum independence, and promotion of sound psychosocial development of the child, parents, and siblings.[1]

In the past 20 years articles concerning children with myelomeningocele have focused on the decreasing mortality of this population with a subsequent increase in their life span.[2] This is the result of improved medical and surgical treatment that controls hydrocephalus and infection and improves kidney function. However, if as adults this population remains unemployed, depressed, and dependent on the care of others, the initial goal of treatment has not been accomplished. To determine the effectiveness of a treatment approach, information concerning the functional status of the adult population is required.

A recent publication edited and written by Dr. David B. Shurtleff,[3] Myelodysplasia Extrophies: Significance, Prevention and Treatment summarizes the most pertinent data currently available about long-term treatment and management issues related to the care of children with spina bifida. It is important to understand evaluation of past data to provide and alter as necessary appropriate treatment modalities, including provision of support services that are needed by children with spina bifida and their families. In a survey of adults born prior to the preshunt era from 1955,[3] 53% were integrated well, had complete self-help skills, and were employed. Fifteen percent partially completed self-help skills, and 32% of this population were under custodial care with no programming. Other studies show employment figures to vary from 17% to 70% of full employment. A more recent study from the Cincinnati population shows[4] none of the young adults followed in the program were gainfully employed. In a more recent study by Shurtleff, 25% of the adult[3] populations were employed. The population who survived to adulthood, and who are now being identified, usually did not have severe hydrocephalus (no shunt procedures were available during that time) and frequently were people who had a lower level of lesions. Urinary continence was achieved by urinary diversions rather than clean intermittent catheterization which was instituted in the early 1970s. In addition to the different medical and surgical approaches, people educated during that period of time were under a different educational and vocational system than were those children who are now in their early adolescence. Public Law No. 94–142, which allows for the least restrictive educational environment for the handicapped child, was not in effect. Of interest, a Cincinnati study showed that as many children were mainstreamed during the early years as are mainstreamed now.

The few studies dealing with young adults also point out their social isolation, few marriages, and social and psychological dependence on family and/or community services. It is important to have such long-term follow-up to identify the problems that the young adults are currently facing. Identification of such problems should allow for establishment of appropriate therapeutic approaches that would be helpful to the young growing child. Some of the current published longitudinal data would lead readers to believe that perhaps the best management of children born with spina bifida is nontreatment. Dr. Lorber's well publicized article in 1971,[5] which elucidates selection criteria for nontreatment, brought to prominence the quality of life issue and the overall purpose of treatment of children with such a multiple handicapping condition. Subsequent articles in the medical literature continue to refine the selective criteria and to pervade the literature. The most recent dramatic case was illustrated by the 1984 case of nontreatment of Baby Jane Doe.[6] The initial decision for nontreatment was made based on the high possibility that Baby Jane Doe would be retarded, emphasizing that retardation is equivalent to a poor quality of life. Those articles that discuss selection criteria and quality of life deal primarily with the physical consequences of the defect; rarely do they discuss what has happened psychologically and emotionally to the child and young adult who have survived. It appears, therefore, that the initial step to management of a child born with spina bifida is the decision to treat or not to treat. Most centers involved with children with spina bifida elect that the first decision should be treatment. However, implicit in this decision (to actively provide for treatment for the infant with spina bifida) is provision of appropriate services from infancy through adulthood. Spina bifida is not an acute medical problem; it is a disorder that involves chronic care with periodic acute medical crises for the person's entire life span. This necessitates that management of the child with spina bifida requires both longitudinal monitoring and provision of acute care for both medical and psychosocial areas.

Multidisciplinary teams have become the established mode of management for children with this complicated disorder. Frequently one of the major efforts of the team coordinator is to coordinate the medical care of the child. The primary concerns of the physicians and families focus on shunt function, ambulation, urinary infection, and incontinence. In addition, the team collects longitudinal information regarding the effectiveness or lack of effectiveness of the various treatment modalities, i.e., shunt vs. intellectual functioning, walking vs. nonwalking, orthopedic treatment results, and urinary continence vs. incontinence. In the age of specialization, the teams now consist not only of nurse/pediatric coordinators, but also of clinical nurse specialists, social workers, psychologists, educators and the various surgical specialties of neurosurgery, orthopedics, and urology. In the past, the neurosurgeon, because of his initial role in the repair of the defect, was the team manager and only occasionally were pediatricians involved. With the changing focus in pediatrics, pediatricians who were trained in developmental pediatrics and care of chronically ill children now serve as team directors. Only a few teams have been able to add special educators and psychologists. Their major focus, however, is evaluating the children and collecting data rather than actively participating in the management of the child's care. This approach has led to the concept of the spina bifida child, the handicapped child, as opposed to the child with spina bifida, the child with a disability. Using the approach that the child is a child first and the handicap comes secondarily, helps focus the professional's attention to view the child as a whole, rather than as the child who has dysfunctioning parts.

An appropriate way for a team to look at the child's management is to consider the developmental periods and those stages known as family life cycle. In considering the child as a whole, it is important to remember that most professionals involved with child development feel that learning follows developmental guidelines, or at least a logical progression that moves the children increasingly to a complex response repertoire. Development, as described by Bricker,[7] can be visualized as an inverse pyramid with the base building blocks acquired by the infant being gradually differentiated to increasingly higher level responses. All individuals grow by a prescribed sequence of locomotor, sensory, and social capacities. Ericson in *Identity—Youth and Crisis*[8] states "personality can be said to develop according to stages predetermined in the human organism's readiness to be driven forward, to be aware of and to interact with a widening radius of significant individuals and institutions".

The treatment team must remember that a developmental model can be modified for the infant with disabilities. We must keep in mind that the infant's outcome is dependent on the organism's integrity (what they come into the world with) and the quality of caregiving environment interaction. Figure 12.1 helps demonstrate the interaction of the child, community, and family.[7]

It is not the intent of this article to describe in detail each developmental area that is important in each period of a child's life, but instead to increase the awareness of teams treating children with spina bifida to a need for using both a developmental and an interactive approach in addition to awareness of the health problems of the child and his family. Evaluations at each clinic visit should include screening for each of the developmental, emotional, and family areas just as well as evaluating kidney function and head size. Where it is appropriate and problems are identified, intervention techniques appropriate to the problem must be prescribed.

Developmental periods that need to be considered include the newborn period as a special entity in a child with a birth defect, infancy, toddler years, preschool, school age, adolescence, and young adulthood. A developmental chart can be helpful to evaluate these various stages. The following illustrates this developmental approach for one of the periods. Developmentally, the newborn arrives in the world with a set of reflexive behaviors that were thought by Piaget to be automatically triggered by either internal states or environmental stimuli. He felt that infants (as they exercise these reflexes) change the form of these reflexes to simple controlled responses. The first few months of life are adjustments toward

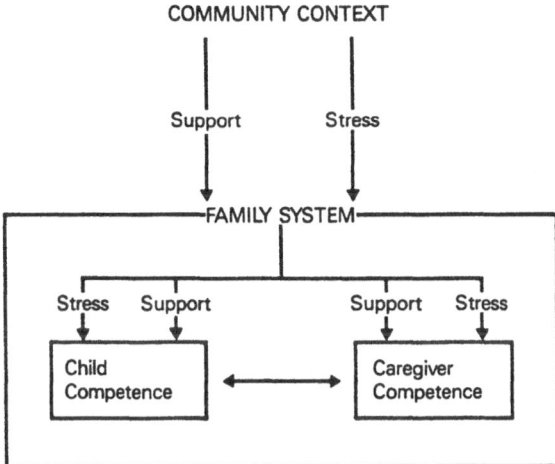

Figure 12.1. Interaction of the child, community, and family in treatment of the child with disabilities. [From Bricker D: Early Education of At-Risk and Handicapped Infants, Toddlers, and Preschool Children, Scott, Foresman and Company, 1986, page 9. Reprinted with permission.]

expanding the reflexive behavior of newborns in terms of the number and characteristics of stimuli that evoke responses of behavior. An example of this is how an infant can attempt to suck any object placed in his mouth. From this the infant begins to discriminate and learn which object will get him or her what consequences. This forms, according to developmental theorists, differential responding of the infant based on feedback from the environment. The newborn infant with spina bifida does not have the normal leg movement but does have appropriate hand, mouthing responses, and visual awareness. Feeding skills can be difficult in the newborn period because usually the infant is on his abdomen for 1 to 2 weeks, necessitating establishment of abnormal feeding patterns. Caretakers, however, can respond to the newborn infant by (1) continuing breast feeding and (2) providing bottles with breast milk until the infant can be held appropriately. The newborn infant can be touched, talked to, and stimulated by visual objects and by vocal recognition of the family. The infant can learn to respond to patting to calm him if he is unhappy though they cannot hold him. The newborn period is perhaps most difficult for the family. Details of the grieving process related to the birth of a child with a defect are elucidated in many articles.[9,10] The family needs to respond to the infant as an infant and begin the bonding process as quickly as possible. Indeed most mothers of children with spina bifida will come to see the infant as soon as they are released from the hospital. A note of concern can be recognized by the professional team if the family tends to avoid touching or looking at the baby. An example of this is one mother who did not come to see her child until the child was over a week old. It was noted throughout her infrequent visits to the infant that she would sit in a chair with her face turned away from the infant, avoiding any contact unless urged to (make contact) by the team.

The mother remained ambivalent for the first 3 years of the child's life. Subsequently, this mother (who had a very chaotic family situation) rejected the infant, the child was admitted to the hospital because of failure to thrive, and was eventually placed in foster care and recently was adopted by the foster parents. The impact of these crucial 3 years could not be minimized; its long-term effect at this point is difficult to distinguish from the child's developmental problems that do exist. Parents need appropriate and accurate information. They need the opportunity to see and hold their infant as soon as possible. Again, the concept that this is a baby first—and secondarily a baby with spina bifida—is important. Sometimes, too much information can be overwhelming to families.

The professional's team role should be to provide effective supportive services during this crucial period, including the provision of accurate data to the parents. Frequently the initial physician who sees the parent, either the obstetrician or the referring physician not familiar with such children, will provide a poor prognosis concluding that the child might not survive, or that if the child does survive he will be paralyzed and retarded. A more positive approach and prognosis is helpful in assisting the family to cope with the initial impact of the child's handicap. Schor and Oppenheimer studied 33 families,[11] comparing families that were given a poor prognosis at birth with those given a more positive prognosis. It was significant that the children whose families were given a poor prognosis achieved a lesser degree of independence than those whose prognosis was more positive. Families stated that all they could remember was that their child probably would not live to be a teenager. The team must also evaluate the presence of family support systems, the preexisting relationships between the family and family members, and (if possible) the individual coping skills and strengths of each parent. Again, many of the observations can be made during those initial few days as the team members begin to meet and know the family better. Too much information can be overwhelming. Time is needed to let the family grieve and to be able to share their feelings with each other and other family members. The availability of other parents can be helpful at this time or soon thereafter. The availability of this resource should be presented to the parents. Repetition of all the information concerning the defect is needed frequently throughout the first few months. Availability of financial support is also a necessity. Cost[12] of the care of the child with spina bifida ranges anywhere from $15,000 to $50,000 during the first 2 years of life. Even those families who have insurance coverage are fearful of the ongoing financial requirements to care for their child. The team members should put the family in touch with appropriate financial resources when available. Giving the family written material (available through a variety of resources, including the Spina Bifida Association of America)[12] is also important during the first few months. The infant with spina bifida may go home, depending on the individual medical problems, anywhere from 2 weeks to more than 1 month. This does not allow the family to become accustomed to the infant's personality and to a specific routine. The infant's schedule has been regulated by the hospital's routine, not by his own inner regulatory system. The surgical scars on the infant's back, possibly deformed legs, and the palpable shunt, serve as constant reminders to the family that this infant is not the "perfectly formed infant" imagined by the parents. These specific issues must be verbalized to allow the family to work through their feelings about the infant who is born with a birth defect. Normal development through the first few months of life allows the infant to expand his reflexive behavior. Infants soon increase the rate of their development if they discover an appropriate consequence to their behavior. They learn to attend to objects in the environment, change their gaze from object to object, and turn their head to locate an object. Motor control is usually jerky and uncoordinated initially, but improves with continual practice and use of the arms and legs in the normal to the extreme positions. The first movement to gain control are eyes and head and then trunk, and eventually sitting. To sit requires that the infant balance without support. This gradually allows the infant to use his or her hands and feet to explore the environment and anything that is in reach. The infant with spina bifida almost always will show delay in head control, rolling and sitting. Range of sitting independently can vary anywhere from 6 months through severe delay of 21 months. This obviously interferes with normal motor development unless compensatory methods are developed to encourage the infant in exploring his environment. Feeding skills also can present a problem in that some children with myelomeningocele have difficulty in swallowing appropriately (secondary to the Arnold Chiari malformation). Again, this needs to be identified to allow feeding to be a pleasurable response. As soon as the child begins to discriminate social smiling, and begins to anticipate a familiar person, he or she can produce a variety of social–emotional responses depending on his or her own internal states.

The emotional behavior of an infant with spina bifida is no different from that of any other infant. It is felt by Emde et al.[13] that three dimensions of emotional expression can be discriminated in infants. They include happy/unhappy, startled/relaxed, curious/interested, and happy/bored. All infants can produce noises and sounds and infant's vocalization can discriminate between cooing and distress sounds. They can locate sound sources at this stage. At times infants with spina bifida can be super sensitive to sound and therefore tune the sound out. Because the infant is unable to perform motor functions in the normal developmental progression and parents focus on motor development, they forget the other above described aspects of development. It is important to provide early infant intervention programs to the families at this time to increase their awareness of these very important developmental aspects. Parents may still be in a grieving state and just begin to become comfortable with their infant only when they can observe the infant make some large developmental milestone. The usual developmental milestones of infancy such as sitting are delayed and increase again the parental anxiety that their child may be mentally retarded. The family frequently is overwhelmed by the initial visits to a medical treatment program, and usually worry throughout the first year about the possibility of shunt malfunctions. Therefore every fretful period or period of lethargy, which may be normal variations of the infant's emotions, can be interpreted by the parents as a shunt malfunction and require visits to the physician. The important role of the team during this period of time is to reiterate the normal aspects of development for the infant and to teach the family to provide a pleasurable response to the infant's needs. At times it can be important to have an early intervention program with other parents of children with spina bifida to allow sharing of feelings and to also learn different compensatory handling of the child's fine and gross motor needs and sensory input. Appropriate team members during this time can be a combination of developmental nurse, physical/occupational therapist, and/or early childhood developmental specialist. Familiarity with these team members also makes the visits to the medical/surgical team easier to handle.

From 6 to 12 months the infant with normal developmental skills continues to gain considerable control over his motor system, sitting independently, shifting into a prone position, beginning to crawl, making a forward motion, and widening the portion of his or her environment for exploration, leading in a culmination of walking. In addition, infants use their hands appropriately to acquire objects. This leads them on to the toddler stages. Functionally an infant can use an adult as a means for obtaining an object and gaining adult attention, respond to the mother using a variety of sounds and gestures, pointing, integrating, showing interest in social interaction, show appropriate distress on separation from the mother, and begin to learn that the mother can return. Communication skills also increase. In the child with spina bifida many of these areas are markedly delayed and indeed many of the infants cannot reach them. Many times various orthopedic procedures and/or braces, which are used in an attempt to prevent contractures and assist in mobility, can hinder the child's mobility. The family may be very involved in having to worry about getting braces on, carrying equipment, and urging the child to make motor progress, and tends to forget that the child's other developmental areas are also important. Beginning independence needs to be stressed to the family by encouraging feeding skills. The parent's role in assisting the child during this crucial period is very important.

Hospitalizations during this time can be very traumatic to both the child and the parent. Many parents tend to elect to stay with their child during the hospitalization and also at times may begin to neglect the siblings who subsequently may resent the infant who requires so much of the parents' time. Families may forget that they have an innate ability to comfort their child if they are tuned into the needs of that child.

It is important for team members to assist families in their adjustment to cope effectively with a child who does not respond in the normal fashion. Again, support the family by providing not only intervention programs but encouraging them to enjoy their infant's development, rather than always being concerned with their infant's physical needs. Therapists working with the infant and the family can combine a variety of modalities when they are trying to encourage movement, introducing toys, language, social responsiveness, avoiding parental overprotectiveness and concern that the child will be hurt and "hit his or her shunt."

The various age periods – toddler, preschool, school years – can be approached in a similar manner as described, with the team identifying normal milestones in the areas of gross–fine motor development, psychosocial development, language development, emotional development, and relating this then to stages of family development and assigning appropriate team responsibility. The following statements will serve only to highlight issues that are pertinent during some of these time periods.

The toddler age normally includes rapid gross motor development with pulling to a stand, cruising, and exploring the environment. In children with spina bifida, in most cases this ability is obviously quite delayed if it ever occurs. Toddlers are frustrated when they are unable to move and if restricted may throw temper tantrums. Many times braces will limit the child's mobility rather than assist mobility, so the managing team and family must allot appropriate time for freedom of movement even if it is scooting about the floor using hand pulls. The Rochester parapodium can be helpful because it frees up hand movements and allows improvement of fine motor skills while the child still can be in an upright position. A scooter board can be appropriate to allow the child to manipulate his environment and to get about. It is at this crucial time that there should be encouragement in self-feeding skills and cooperation in dressing even though this may be difficult because of balance problems. Socially this is the time to express feelings — anger, temper tantrums. This social–emotional outlet is important and sometimes may not occur because the family feels "sorry" for the child and does not want to frustrate the youngster. At age 2 to 3, crucial developmental milestones include again dressing and undressing which families, because it is easier for them, may just continue to do themselves rather than allowing the child to learn and practice even though it takes much longer. Toileting is a crucial stage for children. The child with spina bifida is dependent on the family for continence and frequently takes a very passive role. Despite the fact that the team encourages bowel training throughout this time by putting the child on a potty chair, grunting, etc., few families seem to understand the importance of this and tend to say the child is in diapers anyway so what is the difference. The team need to discuss with the family the importance of this developmental stage, not only because bowel continence can be achieved, but the child can learn very early the importance of self-care techniques and establish the beginning stage of independence. At 3 years of age the biggest stride for all children developmentally is language. Usually children with spina bifida are extremely verbal but because they are so verbal people may not always listen to the content of their statements and think only that "they are cute." Cocktail language has been described as irrelevant and inappropriate language. This language deficit is reported in 24 to 80% of children with hydrocephalus.[14] The relationship of this language problem and other learning deficits of children with spina bifida remains unclear. Cocktail language needs further investigation to provide appropriate intervention techniques.

Preschool years are important for all children to share and develop appropriate peer relationships. Because of this children with spina bifida need to become involved with appropriate peer groups and attend a preschool. The children, if possible, attend a regular preschool where adjustments can be made for their physical handicap. Headstart programs frequently have slots available for children with disabilities regardless of the family income. Emphasis during this time should be the establishment of prekindergarten skills and learning to adapt to a group of children who do not have physical handicaps. Children learn during this time the beginning of independence and peer acceptance, all of which can be difficult for the child with spina bifida. Children establish a daily routine for school, and learn to respond to other children's questions about why they wear diapers and braces. Team members can assist in this adjustment period by providing written information and consultation to the preschool. The school years for a child with spina bifida can present numerous obstacles and require special attention by all concerned. With the passage of Public Law 94–142 (which provides for school placement in the least restrictive environment for children with disabilities), most children with spina bifida are being mainstreamed in the public school systems. The physical adaptive needs of children with spina bifida are the most obvious. The famous Tatro case paved the way to eliminate one of the most common physical limitations for the children. This legal decision provided assistance for the child who achieved continence by intermittent catheterization. Prior to this, children were placed in special orthopedic classes because they would require the assistance of a school nurse to do intermittent catheterization. Schools in the community are becoming more and more physically accessible. Schools have felt if they meet the physical adaptive requirements for the child with spina bifida there will be no other problems. However, special academic concerns are being identified by studies that analyze academic achievement as related to IQ scores. These are described in detail in Spain and Anderson's book.

Spain and Anderson[15] make six major points about the general intellectual development of children with spina bifida. These need to be understood in order for school, parents, and team members to develop the appropriate academic programming assistance.

1. Intelligence mostly tends to be below average but not retarded.
2. Intelligence differs between shunt vs. nonshunt (hydrocephalus vs. nonhydrocephalus).
3. Intelligence does not vary with the severity of the physical handicap unless there is accompanying hydrocephaly.
4. There is always a degree of difference in intellect related to the nature of the lesion.
5. Not all intellectual function is affected equally. Usually verbal development is less impaired than performance.

The phenomena of "cocktail speech and hyperverbalization" makes a false impression of apparent superior verbal ability. Many children with spina bifida appear very chatty and communicative yet on specific testing they will do poorly on abstract reasoning, short- and long-term memory, and may have word-finding problems. This uneven profile that many children with spina bifida demonstrate is similar to that seen with other children who have learning disabilities as described originally in brain-injured children. Children with spina bifida frequently should be considered to have a learning disability which refers to a heterogeneous group of disorders manifested by significant difficulties in listening, thinking, speaking, reading, writing, spelling, or mathematics. Reading[15] scores vary but various controlled studies have shown that children with spina bifida can read at an appropriate level but their comprehension may not be as good as it should be. This may be related to the above language problems including word finding problems. Some educators have recommended a phonic approach rather than a look-and-say approach. This would help use auditory skills which appears to be normal. Most studies agree that math is very difficult for the child with spina bifida. Similar difficulties are seen in other brain-damaged children. Reasons[16] for this may include decreased sensory motor experience, difficulty with visual-motor skills, and distractibility. Perceptual skills, visual/spatial skills, eye–hand coordination, and confusion of figure/ground items are known to be affected in this population. All of these skills play an important role in math ability. Handwriting may be poor.[17] This also may be related to visual/motor difficulties, spatial orientation problems, and speed. Unfortunately because of the physical handicap, the schools will tend not to provide as much special attention for the academic problems. These discrepancies need to be identified early and addressed with appropriate academic support. Distractibility and short attention span interfere with academic performance and sometimes requires learning carrols, smaller classes, immediate feedback through computer learning programming, and when necessary teaching by specialists trained in learning disabilities, self-contained learning disabled classrooms, resource rooms, and tutoring.

The team needs to identify to the parents and to the schools the specific academic difficulties early on and explain that these are not due to motivational problems but are due more to specific neurologic deficits. The team needs to rule out any active neurologic abnormalities, shunt malfunction, chronic increase of intracranial pressure, and decreased arm function suggestive of developing syringomyelia. Physical therapy and ambulation should play less of a role during school time. Surgeries, if possible, should be avoided but if needed should not be scheduled during school hours. The importance of achieving self-help skills should be emphasized as much as possible prior to the beginning of school.

The period of adolescence and young adulthood is the period of development of independence and emotional turmoil. Many times children with spina bifida do not achieve independence because of low parental expectation, protective environment, the adolescent's perception that it is someone else's responsibility to care for them, and the basic problems related to the defect itself such as bowel and bladder incontinence. Articles[18,19] on adolescence frequently deal with self-esteem. Only recently are treatment programs including development of good self-concept as part of their intervention programs. It is known that any interpersonal involvement with an individual affects his environment and also potentially alters his self-concept. The question that should be asked is how should the team approach the teaching of positive self-esteem to ensure the best possible results. This needs to be done not only by parents, school, and medical team, but also by the persons themselves. The normal developmental tasks are complicated by physical limitations, social isolation, physical and emotional dependence on parents, and their ensuing emotional conflicts. The initial mastery of talking,[20] walking, and controlling bowel and bladder results in rewards of social approval and increased independence and contribute to positive self-esteem.

Obviously, children with spina bifida acquire this mastery later and many of these children do not acquire it at all. Also important to remember is that academic success plays an important role in positive self-concept and many children with spina bifida have not had a positive academic experience. Studies by Campbell et al.[21] found the adolescents with spina bifida showed poorer adjustment and lower self-esteem than controls. Acceptance of their own disability is interrelated with self-esteem. Often "management teams" always discusses aspects of treatment with the parents but frequently forgets to discuss it with the child, and the child remains passive throughout his experience with professionals. Family interactions toward the child from the very beginning as we have described play a very important role. The team, child, and family need to increase the child's perception of his own physical competencies and his understanding of the expectations of parents and others.

Psychologic and rehabilitation literature discuss in depth the factors involved in the psychologic adjustment of the physically handicapped vs. those children born with birth defects such as spina bifida. "The person with birth defect has an awareness of his defectiveness at the dawn of the patient's capacity to perceive himself in comparison to others." This leads to poor self-esteem and subsequent anxiety if left untreated. Implicit in the above discussion of adolescents is the shift of the team focus from the parent to the child. The traditional "clinic" setting does not allow this to occur. Adjustments need to be made. If financially available, new consultants, i.e., educators and vocational guidance counsellors, should be added to the team whose expertise is in the adolescent specialty. The team who did well with the younger child must step back and let new team members participate. This allows for the transition from the preadolescent school-age child to the teenage and subsequent role as an independent adult. The same transition must be made by parents and other family members for all adolescents. The "new" professional, however, must be aware of the differences between the adolescent paralyzed from an accident and the child paralyzed because of a birth defect. The adolescent with spinal cord trauma has had a normal perception of himself prior to the injury. He or she has known the importance of mobility, bowel and bladder continence, and academic achievement. Usually this group has established strong peer relationships which has not occurred in many of the adolescents with spina bifida. A recent study by Eckart[22] showed that focusing on children's skills, giving them praise and encouragement for doing their best, may increase feelings of competence. In this study there appeared to be a positive effect on self-esteem when the children perceived they have more control over their situation. Those children who felt external forces had a lot of control over events in their life were less likely to have high self-esteem. It appeared that encouraging children to make decisions when possible would be helpful.

In addition, the sexual development of the adolescent with spina bifida differs from that of the normal adolescent. There is much earlier onset of development of secondary sexual characteristics, at times even at 8 to 9 years of age. Short stature is almost universal. Obesity is a common problem and frequently begins to develop in adolescents when mobility is decreased and where wheelchairs are used as a faster way to get around. These adolescent issues create additional adjustment problems for the adolescent with spina bifida. During the adolescent period the family may have a resurgence of guilt and go through an additional stage of grieving. They are now concerned about the next crisis. Parents wonder whether the adolescent will ever be self-supporting or whether he will always remain dependent. Studies on the effect of the child with the handicap on the family have varied. Some studies[23,24] report the family as being less stable and more socially isolated whereas other studies have stated the reverse. Actually some studies have reported families with children with spina bifida have suffered from less separation and divorce than the overall population. The effect on siblings in the family during all of the life cycles is just recently being explored.

Early adulthood will be discussed very briefly. Adults who belong to the Spina Bifida Association of America are identifying medical needs and requesting teams that will manage adult problems. Several centers have developed techniques of making the transition from the pediatric setting to the adult setting. Once an adult program is identified, the original team can invite them to attend several of the pediatric clinics. Gradually the adult team can overcome both the pediatrician's resistance and the family's resistance to leaving the center that has known them since birth. This allows the young adult to realize that their problems are different and that the young adult must take responsibility for his or her care. Studies of adult concerns sponsored both by Dr. Shurtleff and by the Spina Bifida Association of America illustrate that the major concerns were social, educational, economic, and sexual.[25] Medical concerns include skin breakdown, obesity, urine infections, shunt problems, and degenerative arthritis. The number of employable adults with spina bifida varies. Those adults who were followed from the 1950s, early 1960s, had higher employment and independence (50 to 60%) as compared to our current studies showing employment rates of 25% or less. The effect of society on employment issues, adaption of the job market to the disabled and payment of medical expenses play an important role in employment of the adult with spina bifida. These young adults who have survived in the 70's have not necessarily received appropriate help with school achievement, organizational skills, compensation for the physical handicap, and improved socialization skills.

The problems addressed above illustrate that spina bifida is a defect resulting in a chronic disability. This defect requires availability of appropriate health professionals who are trained in the care of people with chronic disorders. These teams must emphasize evaluation and treatment of all areas of development. Monitoring and intervention must be done for both developmental and medical aspects. It is hoped that the prognosis for the adults of the future will improve with this approach.

References

1. Colgan MT: Child with spina bifida: Am J Dis Child 135:854–858, 1981.
2. Elwood JM, Elwood JH: Epidemiology of Anencephalus and Spina Bifida: Oxford University Press, New York, 1980.

3. Shurtleff DB: Myelodysplasias and Extrophies: Grune & Stratton, Orlando, FL, 1986.

4. McLaurin R, Oppenheimer S (eds): Myelomeningocele: A Multidisciplinary Approach: Greenwood Press, West Port, CT, 1986.

5. Lorber J: Results of treatment of myelomeningocele: an analysis of 524 unselected cases with special reference to possible selection for treatment. Dev Med Child Neurol 13:279–303, 1971.

6. Johnson DE, Thompson TR, Aroskar M: Baby Doe rules: there are alternatives: AJDC, 138:523–529, 1984.

7. Bricker D: Early Education of At-risk and Handicapped Infants, Toddlers and Preschool Children: Scott, Foresman, Glenview, IL, 1986.

8. Erikson E: Identity, Youth and Crisis: Norton, New York, 1968.

9. Olshansky S: Parents Responses to a Mentally Defective Child: Soc Casework, XLIII: 191–193, 1962.

10. Kapke K: Spina bifida: Mother–child relationship. Nursing Forum: IX:310–319, 1970.

11. Schor D, Oppenheimer S: Interpreting Myelomeningocele to Parent: Long-Term Effect of Initial Parent-Physician Contact: Presentation Academy Cerebral Palsy Meeting, October 1980.

12. Spina Bifida Association of America, 343 S. Dearborn St., Chicago, IL 60604.

13. Emde R, Kligman D, Reich J, et al: Emotional expression in infancy: I. Initial studies of social signaling and an emergent model. In: Lewis M, Rosenblum L (eds): Development of Affect: Plenum Press, New York, 1978.

14. Horn D, Lorch E, Lorch R, et al: Distractibility and vocabulary deficits in children with spina bifida and hydrocephalus. Dev Med Child Neurol 27:713–720, 1985.

15. Anderson E, Spain B: The Child with Spina Bifida: London, Methuen & Co, 1977, pp. 117–141, 205.

16. Baron I, Spiegler B: Neuropsychological assessment of the child with spina bifida: Clin Proc CHMC 38:196–201, 1982.

17. Lorton A: Hand preference in children with myelomeningocele and hydrocephalus. Dev Med Child Neurol 18:143–148, 1976.

18. Dorner S: Adolescents with spina bifida: how they see their situation. Arch Dis Child 51:539–544, 1976.

19. Dorner S: The relationship of physical handicap to stress in families with an adolescent with spina bifida. Dev Med Child Neurol 17:765–776, 1975.

20. White W: Motivation reconsidered: the concept of competence. Psychol Rev 297–333, 1959.

21. Campbell W, Hayden PW, Davenport SL: Psychological adjustment of adolescents with myelodysplasia. J Youth Adolesc 6:397–407, 1977.

22. Eckart ML: Correlates of Self Esteem in Children with Myelomeningocele: Masters' Thesis, Department of Psychology, University of Cincinnati, 1986.

23. Bray R, Shurtleff, DB: Psychosocial implications of myelodysplasia: Clin Res 20:82–86, 1972.

24. Dorner S: Psychological and social problems of families of adolescent spina bifida patients: a preliminary report. Dev Med Child Neurol 15:Supp. 129.

25. Dunne KB, Shurtleff DB: The adult with meningomyelocele: A preliminary report: In: McLauren R, Oppenheimer S (eds): Myelomeningocele: A Multidisciplinary Approach. Greenwood Press, West Port, CT, 1986.

Index